# Multidisciplinary Breast Management

*Editors*

GEORGE M. FUHRMAN
TARI A. KING

# SURGICAL CLINICS
# OF NORTH AMERICA

www.surgical.theclinics.com

*Consulting Editor*
RONALD F. MARTIN

April 2013 • Volume 93 • Number 2

**ELSEVIER**

1600 John F. Kennedy Boulevard • Suite 1800 • Philadelphia, Pennsylvania, 19103-2899

http://www.theclinics.com

**SURGICAL CLINICS OF NORTH AMERICA Volume 93, Number 2**
**April 2013 ISSN 0039–6109, ISBN-13: 978-1-4557-7334-3**

Editor: John Vassallo, j.vassallo@elsevier.com
Developmental Editor: Teia Stone

*Surgical Clinics of North America* (ISSN 0039–6109) is published bimonthly by Elsevier Inc., 360 Park Avenue South, New York, NY 10010-1710. Months of publication are February, April, June, August, October, and December. Business and Editorial Offices: 1600 John F. Kennedy Blvd., Suite 1800, Philadelphia, PA 19103-2899. Periodicals postage paid at New York, NY and additional mailing offices. Subscription prices are $353.00 per year for US individuals, $598.00 per year for US institutions, $173.00 per year for US students and residents, $432.00 per year for Canadian individuals, $741.00 per year for Canadian institutions, $487.00 for international individuals, $741.00 per year for international institutions and $238.00 per year for Canadian and foreign students/residents. To receive student/resident rate, orders must be accompanied by name of affiliated institution, date of term, and the *signature* of program/residency coordinator on institution letterhead. Orders will be billed at individual rate until proof of status is received. Foreign air speed delivery is included in all *Clinics* subscription prices. All prices are subject to change without notice. POSTMASTER: Send address changes to *Surgical Clinics*, Elsevier Health Sciences Division, Subscription Customer Service, 3251 Riverport Lane, Maryland Heights, MO 63043. **Customer Service (orders, claims, online, change of address): Telephone: 1-800-654-2452 (U.S. and Canada); 314-447-8871 (outside U.S. and Canada). Fax: 314-447-8029. E-mail: journalscustomerservice-usa@elsevier.com (for print support); journalsonline support-usa@elsevier.com (for online support).**

*Reprints.* For copies of 100 or more, of articles in this publication, please contact the Commercial Reprints Department, Elsevier Inc., 360 Park Avenue South, New York, New York 10010-1710. Tel. (212) 633-3812, Fax: (212) 462-1935, e-mail: reprints@elsevier.com.

*The Surgical Clinics of North America* is also published in Spanish by McGraw-Hill Interamericana Editores S.A., P.O. Box 5-237 06500 Mexico D.F. Mexico; and in Portuguese by Interlivros Edicoes Ltda., Rua Comandante Coelho 1085, CEP 21250, Rio de Janeiro, Brazil; and in Greek by Paschalidis Medical Publications, Athens Greece.

*The Surgical Clinics of North America* is covered in *MEDLINE/PubMed (Index Medicus), EMBASE/Excerpta Medica, Current Contents/Clinical Medicine, Current Contents/Life Sciences, Science Citation Index,* and *ISI/BIOMED.*

Printed and bound by CPI Group (UK) Ltd, Croydon, CR0 4YY
Transferred to Digital Printing, 2013

# Contributors

## CONSULTING EDITOR

**RONALD F. MARTIN, MD, FACS**
Staff Surgeon, Department of Surgery, Marshfield Clinic, Marshfield, Wisconsin; Clinical Associate Professor, University of Wisconsin School of Medicine and Public Health, Madison, Wisconsin; Colonel, Medical Corps, United States Army Reserve

## EDITORS

**GEORGE M. FUHRMAN, MD**
Program Director and Vice Chair, Department of Surgery, Ochsner Clinic Foundation, New Orleans, Louisiana

**TARI A. KING, MD**
Associate Attending Surgeon, Breast Service, Department of Surgery, Jeanne A. Petrek Junior Faculty Chair, Memorial Sloan-Kettering Cancer Center; Associate Professor of Surgery, Weill-Cornell Medical College, New York, New York

## AUTHORS

**AMANDA L. AMIN, MD**
Chief Resident in General Surgery, Department of Surgery, Medical College of Wisconsin, Milwaukee, Wisconsin

**DALLIAH M. BLACK, MD**
Assistant Professor, Department of Surgical Oncology, The University of Texas MD Anderson Cancer Center, Houston, Texas

**RICHARD J. BLEICHER, MD, FACS**
Director, Breast Fellowship Program, Associate Professor, Department of Surgical Oncology, Fox Chase Cancer Center, Philadelphia, Pennsylvania

**ALFRED JOHN COLFRY III, MD**
Department of General Surgery, Atlanta Medical Center, Atlanta, Georgia

**ADRIANA D. CORBEN, MD**
Assistant Attending Breast Pathologist, Director, Breast Pathology Fellowship Program, Department of Pathology, Memorial Sloan-Kettering Cancer Center, New York, New York

**AMY C. DEGNIM, MD**
Associate Professor of Surgery, Department of Surgery, Mayo Clinic, Rochester, Minnesota

**FRANK J. DELLACROCE, MD, FACS**
Director, Department of Plastic Surgery, Center for Restorative Breast Surgery, New Orleans, Louisiana

**DAVID M. EUHUS, MD**
Medical Director, Clinical Cancer Genetics, Simmons Comprehensive Cancer Center; Professor, Department of Surgery, UT Southwestern Medical Center at Dallas, Dallas, Texas

**GEORGE M. FUHRMAN, MD**
Program Director and Vice Chair, Department of Surgery, Ochsner Clinic Foundation, New Orleans, Louisiana

**ANA M. GONZALEZ-ANGULO, MD, MSc**
Associate Professor, Section Clinical Research and Drug Development; Departments of Breast Medical Oncology and Systems Biology, MD Anderson Cancer Center, The University of Texas, Houston, Texas

**LEONEL F. HERNANDEZ-AYA, MD**
Fellow, Division of Hematology/Oncology, Comprehensive Cancer Center, University of Michigan Health System, Ann Arbor, Michigan

**ALICE Y. HO, MD**
Department of Radiation Oncology, Memorial Sloan-Kettering Cancer Center, New York, New York

**TARI A. KING, MD**
Associate Attending Surgeon, Breast Service, Department of Surgery, Jeanne A. Petrek Junior Faculty Chair, Memorial Sloan-Kettering Cancer Center; Associate Professor of Surgery, Weill-Cornell Medical College, New York, New York

**AMANDA L. KONG, MD, MS**
Assistant Professor of Surgery, Division of Surgical Oncology, Department of Surgery, Medical College of Wisconsin, Milwaukee, Wisconsin

**JOANNE D. MATTINGLY, RN, MSN, ANP-BC, CBCN**
Division of Surgical Oncology, Department of Surgery, Medical College of Wisconsin, Milwaukee, Wisconsin

**SARAH A. MCLAUGHLIN, MD**
Assistant Professor, Department of Surgery, Mayo Clinic, Jacksonville, Florida

**ELIZABETH A. MITTENDORF, MD, PhD**
Assistant Professor, Department of Surgical Oncology, The University of Texas MD Anderson Cancer Center, Houston, Texas

**HEATHER B. NEUMAN, MD, MS**
Assistant Professor, Department of Surgery, University of Wisconsin School of Medicine and Public Health, Madison, Wisconsin

**ANNA C. PURDY, RN, MSN, ANP-BC, AOCNP, CBCN**
Division of Surgical Oncology, Department of Surgery, Medical College of Wisconsin, Milwaukee, Wisconsin

**MEREDITH H. REDDEN, MD**
PGY IV Surgery Resident, Atlanta Medical Center, Atlanta, Georgia

**LINDA ROBINSON, MS**
Assistant Director, Clinical Cancer Genetics, Simmons Comprehensive Cancer Center, UT Southwestern Medical Center at Dallas, Dallas, Texas

**DANA H. SMETHERMAN, MD, MPH, FACR**
Vice Chairman for Clinical Affairs, Section Head, Breast Imaging, Department of Radiology, Ochsner Health System, New Orleans, Louisiana

**PAULA M. TERMUHLEN, MD**
Professor of Surgery, Division of Surgical Oncology, Department of Surgery, Medical College of Wisconsin; Medical Director of High Risk Breast Program, Froedtert Hospital and The Medical College of Wisconsin, Clinical Cancer Center, Milwaukee, Wisconsin

**EMILY T. WOLFE, MD**
Department of Surgery, Ochsner Health Care System, Jefferson, Louisiana

**T. JONATHAN YANG, MD**
Department of Radiation Oncology, Memorial Sloan-Kettering Cancer Center, New York, New York

**BARBARA ZAREBCZAN DULL, MD**
Department of Surgery, University of Wisconsin School of Medicine and Public Health, Madison, Wisconsin

# Contents

> This article presents an overview of the benign conditions that affect the breast for the practicing surgeon. The authors discuss the diagnosis and management of a variety of breast pathologic conditions, including those associated with infection and inflammation as well as proliferative and nonproliferative disorders. The authors also offer their experience with the integration of nurse practitioners in the care of patients with benign breast disease.

> Mammography remains the primary modality for breast cancer diagnosis. Other imaging studies, most commonly ultrasonography and magnetic resonance imaging, are also used to characterize breast lesions, stage breast cancer, and aid in surgical planning. Although mammography is the only screening examination demonstrated to decrease breast cancer mortality in the general population, other imaging studies have been shown to be beneficial for screening high-risk patients. In the future, new technologies may also improve the sensitivity and specificity of breast cancer screening and detection.

> High-risk lesions of the breast are lesions that confer an increased risk of breast cancer, either because of an increased probability of finding cancer associated with percutaneous biopsy findings or because of an increased probability of developing breast cancer over the long term. Atypical ductal hyperplasia found on percutaneous biopsy is generally excised, whereas lobular neoplasia lesions, including both atypical lobular hyperplasia and lobular carcinoma in situ, may be observed if radiologic and pathologic findings are concordant and there is no other high-risk lesion present.

> Apart from BRCA1, BRCA2, and TP53, more than a dozen breast cancer susceptibility genes have been identified. Recognizing affected individuals depends on evaluation of cancer family history and recognition of certain phenotypic markers on physical examination. Genetic testing provides a powerful tool for individualized risk stratification. Mutation carriers have several options for managing risk, including lifestyle alterations, enhanced surveillance, chemoprevention, and prophylactic surgery. Genetic counseling and testing should be considered in the initial evaluation of patients with newly diagnosed breast cancer because this information contributes to surgical decisions, radiation therapy options, and systemic therapy choices.

> Invasive breast cancers constitute a heterogeneous group of lesions. Although the most common types are ductal and lobular, this distinction is not meant to indicate the site of origin within the mammary ductal system. The main purpose of the identification of specific types of invasive breast carcinoma is to refine the prediction of likely behavior and response to treatment also offered by the other major prognostic factors, including lymph node stage, histologic grade, tumor size, and lymphovascular invasion.

> Management of ductal carcinoma in situ (DCIS) has evolved from radical surgery to the option of a more minimally invasive approach. Data show that breast conservation surgery performed with administration of radiotherapy, like mastectomy, is feasible and safe. Because efforts to find a safe group for elimination of radiotherapy have resulted in data that conflict, radiotherapy still remains standard of care as a part of breast conservation for DCIS. Tamoxifen has also shown a significant recurrence benefit and has become standard in the treatment of receptor-positive disease. Investigation of other agents, such as anastrazole and trastuzumab, are ongoing.

> The twentieth century has witnessed dramatic changes in the surgical management of breast cancer. Herein we focus on the evolution of breast conservation surgery and current surgical trends of lumpectomy, mastectomy and contralateral prophylactic mastectomy. Margin analysis, specimen localization and processing, and the benefits of magnetic resonance imaging remain controversial. Neoadjuvant chemotherapy can offer prognostic information and aid in surgical planning while radiation therapy continues to reduce the risk of local recurrence after breast conserving surgery. Despite these advances, mastectomy remains a popular choice for many women and the use of nipple sparing procedures is increasing. Overall the low rates of local recurrence are attributed to the combination of surgery and targeted adjuvant and radiation therapies.

# SURGICAL CLINICS
# OF NORTH AMERICA

**FORTHCOMING ISSUES**

*June 2013*
**Modern Concepts in Pancreatic Surgery**
Stephen W. Behrman, MD, FACS, and
Ronald F. Martin, MD, FACS, *Editors*

*August 2013*
**Vascular Surgery and Endovascular Therapy**
Girma Tefera, MD, *Editor*

*October 2013*
**Abdominal Wall Reconstruction**
Michael Rosen, MD, *Editor*

**RECENT ISSUES**

*February 2013*
**Complications, Considerations and
Consequences of Colorectal Surgery**
Scott R. Steele, MD, *Editor*

*December 2012*
**Surgical Critical Care**
John A. Weigelt, MD, *Editor*

*October 2012*
**Contemporary Management of Esophageal
Malignancy**
Chadrick E. Denlinger, MD, and
Carolyn E. Reed, MD, *Editors*

*August 2012*
**Recent Advances and Future Directions in
Trauma Care**
Jeremy W. Cannon, MD, SM, *Editor*

**ISSUE OF RELATED INTEREST**

*Surgical Oncology Clinics of North America* October 2010 (Vol. 19, Issue 4)
**Early-Stage Breast Cancer: New Developments and Controversies**
Eleftherios P. Mamounas, MD, MPH, *Editor*

DOWNLOAD
Free App!

*Review Articles*
THE CLINICS

**NOW AVAILABLE FOR YOUR iPhone and iPad**

# Foreword

# Multidisciplinary Breast Management

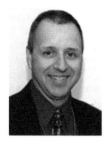

Ronald F. Martin, MD, FACS
*Consulting Editor*

I began as Consulting Editor for the *Surgical Clinics of North America* a number of years ago with 2 basic goals: first, to help produce a series of publications that covered topics of interest and necessity to general surgeons, and second, to try to explore what a general surgeon really is. It doesn't take a grammarian or logician to realize that those 2 goals are either so intertwined as to be one or tautologically impossible. After all, in order to know what matters to a general surgeon, one should probably understand what a general surgeon does. I shall leave it to the readership to decide if the content provided has been useful. As to what constitutes a general surgeon— that, I am still trying to decide.

The American Board of Surgery (ABS), according to its Booklet of Information, requires residency "experience" in 10 areas of surgery, including Alimentary Tract (including Bariatric Surgery); Abdomen and its Contents; Breast, Skin, and Soft Tissue; Endocrine System; Solid Organ Transplantation; Pediatric Surgery; Surgical Critical Care; Surgical Oncology (including Head and Neck Surgery); Trauma/Burns and Emergency Surgery; and Vascular Surgery, for initial certification in surgery. While there are varying degrees of proficiency and exposure required for many of these fields, this is still a pretty daunting list of areas to develop. For the approximately 250 categorical general surgery training programs in the United States, this requirement is consistent throughout. Personally, I don't know of any single person who truly does all these components of surgery in practice, let alone does them well. I know of a few people who *claim* to do them all and perhaps they do—at present I remain skeptical. We do know from the case log data provided to the ABS for recertification examinations that the overwhelming majority of surgeons seeking recertification by the ABS only practice in limited few subsets of these areas.

With all of our categorical general surgery graduates in possession of at least competency skills in all the above-mentioned areas, one would not think that a need for surgical specialization should exist; yet more than two-thirds of our graduates

Surg Clin N Am 93 (2013) xiii–xv
http://dx.doi.org/10.1016/j.suc.2013.01.008
0039-6109/13/$ – see front matter © 2013 Published by Elsevier Inc.

**surgical.theclinics.com**

seek fellowship training. There are only a few reasons one might seek fellowship training. One might wish to expand one's practice opportunities, restrict or alter one's practice opportunities, or might feel inadequately trained during the standard general surgery residency. Let us leave the last of those possibilities out of the equation for now. The first two are a bit more intriguing anyway, especially if we consider workforce issues.

If all those graduates, or even a significant majority—maybe even a significant minority who completed a general surgery residency went into fellowship to expand their capabilities, we probably would not have a shortage of "general surgeons." Yet, we do have a shortage. It would therefore seem reasonable to infer that a significant majority of those who seek fellowship training under these circumstances are, or will, limit or alter their practice spectrum. Some of these disciplines are wholesale departures from what most general surgeons do (cardiothoracic, plastic and reconstructive, pediatric, even vascular, if we are honest with ourselves), while others pry off subsets of what many general surgeons continue to do (minimally invasive, breast, surgical oncology, colorectal, foregut, hepatobiliary, and the latest, "Acute Care," to name a few). The net result is that in some respects general surgery has become what is left over in the land of plentiful specialists or that which one might tackle to avoid transfer of the patient in the land of no specialists. Of course, there are some "in-between" environments but those are seemingly becoming rarer as the older general surgeons retire and are replaced with younger, frequently more specialty interested surgeons. Accountable Care Organizations, "Centers of Excellence" (self-declared or otherwise), hospital and practice consolidations, patient desire and demand, and a large array of other factors will likely accelerate these changes in the immediate future.

This issue of the *Surgical Clinics of North America* on Multidisciplinary Breast Management is dedicated to a topic that used to be in the wheelhouse of nearly every general surgeon. Depending on where one lives, many patients who require breast surgery are still cared for by general surgeons but increasingly this care is being shifted to those who have advanced oncologic training or advanced specialty training in breast surgery, and also to some who simply "limit" their practice to surgery of breast conditions and declare expertise. There are a myriad of factors from both the provider side and the consumer side of this equation that foster this change. For providers, some of the benefit may be that surgery of breast disorders comes with a scope of knowledge that can be perhaps more easily managed, less (if any) night calls, few emergencies, and a certain predictability of workflow. For patients, there appears to be an increasing desire for increased specialization by surgeons in breast surgery that is not as heavily expected for some other areas of general surgery.

Breast surgery, while perhaps a bit of an outlier discipline at present, is probably more of a harbinger of things to come than it is a departure from business as usual. Breast surgery resides at the intersection of multispecialty care, intense basic science and clinical research, patient advocacy, financial support, political pressure, and emotionality. If I had to pick a bellwether for the future direction in American medicine, I can't think of one more likely than breast surgery right now. It is up to you, dear reader, to decide if that would be good news or not.

No matter what the future holds for our discipline, at present we must know and understand the relevant topics to breast surgery. To that we have once again turned to a most valued colleague, Dr George Fuhrman, who has with Dr Tara King provided us with a comprehensive and most useful collection of information to help us sort through this topic. They and their colleagues' work should be invaluable to any who participate in the care of these patients.

What is in store for general surgery is anybody's guess, but as Yogi Berra is attributed as saying, "The future ain't what it used to be." So whichever path we take, we are all better off if we are better informed.

Ronald F. Martin, MD, FACS
Department of Surgery
Marshfield Clinic
1000 North Oak Avenue
Marshfield, WI 54449, USA

E-mail address:
martin.ronald@marshfieldclinic.org

# Preface

# Multidisciplinary Breast Management

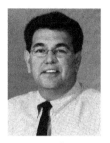 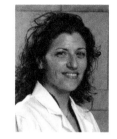

George M. Fuhrman, MD    Tari A. King, MD
*Editors*

This issue of *Surgical Clinics of North America* is focused on the management of breast disease. Over the past several decades, the management of both benign and malignant breast disease has become more specialized, as evidenced by the accreditation of at least 32 dedicated breast fellowships. Despite the shift toward specialization, general surgeons continue to provide the majority of care for women with breast disease. The goal of this issue is to provide an up-to-date resource for both surgeons in training and general surgeons involved in the rapidly evolving multidisciplinary management of benign and malignant breast disease. The topics have been selected to provide the surgeon with evidence-based approaches to the breast and the axilla, detailed information regarding postmastectomy reconstruction, and insights into the nonsurgical specialties that collaborate with the surgeon in providing multidisciplinary care. Articles focused on medical oncology, radiation oncology, pathology, and radiology illustrate the importance of the relationships between the breast surgeon and other specialists involved in the care of women with breast disease.

Perhaps the most important aspect of providing high-quality care for women with breast disease is the relationship between the surgeon and the patient. Women fear breast cancer more than any other disease and the stress associated with this fear can dramatically impact a woman's quality of life. A well-informed surgeon can provide the information necessary to counsel a patient regarding all aspects of their disease management, enabling patients to navigate often complex treatment choices better and thereby reducing anxiety. A well-informed surgeon can also actively participate in multidisciplinary treatment planning and act as an advocate for their patient. Surgeons that simply function as technicians for their nonsurgical colleagues will find that their role in the management of breast disease will decline as patients seek more information than ever before and treatment choices become more individualized.

Surg Clin N Am 93 (2013) xvii–xviii
http://dx.doi.org/10.1016/j.suc.2013.01.007
0039-6109/13/$ – see front matter © 2013 Published by Elsevier Inc.

**surgical.theclinics.com**

We hope that this issue will provide our readers with an opportunity to more fully engage in the care of patients with breast disease by fostering important relationships with other surgical and nonsurgical colleagues as well as with patients.

As coeditors we appreciate the contributions from our author colleagues. They are a talented group of friends that we respect and frequently turn to for advice and care of our patients. These are the doctors that we would choose to care not only for our breast patients but also for our family members if needed.

Finally, as coeditors, we appreciate the opportunity to rekindle a collaboration that produced a multitude of scholarly activity over a decade ago at The Ochsner Clinic in New Orleans. The professional relationships established in surgical training programs are often the relationships that carry one through a career in surgery. The mentor/mentee relationship between faculty and residents provides motivation for the attending surgeon and serves as a lifelong example to the trainee to pay it forward in mentoring the next generation of surgeons.

George M. Fuhrman, MD
Department of Surgery
Ochsner Clinic Foundation
1514 Jefferson Highway
New Orleans, LA 70121, USA

Tari A. King, MD
Department of Surgery
Memorial Sloan-Kettering Cancer Center
300 East 66th Street
New York, NY 10065, USA

E-mail addresses:
gfuhrman@ochsner.org (G.M. Fuhrman)
kingt@mskcc.org (T.A. King)

# Benign Breast Disease

Amanda L. Amin, MD[a],
Anna C. Purdy, RN, MSN, ANP-BC, AOCNP, CBCN[b],
Joanne D. Mattingly, RN, MSN, ANP-BC, CBCN[b],
Amanda L. Kong, MD, MS[b], Paula M. Termuhlen, MD[c,d],*

## KEYWORDS

- Benign breast disease • Nurse practitioner • Papilloma • Fibroadenoma • Mastitis

## KEY POINTS

- Benign breast conditions are often underdiagnosed.
- Malignancy is not commonly associated with benign conditions.
- Management of benign breast disease depends on accurate diagnosis.
- Knowledge of benign breast pathologic conditions continues to grow.
- Most benign breast conditions can be managed without surgery.

## INTRODUCTION

Benign breast diseases includes all nonmalignant conditions of the breast and typically do not convey an increased risk of malignancy. Patients with benign breast conditions are often first seen by their primary care physician or their gynecologist. Benign breast diseases are often misdiagnosed and misunderstood because of their variety in presentation and anxiety about the possibility of malignancy. Physicians that interface with patients with benign breast disease must have a complete understanding of the conditions discussed in this article to competently evaluate these disorders and calm concerns regarding the possibility of breast cancer.

In recent years, breast care has become an established specialty throughout our health care system as evidenced by the existence of breast surgical fellowships and dedicated breast care centers. The care of women who have concerns about their

The authors have nothing to disclose.
[a] Department of Surgery, Medical College of Wisconsin, 9200 West Wisconsin Avenue, FWC 3691, Milwaukee, WI 53226, USA; [b] Department of Surgery, Division of Surgical Oncology, Medical College of Wisconsin, 9200 West Wisconsin Avenue, Milwaukee, WI 53226, USA; [c] Department of Surgery, Division of Surgical Oncology, Medical College of Wisconsin, 9200 West Wisconsin Avenue, FWC 3691, Milwaukee, WI 53226, USA; [d] Froedtert Hospital and The Medical College of Wisconsin Clinical Cancer Center, 9200 West Wisconsin Avenue, Milwaukee, WI 53226, USA
* Corresponding author. Department of Surgery, Medical College of Wisconsin, 9200 West Wisconsin Avenue, Milwaukee, WI 53226.
E-mail address: ptermuhlen@mcw.edu

breast health or breast abnormalities is a complex process that is best addressed by an interdisciplinary, collaborative model of care.[1] These models of breast care often include surgeons with a practice focused on breast diseases, a dedicated team of imaging specialists, and nurse practitioners. Nurse practitioners can play an important role in helping women with breast concerns by incorporating clinical expertise with teaching and counseling skills.[1] Nurse practitioners with specialized training are well qualified to assess, diagnose, and manage all aspects of benign breast diseases, including breast cysts, masses, nipple discharge, mastitis, abscess, breast pain, and abnormal mammograms. The value of incorporating nurse practitioners in a breast care setting has been well documented to include reduced wait times to consultation, expedited diagnosis, and decreased anxiety for patients.[2] At the Medical College of Wisconsin, 2 of the authors' nurse practitioners (authors A.C.P and J.L.M.) have independent practices that manage most patients who come to their facility with benign breast disorders and serve as a triage for patients with abnormal mammograms.

The following information is organized to allow for easy reference. Diagnoses are grouped by whether or not patients are lactating women, presence or absence of infection/inflammation, and nonproliferative or proliferative disorders.

## BREAST INFECTIONS IN LACTATING WOMEN
### Mastitis and Abscess

Mastitis is a complication often encountered in primiparous women and develops in 1% to 24% of breastfeeding women. A breast abscess develops as a complication of mastitis in 5% to 11% of cases.[3] The most common bacteria is *Staphylococcus aureus*. Bacteria enter the skin by a small laceration or proliferate in a stagnant lactiferous duct. Common clinical symptoms of breast infection include pain, redness, and heat.[4] Differentiating between mastitis and abscess can be difficult; when there is suspicion for abscess, the woman should be referred for ultrasound evaluation. Mastitis on ultrasound will appear as an ill-defined area of altered echotexture with increased echogenicity in the infiltrated and inflamed fat lobules. The diagnosis of abscess requires identification of a hypoechoic collection, often with a thick echogenic periphery. Ultrasound is the first-line investigation because it is relatively painless and provides guidance for percutaneous drainage. Antibiotics should always be offered in addition to percutaneous drainage for lesions with well-defined fluid collections. A drain may be placed as needed for full evacuation of the cavity. Aspirates should be sent for culture and sensitivity testing with antibiotic therapy directed accordingly. Oral cephalosporins or clindamycin hydrochloride (Cleocin) are excellent choices to cover the most common organisms.

Women should be encouraged to continue to breastfeed throughout the treatment to keep the ducts from becoming engorged. The only reason to cease breastfeeding would be when treatment with an antibiotic is contraindicated for the newborn or after surgical drainage.

Open surgical drainage may be necessary for patients with loculated collections or for those who have failed conservative management with antibiotic therapy and percutaneous drainage. In general, open surgical drainage should be reserved as a last resort in lactating patients to avoid the potential for milk fistula development.

## BREAST INFECTIONS IN NONLACTATING INDIVIDUALS
### Mastitis and Abscess

Breast abscess not associated with lactation, termed *nonpuerperal*, can be a challenging clinical problem that often recurs despite surgical treatment. They are classified according to location, either central (periareolar) or peripheral. Tobacco smoking is significantly associated with the development of primary abscesses, and smokers are 15 times more likely to develop recurrence than nonsmokers.[5] Nipple piercing also seems to be associated with an increased risk and may be as high as 10% to 20% after the procedure.[5] Other risk factors include diabetes, black race, and obesity.[3]

Abscesses in nonlactating women form as a complication of periductal mastitis. The first step is squamous metaplasia of the cuboidal epithelium leading to keratin plug formation. Cellular debris distends and obstructs the lactiferous ducts, leading to ductal dilation. Secondary infection occurs with stagnation of bacterial laden debris. Central nonpuerperal abscesses are the most difficult to treat and recur in 25% to 40% of women. Cutaneous fistulae occur in one-third of patients.[3] These abscesses are often caused by mixed flora (*Staphylococcus* and *Streptococcus*) and include anaerobes.[3] Antibiotic therapy should be instituted with a broad-spectrum drug that the most common organisms and may require an extended period of treatment (2 weeks or longer) to clear the infection.

Up until the early 1990s, surgical incision and drainage was the recommended treatment of almost all breast abscesses. With the common use of ultrasound, treatment is now typically percutaneous drainage with repeated aspirations as needed and may include saline lavage of the cavity. In up to 54% to 100% of patients, an abscess can be adequately managed using this process. Occasionally, an indwelling catheter may be left in place for collections larger than 3 cm, but even this is seldom necessary.[6] Patients should be encouraged to stop smoking. Mammography is recommended in women older than 35 years to rule out malignancy once the symptoms have calmed sufficiently to allow for compression of the breast. If there is any doubt, a tissue sample should be sent for cytology.

Peripheral nonpuerperal abscesses are less common and can occur with underlying chronic medical conditions, such as diabetes or rheumatoid arthritis.[3] The most common pathogen is *Staphylococcus aureus*, but mixed flora can also be encountered. These abscesses respond well to drainage and antibiotics and recurrences are rare.[3]

## INFLAMMATORY CONDITIONS OF THE BREAST
### Mondor Disease

Mondor disease is a rare benign condition defined as superficial thrombophlebitis of the anterolateral thoracoabdominal wall, most commonly the thoracoepigastric, lateral thoracic, or superior epigastric veins.[7] The exact cause is unclear. The clinical presentation is a painful palpable cordlike structure that can last several weeks. This condition is usually self-limiting and responds to application of heat, systemic antiinflammatory medications, and physical support with a brassiere.[8]

### Lymphedema After Breast Radiation

For many women with breast cancer, the breast can be conserved with a partial mastectomy (lumpectomy). However, lumpectomy alone is associated with a high incidence of local recurrence. The introduction of adjuvant radiation therapy has improved local control rates that are similar to those of a mastectomy.[9] Despite the high rate of local control, some women are left with breast edema after radiation therapy that causes discomfort and reduced satisfaction with the cosmetic appearance of the breast. Risk factors associated with the development of breast edema after postlumpectomy radiation include the extent of axillary dissection, large breast size, and a shorter time between surgery and the start of radiotherapy.[9] The type of nodal dissection, the need to treat the axilla with radiotherapy, and/or the presence of a wound infection postoperatively significantly impact the time course of breast edema. Patients who undergo no nodal sampling and those with uncomplicated sentinel lymph node biopsy experience similar rates of breast edema after radiation. The addition of a wound infection or axillary dissection results in significantly more edema that peaks around 4 months after radiation but returns to baseline around 12 months after treatment.[9]

Postradiation breast edema following may present with erythema, warmth, heaviness, and peau d'orange. It may mimic mastitis or inflammatory breast cancer. If there is any question of infection, a course of antibiotics should be prescribed and imaging performed. If there is a concern for the possibility of inflammatory carcinoma, then a skin biopsy looking for a dermal lymphatic tumor should be performed. Otherwise, breast edema can be treated with lymphatic massage, also known as decongestive therapy, by a physical therapist or lymphedema specialist.[10] Wearing a supportive brassiere may improve the physical symptoms.

### Fat Necrosis

Fat necrosis is associated with some form of injury to the breast, such as trauma or surgery. It typically presents as an irregular mass which is not tender to palpation. Imaging studies are usually insufficient to distinguish fat necrosis from malignant lesions, as fat necrosis typically appears as an undefined, spiculated, dense mass. Biopsy is recommended for definitive diagnosis to rule out malignancy. Fat necrosis does not increase the risk of developing a subsequent breast cancer.[4]

## NONPROLIFERATIVE DISORDERS OF THE BREAST
### Cystic Disease

Cystic disease of the breast is the most frequent female benign breast disease. Up to one-third of women aged 30 to 50 years have cysts in their breasts.[4,11] It most commonly presents in the third decade, peaks in the fourth decade when hormonal function is at its peak, and sharply diminishes after menopause. Cystic disease is caused by dilation of ducts and acini to form cysts, proliferation and metaplasia of their epithelial lining, and multiplication of ducts and acini (adenosis) resulting in obstruction of the terminal ductal lobular unit.[11]

Cysts greater than 3 mm can be visualized by ultrasound and are potentially palpable on breast examination. Ultrasound findings of a simple cyst include round or oval shape, anechoic with posterior enhancement, sharp demarcation, and relative mobility in the surrounding tissue. Cysts with these findings can be classified as benign breast imaging-reporting and data system (BI-RADS 2). Ultrasound has 98% accuracy for diagnosing simple cysts.[4] Complicated cysts often have septations within the cyst, homogeneous low-level internal echoes, and brightly echogenic foci. Cysts that have thickened walls, thick internal septations, and are a mixture of cystic and solid components are at a high risk for cancer and should undergo biopsy. Patients are often asymptomatic. If patients are symptomatic with pain or have a very large cyst, aspiration can be performed electively with ultrasound guidance. Aspirated cyst fluid that is clear, yellow, or green may be discarded. Aspirated cyst fluid that is bloody or has floating debris should be sent for cytology. Complex cysts that have been aspirated and have negative cytology can be managed with 6-month follow-up imaging studies instead of intervention, if asymptomatic.[11] However, cysts that do not completely collapse after aspiration or that have asymmetric wall thickening should undergo an image-guided biopsy of the cyst wall to exclude the possibility of malignancy. Any lesion that has atypical cellularity noted in the aspirate should also be excised.

### Duct Ectasia

Most nipples contain 5 to 9 ductal orifices. Duct ectasia predominantly affects the ducts in the retroareolar region and is defined as a nonspecific dilation of one or more ducts, typically larger than 2 mm in diameter.[12] This finding may be palpable and may be associated with nipple discharge. The cause of the duct dilation is not well understood but is often seen in conjunction with periductal inflammation.[4] On imaging with mammography, duct ectasia appears as radiodense serpentine tubular structures converging on the nipple-areolar complex. On ultrasound, the duct is an anechoic smooth-walled branching structure that tapers peripherally. The duct is usually filled with fluid or cellular debris but can occasionally contain calcifications.[12] These findings centrally located favor a benign process, but duct ectasia can also be seen in a spectrum of malignant diseases. When located more peripherally with irregular duct margin and focal thickening of the duct wall, malignancy should be considered and appropriate sampling performed.[12]

### Metaplasia, Squamous, and Apocrine

Apocrine metaplasia is dilated ducts and adjacent cysts that contain inspissated secretions, which can calcify and manifest as heterogeneous calcifications. It is thought that this entity arises from the lobular cells of the terminal duct-lobular unit of the breast. Apocrine metaplasia is present in the epithelial lining of the cysts. Clinically, women may have breast tenderness or irregular nodularity, which may vary during the menstrual cycle. The presence of apocrine metaplasia is not thought to elevate the risk for breast carcinoma.[12]

## PROLIFERATIVE DISORDERS OF THE BREAST
### Mild Hyperplasia (Usual Hyperplasia)

Hyperplasia is abnormally increased cell proliferation and can be present with or without atypia. Hyperplasia with atypia is also known as atypical hyperplasia and can be present as atypical ductal or lobular hyperplasia. These entities are covered elsewhere in this monograph.

The ducts in the breast normally contain 2 layers of epithelial cells. When the number of layers increases, this is known as ductal hyperplasia. Mild ductal hyperplasia has 3 or 4 epithelial layers.[4] It is typically noted as an incidental finding after tissue sampling and does not require any further intervention.

### Fibroadenoma

Fibroadenoma is the most common benign tumor of the breast and typically occurs in women younger than 30 years. It originates in the breast lobules and can be comprised of stromal and epithelial cells. Fibroadenomas are firm, rubbery masses with a well-circumscribed border. Usually fibroadenomas form as a single tumor. However, in up to 15% of patients, multiple tumors are present, and 10% will be bilateral.[4] Fibroadenomas may grow rapidly during pregnancy or whenever there is an increase in hormonal influence. Those larger than 5 cm are termed *giant fibroadenomas*. Ultrasound can be used to differentiate a fibroadenoma from a cyst. Fibroadenomas are well-defined, usually oval masses with weak, uniformly distributed internal echoes. If imaging cannot conclusively confirm the diagnosis, the mass should be biopsied.[4]

Fibroadenomas carry little to no increased risk of breast cancer. However, on rare occasions, intraductal or invasive cancer can develop in a fibroadenoma, just as it can in any other part of the breast. In addition, multiple fibroadenomas are associated with some rare cancer syndromes, such as Maffucci syndrome, Cowden syndrome, and Carney complex. Fibroadenomas that develop in these kindred should be excised.[13]

In many instances, fibroadenoma may be observed and managed conservatively. Criteria for excision include a size greater than 2 to 3 cm, symptomatic tumors, or when the diagnosis is in question such as with imaging findings of vascularity or irregular borders on ultrasound. Additionally, an increase in size documented by ultrasound measurements or clinical examination raises the potential for an alternative diagnosis and warrants removal of the lesion.[13] When performed, excision is focused on removing the tumor without additional surrounding breast tissue. Because these lesions are not infiltrative, they usually do not cause deformities of the breast after removal.

Recently an alternative to excision has been developed. Lesions that have undergone the triple test of clinical examination, ultrasound imaging, and tissue sampling with benign findings are candidates for cryoablation. Cryoablation is performed percutaneously and destroys the lesion by freezing. Excellent long-term cosmetic results are possible with the use of cryoablation, but its use requires specialized training and equipment to perform.[14] Patients nearing menopause with fibroadenoma should be educated as to the likely involution of these lesions with aging and a changing hormonal environment, which would argue against consideration of either excision or ablation for most patients.

### Papillomas and Nipple Discharge

Papillomas occur in major ducts and consist of epithelial proliferation on a fibrovascular stalk. They are typically located within a few centimeters of the nipple and grow within the duct, occasionally resulting in obstruction. Clinically, they may be asymptomatic or manifest as serous or serosanguinous nipple discharge. The classic presentation is one of spontaneous nipple discharge noted by patients on their undergarments. Discharge may also be identified during a clinical breast examination or during mammography. Papillomas may also present as an asymmetric density on mammography or found incidentally during ultrasonography for other reasons. A papilloma can be visualized on galactography as a focal filling defect and may completely obstruct further filling beyond the level of obstruction. On ultrasound, a papilloma typically appears as an ovoid solid mass associated with ductal dilation. These imaging abnormalities will often trigger a need for tissue sampling.

When papillomas are diagnosed via a core needle biopsy, whether or not to excise the entire lesion remains controversial. Some investigators have reported large series with a low risk of malignancy (3%) associated with benign papillomas, and those institutions advocate observation for these lesions, reserving excision for lesions with atypia.[15,16] Other series have noted a much higher false-negative biopsy rate of benign papillomas, with upstaging up to 19% of the time and rates of malignancy in the range of 14%.[17,18] At the Medical College of Wisconsin, the authors have observed a malignancy rate of up to 7.4%, with some variability among racial groups. (Amanda L. Kong, MD, Milwaukee, Wisconsin, personal communication, September 2012) Thus, the authors, like most institutions, recommend excising papillomas diagnosed on core needle biopsy. Higher-risk lesions include a papilloma greater than 1 cm and those located more than 3 cm from the nipple in patients older than 50 years.[12] All investigators agree that lesions demonstrating atypia should be excised for a definitive diagnosis.[15,17,18]

Papillomatosis, or multiple papillomas, may occur in the distal ducts of the terminal duct-lobular unit. This entity is more often associated with hyperplasia, atypia, ductal carcinoma in situ, invasive cancer, sclerosing adenosis, and radial scars. Patients with papillomatosis are at an increased lifetime risk of breast cancer, although the reason for this is unclear. Most patients with papillomatosis are asymptomatic, although some may present with spontaneous nipple discharge.[12]

Nipple discharge is the third most common presenting symptom to a breast clinic, after palpable masses and pain. It can be a source of considerable anxiety but is rarely the presenting symptom of a breast cancer. Discharge that is more suspicious is unilateral, from a single duct, spontaneous, persistent, and clear, serous, sero-sanguinous, or bloodstained in character.[4] Approximately 55% of patients presenting with nipple discharge have an associated mass, 19% of which are malignant.[19] Milky discharge (galactorrhea) can be caused by benign breast conditions or by some medications, including oral contraceptives, serotonin reuptake inhibitors, tricyclic antidepressants, methyldopa, and morphine. Galactorrhea can also result from increased production of prolactin from a tumor in the pituitary gland or hypothyroidism.[4] Patients who present with bilateral breast discharge warrant an endocrine evaluation.

Modalities to investigate nipple discharge include discharge cytology, fluorescent in situ hybridization (FISH) analysis of discharge, ductography, and ductoscopy. Cytology has a low sensitivity for detection of breast cancer and is unlikely to alter the management of patients with nipple discharge. There is a small pilot study using FISH that demonstrates 100% specificity in making a definitive diagnosis of malignancy in patients with indeterminate cytology, and may serve as a good adjunct to cytology, but is not routinely used in clinical practice at this time.[20] Ductography has a high-positive predictive value for the diagnosis of intraductal lesions, papillomas, and carcinoma; but it has a low sensitivity and is painful for patients. Ductoscopy is a promising tool that can be used to localize the lesion to one duct, sparing the others in young women, allowing them to retain the ability to lactate. Duct excision is the only modality that provides a definitive histologic diagnosis and remains the gold standard.[19] When excision is required, a selective excision of the draining duct versus complete excision of the retroareolar major ducts should be discussed. Complete major duct excision has the advantage or reducing the risk of recurrence of discharge while eliminating the potential for future breastfeeding. Patients' likelihood of future child bearing should be the deciding factor because when performed through a small areolar edge incision, complete excision has no impact on breast sensation or appearance.

### Sclerosing Adenosis

Adenosis is a fibrocystic change in the breast resulting from an increase in the number of acini in the lobules. Sclerosing adenosis is a proliferative disease whereby the number of acini more than double and the acini lose their normal appearance. The cause is unknown, but the theory is that it is caused by an abnormality in the involution process. It may present as a mass or architectural distortion. On mammogram, calcifications may be present. Biopsy is necessary to diagnose this benign condition.[4]

### Radial Scar/Complex Sclerosing Lesions

Radial scars and complex sclerosing lesions are benign clinical entities that are rare findings most often identified during screening mammography as an asymmetric density or a distortion with spiculation emanating from a central lucency.[21] Both lesions have a characteristic microscopic appearance of slender, radially arranged bands around a fibroelastic core with entrapped ducts and lobules.[22] *Complex sclerosing lesion* is the term used for lesions greater than 1 cm in diameter and *radial scar* is used for lesions less than 1 cm in diameter.

Radial scars and complex sclerosing lesions are associated with malignancy or another high-risk lesion up to 28% of the time.[22] Thus, most institutions have recommended complete excision of these lesions for diagnosis. However, some institutions have taken a more conservative approach and only excise lesions that demonstrate atypia. Long-term follow-up of patients with a history of a radial scar that has been excised has not demonstrated any greater risk of developing cancer, regardless of the size of the lesion, unless other high-risk lesions were identified.[21]

## BREAST PAIN/MASTALGIA

Mastalgia or breast pain is a common symptom among patients seeking treatment in a breast clinic. About 90% of conditions that cause breast pain are benign.[4] The key to management of breast pain lies in a determination of the cause and whether or not it is cyclic or noncyclic in nature. Cyclic breast pain usually starts within 2 weeks before menses and resolves or diminishes with the onset of menses. It recurs at roughly the same time each month during a woman's cycle. Although commonly thought to be related to a variety of factors, caffeine intake, iodine deficiency, and dietary fat intake have not been definitively established as causal factors in cyclic breast pain.[23] In most instances, cyclic breast pain can be managed by watchful waiting without treatment once it is established that there is no associated malignant process present. Other modifying factors to try include improving support for pendulous breasts, ensuring proper fit of a brassiere, and a trial of nonsteroidal antiinflammatory agents.

Noncyclic breast pain usually occurs in postmenopausal women and can be caused by certain medications, such as antidepressants, digoxin, thiazide-class diuretics, and methyldopa.[4] However, it is frequently associated with underlying musculoskeletal issues with the chest wall, such as arthritis and costochondritis. Breast pain resulting from musculoskeletal conditions is best appreciated on physical examination and patients' pain reproduced with palpation of the pectoralis major muscle separated from the breast with patients in the sitting position or palpation of the intercostal muscles through the axilla. The pain is often burning or sharp in nature and may localize to a specific area.[23]

Several agents have been tried for the treatment of cyclical and noncyclical breast pain, including hormonal manipulation, nonsteroidal antiinflammatory agents, and plant derivatives like evening primrose oil (EPO). Srivastava and colleagues[24] published a meta-analysis of the randomized trials using different treatments for mastalgia and assessing their effectiveness on breast pain. The most common treatments included bromocriptine mesylate (Cycloset, Parlodel), danazol (Danocrine), tamoxifen citrate (Nolvadex, Soltamox) and EPO. They found women received significant pain relief using bromocriptine mesylate, danazol, and tamoxifen citrate; but there was no significant difference in pain scores in women treated with EPO. There is a lack of strong data comparing the 3 drugs. However, tamoxifen citrate was associated with the fewest side effects and should be the first drug of choice. The natural history of mastalgia seems to be that in some women that achieve good control of pain, they will remain in remission for a long time regardless of whether they receive any medication or not.[24]

## SUMMARY

Benign breast disorders are a group of conditions that are commonly managed by surgeons. Benign breast pathologic conditions rarely increases the risk of malignancy. As knowledge of benign breast pathologic conditions improves, many conditions can be managed without the need for open surgery. Collaborative care models including nurse practitioners can improve patient experience and education about their breast health.

# REFERENCES

1. Dontje KJ, Sparks BT, Given BA. Establishing a collaborative practice in a comprehensive breast clinic. Clin Nurse Spec 1996;10(2):95–101.
2. Garvican L, Grimsey E, Littlejohns P, et al. Satisfaction with clinical nurse specialists in a breast care clinic: questionnaire survey. BMJ 1998;316(7136): 976–7.
3. Trop I, Dugas A, David J, et al. Breast abscesses: evidence-based algorithms for diagnosis, management, and follow-up. Radiographics 2011;31(6):1683–99.
4. Ferrara A. Benign breast disease. Radiol Technol 2011;82(5):447M–62M.
5. Gollapalli V, Liao J, Dudakovic A, et al. Risk factors for development and recurrence of primary breast abscesses. J Am Coll Surg 2010;211(1):41–8.
6. Karstrup S, Solvig J, Nolsoe CP, et al. Acute puerperal breast abscesses: US-guided drainage. Radiology 1993;188(3):807–9.
7. Salemis NS, Merkouris S, Kimpouri K. Mondor's disease of the breast. A retrospective review. Breast Dis 2011;33(3):103–7.
8. Paniagua CT, Negron ZD. Mondor's disease: a case study. J Am Acad Nurse Pract 2010;22(6):312–5.
9. Wratten CR, O'brien PC, Hamilton CS, et al. Breast edema in patients undergoing breast-conserving treatment for breast cancer: assessment via high frequency ultrasound. Breast J 2007;13(3):266–73.
10. Degnim AC, Miller J, Hoskin TL, et al. A prospective study of breast lymphedema: frequency, symptoms, and quality of life. Breast Cancer Res Treat 2012;134(3): 915–22.
11. Rinaldi P, Ierardi C, Costantini M, et al. Cystic breast lesions: sonographic findings and clinical management. J Ultrasound Med 2010;29(11):1617–26.
12. Ferris-James DM, Iuanow E, Mehta TS, et al. Imaging approaches to diagnosis and management of common ductal abnormalities. Radiographics 2012;32(4): 1009–30.
13. Jayasinghe Y, Simmons PS. Fibroadenomas in adolescence. Curr Opin Obstet Gynecol 2009;21(5):402–6.
14. Kaufman CS, Littrup PJ, Freeman-Gibb LA, et al. Office-based cryoablation of breast fibroadenomas with long-term follow-up. Breast J 2005;11(5):344–50.
15. Sydnor MK, Wilson JD, Hijaz TA, et al. Underestimation of the presence of breast carcinoma in papillary lesions initially diagnosed at core-needle biopsy. Radiology 2007;242(1):58–62.
16. Cuneo KC, Dash RC, Wilke LG, et al. Risk of invasive breast cancer and ductal carcinoma in situ in women with atypical papillary lesions of the breast. Breast J 2012;18(5):475–8.
17. Rozentsvayg E, Carver K, Borkar S, et al. Surgical excision of benign papillomas diagnosed with core biopsy: a community hospital approach. Radiol Res Pract 2011;2011:679864.
18. Liberman L, Tornos C, Huzjan R, et al. Is surgical excision warranted after benign, concordant diagnosis of papilloma at percutaneous breast biopsy? AJR Am J Roentgenol 2006;186(5):1328–34.
19. Foulkes RE, Heard G, Boyce T, et al. Duct excision is still necessary to rule out breast cancer in patients presenting with spontaneous bloodstained nipple discharge. Int J Breast Cancer 2011;2011:495315.
20. Yamamoto D, Senzaki H, Nakagawa H, et al. Detection of chromosomal aneusomy by fluorescence in situ hybridization for patients with nipple discharge. Cancer 2003;97(3):690–4.

21. Bunting DM, Steel JR, Holgate CS, et al. Long term follow-up and risk of breast cancer after a radial scar or complex sclerosing lesion has been identified in a benign open breast biopsy. Eur J Surg Oncol 2011;37(8):709–13.
22. Andacoglu O, Kanbour-Shakir A, Teh YC, et al. Rationale of excisional biopsy after the diagnosis of benign radial scar on core biopsy: a single institutional outcome analysis. Am J Clin Oncol 2013;36(1):7–11.
23. Santen RJ, Mansel R. Benign breast disorders. N Engl J Med 2005;353(3): 275–85.
24. Srivastava A, Mansel RE, Arvind N, et al. Evidence-based management of mastalgia: a meta-analysis of randomised trials. Breast 2007;16(5):503–12.

# Screening, Imaging, and Image-Guided Biopsy Techniques for Breast Cancer

Dana H. Smetherman, MD, MPH

## KEYWORDS

- Mammography • Screening • Breast ultrasonography • Breast MRI

## KEY POINTS

- Multidisciplinary care requires careful integration of imaging and pathologic information both prospectively and throughout the course of treatment of the patient with breast cancer.
- A thorough understanding of the appropriate strategies for breast cancer screening based on risk factors is essential to identify breast cancer in its earliest and most treatable stages.
- Although mammography remains the cornerstone imaging study for breast cancer diagnosis, other examinations, currently in use and still in development, may provide additional information that results in earlier detection, better staging and surgical planning, more precise assessment of response to treatment, earlier identification of recurrent carcinoma, and, hopefully, better patient outcomes.

## INTRODUCTION

Diagnostic imaging and image-guided needle biopsies play a central role in the diagnosis, treatment planning, and staging of patients with breast cancer. Mammography remains the mainstay in breast cancer detection. Most patients with newly diagnosed breast cancer will have been imaged with mammography, ultrasonography, or both.

Breast cancer most often presents as a mass, calcifications, or both on imaging. Usually, masses indicate invasive breast carcinoma, whereas calcifications suggest ductal carcinoma in situ (DCIS). When breast cancer presents as a mass, initial evaluation generally includes characterization with mammogram and ultrasonogram plus an evaluation to identify satellite lesions and associated calcifications. As an example of the importance of breast imaging, when DCIS associated with a mass meets the criteria for extensive intraductal component, the likelihood of obtaining clear surgical margins is decreased and therefore the risk of local recurrence is increased.[1,2] Carcinomas that

Breast Imaging, Department of Radiology, Ochsner Health System, 1516 Jefferson Highway, New Orleans, LA 70121, USA
E-mail address: dsmetherman@ochsner.org

Surg Clin N Am 93 (2013) 309–327
http://dx.doi.org/10.1016/j.suc.2013.01.004
0039-6109/13/$ – see front matter © 2013 Elsevier Inc. All rights reserved.

surgical.theclinics.com

present solely with calcifications should be imaged with mammographic magnification images to evaluate the extent of disease and, in some instances, with ultrasound to document the presence of underlying masses, which may indicate coexistent invasive carcinoma. Diagnostic imaging is also used to identify axillary adenopathy, involvement of the skin, pectoralis muscles and chest wall, and, when appropriate, distant metastases. Establishment of multifocal and multicentric carcinoma, which may not be apparent on initial imaging with mammography and ultrasonography, is also critical for optimal surgical management and ultimately successful treatment.

Preoperative magnetic resonance imaging (MRI) has been shown to detect unsuspected additional disease and change surgical management in patients diagnosed with breast cancer.[3] MRI can also identify unsuspected, mammographically occult contralateral synchronous breast cancers in 3% to 5% of patients with newly diagnosed breast cancer.[4,5] Nonetheless, the routine use of preoperative MRI remains controversial. There are little data about improvement in recurrence and mortality rates if preoperative MRI is used at the time of breast cancer diagnosis. In addition, false-positive findings on MRI may lead to unnecessary, additional workup and biopsies and, thus, delay treatment.[6–8]

## MAMMOGRAPHY

A mammogram is a radiographic examination of the breast, either displayed on a film or on a computer monitor. Screening mammograms are performed on women who are asymptomatic and include images of each breast in the CC (craniocaudad) and MLO (mediolateral oblique) projections (**Fig. 1**). Diagnostic mammograms are performed in women who have a clinical problem, such as a palpable mass or other symptom of breast disease, a history of breast cancer within the preceding 5 years, or have been recalled for additional imaging from an abnormal screening mammogram. Diagnostic mammograms may include special views such as focal compression of one area of the breast tissue or magnification images. Another variation on special mammographic views includes women with breast implants that should be evaluated with Eklund views. These views displace the implants and allow for an increase in the amount of imaged breast tissue compared with traditional mammographic views.

During a mammogram, the breast tissue is compressed between 2 plates, one a plastic compression paddle and the other an x-ray detecting plate. Compression is necessary to prevent the image from appearing unsharp due to motion, to physically spread out the glandular tissue, and to decrease the thickness of the breast tissue by reducing overlapping dense tissue. The average radiation dose from a 4-view mammogram is 0.4 mSv or roughly equal to 7 weeks of natural background radiation.

Full-field digital mammography (FFDM) replaces x-ray film with solid-state detectors that convert x-rays into electrical signals to produce images of the breasts. Digital mammography images can be viewed on a computer screen or on printed films. Computer-aided detection (CAD) assesses the data from a digital or digitized film-screen mammogram for signs of increased density or calcifications. CAD programs superimpose markings on mammographic images, drawing the radiologist's attention to a potential abnormal. Early, retrospective studies demonstrated improved cancer detection when radiologists used CAD programs when interpreting mammograms.[9–14] Subsequent research has shown more modest results and even decreased diagnostic accuracy and increased rate of biopsy without improvement in detection of invasive breast carcinoma.[15]

The Mammography Quality Standards Act (MQSA) was passed in 1992. MQSA was intended to ensure that mammography performed in the United States for detection of

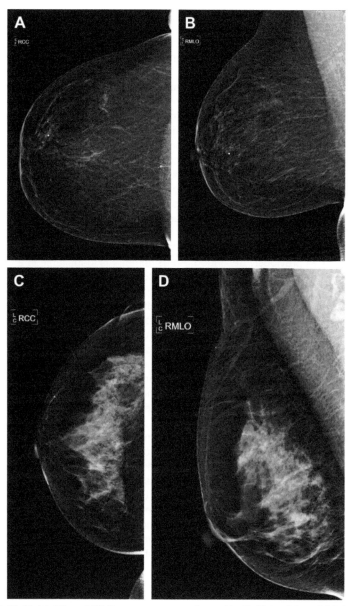

**Fig. 1.** (A–D) Right CC and MLO mammograms, fatty. (A, B) Right CC and MLO mammograms, dense (C, D).

early breast cancer is safe and of reliable quality. Under MQSA, all facilities performing mammography in the United States must be certified by the US Food and Drug Administration (FDA) or an FDA-approved Certifying State. MQSA requirements address the quality of mammographic equipment, personnel who perform and interpret mammography, and reporting. MQSA also stipulates that all facilities that perform mammograms must have a quality assurance program and procedures for following abnormal findings and obtaining and tracking pathologic results from biopsy procedures. Annual inspection by appropriately trained FDA or state inspectors is mandatory, and facilities are required to display their FDA certificates. The result of MQSA has been improved mammographic technique, lower radiation dose, and better training of personnel.[16]

The Breast Imaging Reporting and Database System (BI-RADS) is the standardized method for reporting of mammographic findings.[17] The BI-RADS lexicon is used to describe and classify findings on breast imaging studies. Originally developed for mammographic findings, the BI-RADS lexicon has been expanded to encompass findings on ultrasonography and MRI. Mammography reports also include an estimation of the relative fatty and fibroglandular composition of the breast tissue (Table 1).

On mammograms, carcinomas present as masses, asymmetries, and calcifications. By definition, a mass is a space-occupying lesion seen in 2 different planes. This is distinguished from a density, which is seen only in a single plane. The shape of masses is described as round, oval, lobular, or irregular, while the margins are identified as circumscribed (with well-defined margins), indistinct, and spiculated (with lines radiating from the margins) (Fig. 2). An asymmetry cannot be accurately described as any of the shapes previously described. An asymmetry is identifiable in 2 planes but lacks the borders and conspicuity of a mass and may simply represent an island of normal glandular tissue. Additional mammographic imaging of an asymmetry may identify a mass or architectural distortion. Architectural distortion, which can occur with or without a central mass, is used to describe spiculations radiating from a point and focal retraction at the edge of parenchyma. Architectural distortion can be seen in association with a mass or as an isolated finding.

Calcifications associated with benign disease are generally larger than those seen with malignancy and typically are coarse (round, lucent centered, or "layering" on 90° medial lateral or lateral medial images). Amorphous, indistinct, pleomorphic (or heterogeneous), fine, linear, or branching calcifications are more typical of carcinomas (Fig. 3).

DCIS typically presents with calcifications on mammography. In the past 30 years, there has been a large increase in the frequency of DCIS diagnosed in the United States because of the widespread adoption of screening mammography.

Finally, the BI-RADS lexicon requires a final assessment of one of 7 categories (0–6) and recommended follow-up plan (Table 2). Using the lexicon and assessment system, a quality audit is generated identifying the number of false-negative (ie, missed cancers) and false-positive findings, positive and negative predictive values, sensitivity, and specificity for each practice as a whole and for individual radiologists. The report of a breast imaging study must be sent to the referring health care provider,

| Table 1 Breast imaging reporting and database system method for reporting of mammographic finding | |
|---|---|
| BI-RADS Description | Glandular Tissue (%) |
| The breast is almost entirely fat | <25 |
| Scattered fibroglandular tissue | 25–50 |
| Heterogeneously dense breast tissue | 51–75 |
| Extremely dense | >75 |

*Data from* American College of Radiology. Breast imaging reporting and data system (BI-RADS). 4th edition. Reston (VA): American College of Radiology; 2003.

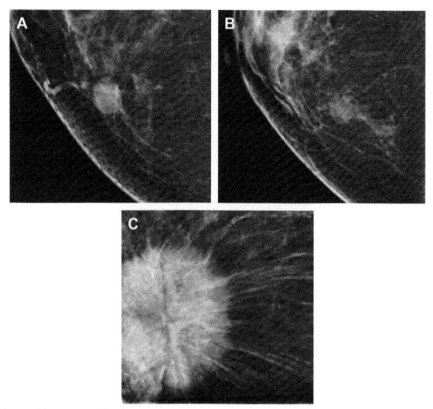

**Fig. 2.** (*A*) Circumscribed mass on mammogram. (*B*) Indistinct mass on mammogram. (*C*) Spiculated mass on mammogram.

and a written report in lay language must be sent to the patient within 30 days of the mammographic study. If the assessment is "suspicious" or "highly suggestive of malignancy," the report should be communicated to the health care provider and patient as soon as possible (ideally within 3–5 days).

### Full-Field Digital Mammography

In 2000, the FDA approved the use of FFDM in the United States. In 2005, the Digital Mammographic Imaging Screening Trial studied 49,528 women who presented for screening mammography in the United States and Canada.[18] The overall diagnostic accuracy was found to be similar for digital and film mammography. The accuracy of digital mammography exceeded that of film mammography in women younger than 50 years, women with heterogeneously or extremely dense breasts, and premenopausal and perimenopausal women.

Since 2000, FFDM has largely replaced film-screen mammography. Based on the MQSA National Statistics as of June 1, 2012, from the US FDA, 7313 of 8626 (84.8%) mammography facilities and 10,639 of 12,367 (86%) mammography units in the United States are FFDM units.[19] Nonetheless, the transition to digital mammography has not eliminated the issues with mammography as a screening tool. Overall, the sensitivity and specificity of mammography are 79% and 90%, respectively, and both are lower in younger women and women with dense breast tissue.

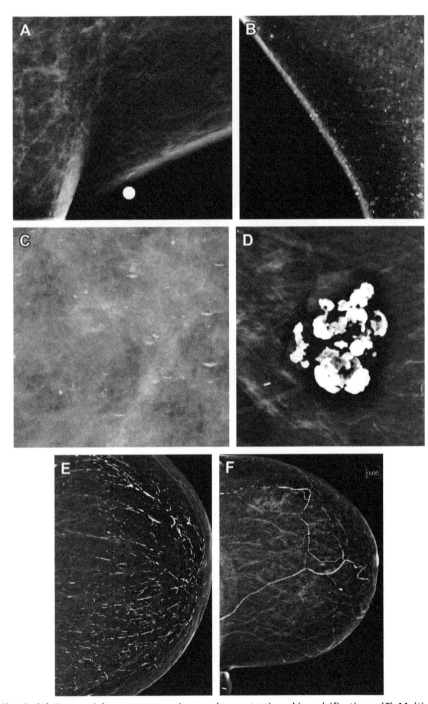

**Fig. 3.** (*A*) Tangential mammogram image demonstrating skin calcifications. (*B*) Multiple skin calcifications. (*C*) Layering milk of calcium on 90° lateral mammogram image. (*D*) Coarse, popcorn-type calcifications in a fibroadenoma. (*E*) Coarse linear and branching secretory type calcifications. (*F*) Vascular calcifications. (*G*) Linear branching calcifications in DCIS. (*H*) Linear branching calcifications in DCIS.

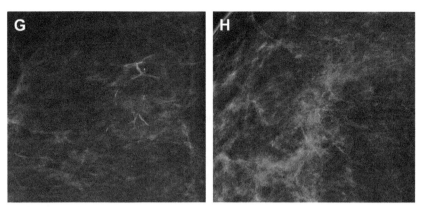

**Fig. 3.** (*continued*)

## ULTRASOUND IMAGING

Ultrasound imaging uses high-frequency sound waves to generate images without the use of ionizing radiation. The current indications for breast ultrasonography include palpable findings (including as the initial imaging test of palpable findings in patients who are younger than 30 years, pregnant, or lactating), abnormalities or suspected abnormalities on mammography or MRI, problems with breast implants, suspected underlying mass in the setting of microcalcifications or architectural distortion on mammography, supplemental screening in women at high risk for breast cancer who are not candidates for or do not have easy access to MRI, and suspected axillary lymphadenopathy. Real-time imaging is also possible with ultrasonography, making it ideal for interventional procedures. Breast ultrasound imaging should be performed with a high-resolution real-time linear array transducer with a center frequency of at least 10 MHz, using the highest frequency with which adequate penetration of the tissue is feasible.

**Table 2**
**Breast imaging reporting and database system assessment categories**

| Category | Assessment | Follow-up |
|---|---|---|
| 0 | Need additional imaging evaluation | Additional imaging needed before a category can be assigned |
| 1 | Negative | Continue annual screening mammograms (women older than 40 y) |
| 2 | Benign finding | Continue annual screening mammograms (women older than 40 y) |
| 3 | Probably benign | Initial short term follow-up (usually six month) mammogram (<2% chance of malignancy) |
| 4 | Suspicious abnormality | Biopsy should be considered (2%–95% chance of malignancy) |
| 5 | Highly suggestive of malignancy | Requires biopsy (>95% chance of malignancy) |
| 6 | Known cancer | Biopsy-proven malignancy |

*Data from* American College of Radiology. Breast imaging reporting and data system (BI-RADS). 4th edition. Reston (VA): American College of Radiology; 2003.

BI-RADS descriptors for ultrasound lesions include morphologic descriptors that are similar to those used in mammography. Masses are described by shape (oval, round, or irregular) and margins (circumscribed, indistinct, angular, or spiculated) (**Fig. 4**A–D). The ultrasound imaging lexicon also includes features unique to sonography, including orientation relative to the skin line (parallel or not parallel), lesion boundary (sharp or with an echogenic halo), posterior acoustic features (enhancement or shadowing), and vascularity. The echogenicity (shade of gray) of masses on ultrasound imaging is compared with normal fat lobules and described as hypoechoic, isoechoic, hyperechoic, or mixed echogenicity.

Elastography, the measurement of the elastic properties of tissues, is another method to evaluate breast lesions that can be performed with adaptation of sonographic equipment. Interest in using elastography arose from the observation that malignant tissues are firmer than benign tissues and, thus, less compressible. Elastography uses data before and after the application of compression (either manually applied "static" elastography or "shear wave" elastography where waves are emitted perpendicular to the ultrasound transducer).

## MAGNETIC RESONANCE IMAGING OF THE BREAST

Breast MRI has evolved to become an integral part of breast cancer diagnosis and management. Current indications for breast MRI include screening of the contralateral breast in patients with newly diagnosed breast carcinoma, evaluation of patients in whom mammographic evaluation is limited by augmentation (including silicone and

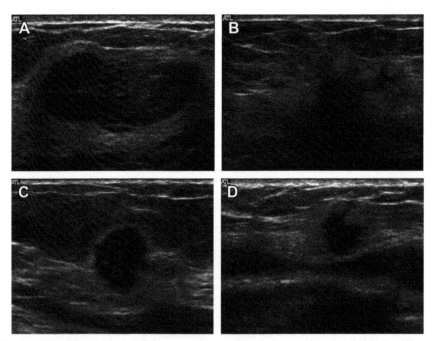

**Fig. 4.** (*A*) Oval, hypoechoic solid mass with smooth margins on ultrasound imaging (fibroadenoma). (*B*) Irregular hypoechoic solid mass with irregular margins and posterior acoustic shadowing on ultrasound imaging (IDC). (*C*) Irregular nonparallel hypoechoic solid mass with spiculated margins on ultrasound imaging (IDC). (*D*) Irregular hypoechoic solid mass with angulated margins on ultrasound imaging (IDC). IDC, invasive ductal carcinoma.

saline implants and silicone injections), determining the extent of disease at the time of initial diagnosis of breast cancer (including identification of invasion of the pectoralis major, serratus anterior, and intercostal muscles), evaluation of inconclusive findings on clinical examination, mammography, and/or ultrasonography, and asymptomatic screening of patients at very high risk of breast carcinoma (in conjunction with routine mammography). Other uses of breast MRI include evaluation of response to neoadjuvant chemotherapy with imaging before, during, and/or after treatment, and identification of residual disease in patients with positive margins after lumpectomy. MRI may be useful in patients who present with metastatic disease or axillary adenopathy suspicious for breast origin with no primary identified on mammography.

According to the American College of Radiology Practice Guideline for the Performance of Contrast-Enhanced Magnetic Resonance Imaging (MRI) of the Breast, facilities that perform diagnostic breast MRI should either have the capability to perform MRI-guided biopsies for lesions seen only on MRI or have arrangements with another facility that can perform these services. This arrangement is necessary to ensure that findings seen on MRI can be biopsied.

Breast MRI is generally performed with a dedicated breast coil on a magnet of 1.5 T field strength or greater, using slice thickness of 3 mm or less, and in plane resolution of 1 mm or less. To detect small abnormalities, high spatial and temporal resolution is necessary, as well as optimization of contrast between normal tissue and carcinoma. T1- and T2-weighted images are obtained. Chemical fat suppression techniques and subtraction are often used. Kinetic curves are generated by measuring lesion enhancement at scan intervals separated by 3 minutes or less. Dynamic scanning is usually performed with T1-weighted images (with or without fat suppression). Both breasts should be imaged simultaneously unless the patient has undergone mastectomy. Gadolinium contrast (0.1 mmol/kg) is used unless the examination is performed solely for the evaluation of implant integrity, which does not require contrast enhancement.

MRI evaluation of breast lesions includes assessment of morphologic features, signal characteristics, and enhancement patterns. As with mammographic and sonographic lesions, morphology is described using a BI-RADS lexicon. Masses are described as round, oval, lobulated, or irregular, with smooth, irregular, or spiculated margins. Enhancement patterns are described as homogeneous, heterogeneous, central or rim enhancing, or with dark (nonenhancing) or enhancing internal septations. Generally, benign lesions such as cysts, lymph nodes, and fibroadenomas with myxomatous contents have high (bright) signal on T2-weighted images. Most malignant masses have low signal on T2-weighted images (**Fig. 5**A).

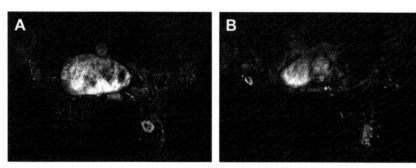

**Fig. 5.** (*A*) Irregular rim enhancing mass on MRI (IDC). (*B*) Stippled and clumped nonmass enhancement on MRI (DCIS).

Unlike the BI-RADS classification for mammographic and sonographic findings, the American College of Radiology (ACR) lexicon for MRI includes so-called nonmass enhancement. With nonmass enhancement, there is enhancement of the breast tissue without the presence of a defined mass. Nonmass enhancement can be symmetric or asymmetric. The distribution of nonmass enhancement is described as a focal area, linear, ductal, regional, segmental (triangular, apex toward the nipple), or diffuse. The pattern of nonmass enhancement is characterized as homogeneous, heterogeneous, stippled, clumped, or reticular. Linear, clumped, or irregular nonmass enhancement suggests DCIS (see **Fig. 5B**).

Enhancement of lesions on dynamic MRI is quantified and displayed as kinetic curves, demonstrating initial uptake and subsequent washout or accumulation of contrast over time. Initial enhancement (within the first 2 minutes usually) is described as rapid, medium, or slow. Enhancement after the first 2 minutes follows a pattern of decreasing enhancement (washout), stable enhancement (plateau), or gradually increasing enhancement (persistent). Breast carcinomas typically demonstrate rapid uptake and washout. Normal tissue and benign lesions generally have slow uptake and persistent delayed enhancement (**Fig. 6**). There is considerable overlap between the enhancement curve characteristics of benign and malignant lesions, however, and use of both morphologic features and kinetic curves is thought to be preferable to relying solely on enhancement characteristics.[20]

The sensitivity of MRI for detection of breast cancer is high, generally reported in the range of 90%. Nonetheless, the sensitivity is considerably lower for DCIS than for invasive carcinoma, and the specificity of breast MRI is only in the range of 50% to 70%.[21–23]

Breast MRI has also been shown to be the best predictor of response in patients who have undergone neoadjuvant chemotherapy. In the American College of Radiology Imaging Network (ACRIN) 6657/I-SPY Trial, MRI imaging findings were found to be a stronger predictor of response to chemotherapy at pathologic evaluation than clinical assessment for locally advanced breast cancer. The most useful sign of response was change in volumetric measurement early in treatment.[24]

## IMAGING-GUIDED BREAST INTERVENTIONAL PROCEDURES

In the current practice of breast cancer diagnosis, one important objective is to reduce unnecessary surgical excisional biopsies. Percutaneous needle biopsies have become the procedure of choice for diagnosis of image-detected abnormalities. In addition to distinguishing benign from malignant causes, percutaneous biopsy facilitates surgical planning. In many cases, all necessary surgical procedures can be performed in a single setting with attention to surgical margins, appropriate selection of patients for breast conservation versus mastectomy, and performance of sentinel node biopsy, if indicated.

Interventional procedures can be guided by mammographic, ultrasonographic, or magnetic resonance images. Percutaneous sampling is conducted with core needle biopsy (using "gun type" or vacuum-assisted needles) or fine needle aspiration. Core biopsy needle sizes range from 7 to 14 gauge for most breast lesions. MRI-guided biopsies generally require intravenous gadolinium contrast to identify the lesion to be biopsied. With core needle biopsy, a radiopaque, usually metal marker is frequently placed at the biopsy site, particularly for small lesions, to document the location of the area sampled.

Image guidance is also used for preoperative needle localization. With needle localization, a hook wire is placed at the area of interest. Surgical removal of the lesion is confirmed with a radiographic or sonographic image of the specimen.

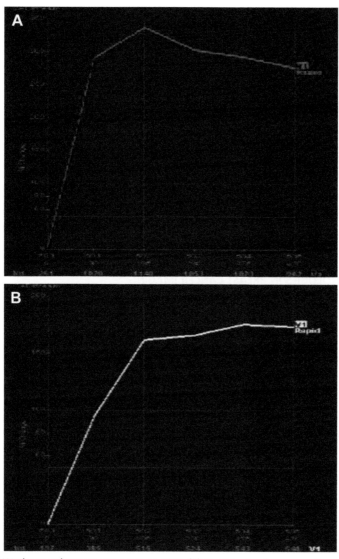

Fig. 6. (A) Washout enhancement curve on MRI. (B) Persistent enhancement curve on MRI.

Correlation of imaging and pathologic findings is necessary for all image-guided percutaneous biopsies to ensure radiologic-pathologic correlation. Presuming there is no discordance, surgical removal of lesions found to be benign at core needle biopsy is usually unnecessary.

Breast cancer is most likely to spread to the ipsilateral axillary lymph nodes first (**Fig. 7**). Pathologic evaluation of axillary lymph nodes is necessary to stage breast cancer. Image-guided breast biopsy can be used to perform fine or core needle biopsies on suspicious axillary mode identified by imaging. A positive finding on image-guided axillary biopsy can be incorporated into the selection and sequencing of multidisciplinary treatment planning.

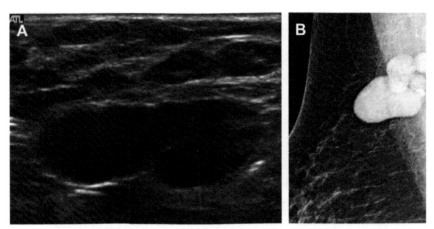

**Fig. 7.** (*A*) Axillary adenopathy on ultrasound imaging. (*B*) Axillary adenopathy on mammography.

## NEW TECHNOLOGIES IN BREAST CANCER IMAGING
### Tomosynthesis

Digital breast tomosynthesis (DBT) is a 3-dimensional (3D) technique in which radiographic images are acquired at multiple angles during a sweep of the x-ray tube. DBT uses FFDM units as a platform. Much like conventional tomography, DBT produces thin slices at different depths through the breast tissue, removing normal overlying structures that can overlap and obscure abnormal tissue on standard, 2-dimensional (2D) mammograms. Compression is required for DBT, and the radiation dose from the combination of DBT and mammography is higher than that from mammography alone. If DBT is used for screening, the radiation dose should decrease for those patients who avoid being recalled. Most women are not recalled from screening mammography, however.

The FDA approved the first DBT device as an adjunct to mammography for diagnostic and screening breast imaging in 2011. The use of 2D and 3D images has been shown to improve the radiologists' ability to differentiate cancerous from noncancerous lesions and to reduce the number of patients recalled from screening studies when compared with mammography alone.[25]

Lack of reimbursement has prevented large-scale adoption of DBT in the United States at the current time. In addition, the larger number of images when DBT is added to mammography may be a challenge for radiologists, for whom it takes more time to review images from both the mammogram and the DBT.

### Contrast-enhanced Mammography

Contrast-enhanced mammography, like contrast-enhanced MRI, uses both anatomic and physiologic information based on enhancement with contrast. Neovascularity in malignancies leads to rapid uptake and washout of contrast in both MRI and contrast-enhanced mammography. In 2011, contrast-enhanced mammography received approval from the FDA. Originally, contrast-enhanced mammography was envisioned as an alternative to MRI in places where MRI is not readily available or in patients for whom there is a contraindication to MRI.

Like DBT, contrast-enhanced mammography is performed using digital mammographic technology. The same type and dose of iodinated contrast are used for contrast-enhanced mammography as for computed tomography. With contrast-enhanced mammography, 2 images of each breast are acquired in the standard CC and MLO positions, a low-energy image and a high-energy image. The 2 images are combined and processed. Then, the background, nonenhancing structures are subtracted, making areas of enhancement more conspicuous (similar to subtracted images from MRI studies). The radiation dose is 20% greater than a standard mammogram. Sensitivity is higher than mammography (93% compared with 78% for mammography alone), with no loss of specificity.[26]

### Radionuclide Breast Imaging—Positron Emission Mammography and Breast-specific Gamma Imaging

Over the years, many breast cancers were incidentally identified on nuclear medicine studies of other parts of the body (such as cardiac studies) using the radionuclide Technetium 99m (Tc 99m). In the past, however, breast cancer detection with nuclear medicine imaging was limited by poor spatial resolution. The recent development of higher-resolution detectors has made nuclear medicine imaging a viable option for breast cancer diagnosis.

Breast-specific gamma imaging (BSGI) uses a scintillating crystal detector to identify uptake of Tc 99m in breast lesions. Two views of each breast are obtained. Studies report an overall high sensitivity (91%–96%) for detection of breast cancer, although sensitivity is less for small lesions measuring less than 1 cm. The specificity (in the range of 60%) is not a significant improvement over MRI.[27–29]

Positron emission mammography (PEM) uses $^{18}$F fluorodeoxyglucose ($^{18}$F FDG), the same agent used for whole-body positron emission tomography (PET). Unlike whole-body PET, PEM studies are imaged with a special detector whose design mimics a mammographic unit. A total of 12 images of each breast are acquired. Originally, the same dose of FDG was used as for whole-body PET. This method showed high sensitivity and specificity (both exceeding 90%) for breast cancer detection. In general, PEM has been shown to be as sensitive as MRI for detection of breast cancer with better specificity.[30,31] Widespread acceptance of both BSGI and PEM has been limited by the high radiation dose associated with these studies, 50 mGy to the lower colon and 59 mGy to the bladder for PEM. Research has been directed to reducing the radiation dose for PEM and BSGI.

## SCREENING MAMMOGRAPHY CONTROVERSIES

Since the early 1990s, when mammographic screening was widely adopted, the mortality rate from breast cancer has dropped more than 30% in the United States. The largest and longest studies of breast cancer screening with mammography have demonstrated a reduction in breast cancer deaths in women starting at age 40 years.[32,33] In June 2012, the American Medical Association joined the American Congress of Obstetricians and Gynecologists, American Society of Breast Surgeons, American Cancer Society, and the American College of Radiology in endorsing mammographic screening for women with average risk of breast cancer starting at age 40 years.

Nonetheless, these recommendations have frequently been challenged, particularly for women from ages 40 to 49 years.[34] In November 2009, the United States Preventive Services Task Force (USPSTF) recommended against routine mammographic screening in women of average risk of breast cancer before age 50 years.[35] Instead, the USPSTF recommended screening between the ages of 50 and 74 years and only every other year. In making this recommendation, the USPSTF reviewed randomized controlled trials on screening mammography but not any information from other peer-reviewed studies, including service screening trials.[32,36] The USPSTF cited the potential harms from screening mammography including radiation exposure, pain during procedures, anxiety and other psychological responses, consequences of false-positive and false-negative findings, and overdiagnosis of breast cancer.

It has been demonstrated that roughly 6500 additional women would die each year in the United States if USPSTF guidelines were used.[37] In June 2012, Mayo Clinic researchers presented data indicating that the USPSTF recommendation had resulted in a 5.72% decrease in mammograms performed in women aged 40 to 49 years. Mammography rates in almost 8 million women were reviewed before and after the announcement of the USPSTF guidelines.[38]

## Screening with Ultrasonography

The limitations of mammography are well documented, with false-negative rates as high as 20%.[39–48] Cancers are more difficult to detect on mammography if the breast tissue is dense, which is more common in younger women. In addition, the density of breast tissue on mammography may be an independent risk factor for the development of breast cancer. Increased breast density is associated with a higher risk of the proliferative lesions that are precursors of breast cancer.[49–52] Thus, much effort has been spent trying to find more accurate methods to detect breast cancer either in addition to or in the place of mammography.

ACRIN trial 6666 is the largest study to date of screening ultrasonography.[53] A total of 2637 women at high risk for breast cancer were screened with mammography and ultrasonography. Forty breast cancers (in 1.5% of participants) were diagnosed. Twenty of the cancers were found with mammography alone (cancer detection rate of 7.6 per 1000 women screened; diagnostic accuracy, 78%). The combination of ultrasound imaging and mammography detected 31 cancers (a detection rate of 11.8 cancers per 1000 women screened; diagnostic accuracy, 91%). Of the 40 total cancers, 8 identified were not seen on initial mammographic or sonographic screening but were identified later in the 12-month period of the study. Both modalities together detected 28% more breast cancers than were identified by mammography alone.

The false-positive rate for findings seen only on ultrasound imaging was greater than for findings seen only on mammography. More than routine follow-up was recommended in 13% of the mammographic screening examinations and 28% of combined mammographic and sonographic screening examinations.

Biopsy was recommended in 241 cases. Findings identified on mammography alone resulted in an unnecessary biopsy for 1 in every 40 women in the study. Findings identified with the combination of mammography and ultrasound screening resulted in an unnecessary biopsy for 1 in 10 women in the study. A total of 168 biopsies were recommended for findings seen with ultrasound imaging only (results: 7.1% carcinoma, 3.6% atypical, 89% benign); 46 biopsies were recommended for findings seen with mammography only (results: 26% carcinoma, 2% atypical, 72% benign).

In a follow-up study, Berg and colleagues[54] examined the impact of adding yearly screening ultrasonography or a single screening MRI to mammography in women at high risk for breast cancer. In 2662 women, 111 breast cancers were detected in 110 women. Of the breast cancers identified on imaging screening studies, there were 33 detected by mammography only, 32 detected by ultrasound imaging only, 26 detected by both mammography and ultrasound imaging, and 9 detected by MRI only (after negative mammography and ultrasound imaging). Eleven breast cancers were not detected by any screening imaging modality.

The increase in cancer detection with supplemental annual screening ultrasound imaging persisted after the first screening ultrasound imaging. With subsequent annual screening ultrasound imaging, the risk of false-positive results decreased but remained higher than for mammography. The positive predictive value (PPV) for lesions seen only on ultrasonography was 9% for the first screening ultrasound imaging and 11.7% for the second and third. The PPV for lesions seen only with mammography was 29.2% for the first screening study and 38.1% for the second and third.

The addition of ultrasound imaging to mammographic screening increased cancer detection by 5.3 cancers per 1000 women in the first year and 3.7 cancers per 1000 women in the second and third years. The addition of MRI screening resulted in a supplemental cancer detection of 14.7 cancers per 1000 women screened. Although the addition of MRI to screening with mammography alone or to mammography plus ultrasonography significantly increased detection of early breast cancer, there was a low rate of interval cancers (8%) in the main ACRIN 6666 study and all interval cancers were node negative. Thus, the benefit of adding screening MRI (rather than ultrasound imaging) to mammographic screening was unclear in patients who are not at high risk.

Under MQSA, all mammography reports sent to clinicians are required to include one of the 4 categories addressing the density of the breast parenchyma. In 2009, Connecticut became the first state to require that all mammography reports given to patients include information regarding the density of the breast tissue also. Since then, other states have followed suit. Almost certainly, this will lead to increased demands for nonmammographic screening tests. These additional tests (most commonly ultrasonography and MRI) may not be readily available and could also result in a high number of false-positive examinations, generating unnecessary follow-up studies and biopsies. Supplemental screening studies may not be cost-effective or reimbursed by insurers. In addition, there may be insufficient resources (equipment and personnel) to implement large-scale screening with modalities other than mammography.

Breast ultrasound imaging is traditionally performed using hand-held equipment, which is time and labor intensive. In ACRIN Trial 6666, physicians performed the screening ultrasound examinations. Reproducibility of that study's results using technologists or automated breast ultrasound systems (although certainly feasible) is still under investigation. In June 2012, an automated breast ultrasound machine was approved by the FDA for use in breast cancer screening.

### Screening with MRI

In March 2007, the American Cancer Society recommended that women with an especially high risk (greater than 20% lifetime) of developing breast cancer undergo screening with MRI in addition to mammography.[55] Women were considered to meet the criteria for additional screening with MRI if they had a BRCA1 or 2 mutation, a first-degree relative with a BRCA1 or 2 mutation and had not undergone genetic testing, a greater than 20% lifetime risk of breast cancer based on risk-assessment tools that take family history and other factors into consideration, undergone radiation therapy to the chest between ages 10 and 30 years, or a history of Li-Fraumeni, Cowden, or Bannayan-Riley-Ruvalcaba syndrome.

There was not believed to be sufficient evidence to recommend for or against screening with MRI in women with a 15% to 20% lifetime risk of breast cancer. Women with a 15% to 20% lifetime risk of breast cancer include those with lobular carcinoma in situ or atypical lobular hyperplasia, atypical duct hyperplasia, very dense or unevenly dense breasts, and a personal history of breast cancer. Finally, the American Cancer Society did not recommend screening for breast cancer with MRI in women with a lifetime risk of breast cancer less than 15%. In addition, although ultrasound can detect additional cancers, it should not take the place of screening with MRI in addition to mammography in women at very high risk of developing breast cancer.

## SUMMARY

Multidisciplinary care requires careful integration of imaging and pathologic information both prospectively and throughout the course of treatment of the patient with breast cancer. A thorough understanding of the appropriate strategies for breast cancer screening based on risk factors is essential for identifying breast cancer in its earliest and most-treatable stages. Although mammography remains the cornerstone imaging study for breast cancer diagnosis, other examinations, currently in use and still in development, may provide additional information that results in earlier detection, better staging and surgical planning, more precise assessment of response to treatment, earlier identification of recurrent carcinoma, and, hopefully, better patient outcomes.

## REFERENCES

1. Schnitt SJ, Connolly JL, Recht A, et al. Breast relapse following primary radiation therapy for early breast cancer. II. Detection, pathologic features and prognostic significance. Int J Radiat Oncol Biol Phys 1985;11:1277–84.
2. Bartelink H, Borger JH, van Dongen JA, et al. The impact of tumor size and histology on local control after breast conserving treatment. Radiother Oncol 1988;11:297–303.
3. Bedrosian I, Mick R, Orel SG, et al. Changes in the surgical management of patients with breast carcinoma based on preoperative magnetic resonance imaging. Cancer 2003;98:468–73.
4. Liberman L, Morris EA, Kim CM, et al. MR imaging findings in the contralateral breast of women with recently diagnosed breast cancer. AJR Am J Roentgenol 2003;180:333–41.
5. Lehman CD, Gatsonis C, Kuhl CK, et al, ACRIN Trial 6667 Investigators Group. MRI evaluation of the contralateral breast in women with recently diagnosed breast cancer. N Engl J Med 2007;356(13):1295–303.
6. Morrow M. Magnetic resonance imaging in the pre-operative evaluation breast cancer: primum non nocere. J Am Coll Surg 2004;198:240–1.
7. Morrow M. Magnetic resonance imaging in breast cancer: one step forward, two steps back? JAMA 2004;292:2779–80.
8. Morrow M. Magnetic resonance imaging in breast cancer: is seeing always believing? Eur J Cancer 2005;41:1368–9.
9. Warren Burhenne LJ, Wood SA, D'Orsi CJ, et al. Potential contribution of computer-aided detection to the sensitivity of screening mammography. Radiology 2000;215(2):554–62.
10. Brem RF, Baum J, Lechnter M, et al. Improvement in sensitivity of screening mammography with computer-aided detection: a multi-institutional trial. AJR Am J Roentgenol 2003;181(3):687–93.
11. Birdwell RL, Ikeda DM, O'Shaughnessy KF, et al. Mammographic characteristics of 115 missed cancers later detected with screening mammography and the potential utility of computer-aided detection. Radiology 2001;219(1):192–202.

12. Freer TW, Ulissey MJ. Screening mammography with computer-aided detection: prospective study of 12,860 patients in a community breast center. Radiology 2001;220(3):781–6.

13. Gilbert FJ, Astley SM, McGee MA, et al. Single reading with computer-aided detection and double reading of screening mammograms in the United Kingdom National Breast Screening Program. Radiology 2006;241(1):47–53.

14. Ikeda DM, Birdwell RL, O'Shaugnessy KF, et al. Analysis of 172 subtle findings on prior mammograms in women with breast cancer detected at follow-up screening. Radiology 2003;226(2):494–503.

15. Fenton JJ, Taplin SH, Carney PA, et al. Influence of computer-aided detection on performance of screening mammography. N Engl J Med 2007;356:1399–409.

16. Lillie-Blanton M. Mammography Quality Standards Act: x-ray quality improved, access unaffected, but impact on health outcomes unknown: testimony before the Subcommittee on Health and the Environment, Committee on Commerce, House of Representatives. Washington, DC: Committee on Commerce; 1998.

17. American College of Radiology. Breast imaging reporting and data system (BI-RADS). 4th edition. Reston (VA): American College of Radiology; 2003.

18. Pisano ED, Gastonis C, Hendrick E, et al. Diagnostic performance of digital versus film mammography for breast cancer screening – the results of the American College of Radiology Network (ACRIN) Digital Mammographic Imaging Screening Trial (DMIST). N Engl J Med 2005;353(17):1773–83.

19. MQSA National Statistics. Available at: http://www.fda.gov/. Accessed June 1, 2012.

20. Schnall MD, Blume J, Bluemke DA, et al. Diagnostic architectural and dynamic features at breast MR imaging: multicenter study. Radiology 2006; 238:42–53.

21. Lee CH. Problem solving MR imaging of the breast. Radiol Clin North Am 2004; 42:919–34.

22. Bluemke DA, Gatsonis CA, Chen MH, et al. Magnetic resonance imaging of the breast prior to biopsy. JAMA 2004;292:2735–42.

23. Ikeda DM, Birdwell RL, Daniel BL. Potential role of magnetic resonance imaging and other modalities in ductal carcinoma in situ detection. Magn Reson Imaging Clin N Am 2001;9:345–56, vii.

24. Hylton NM, Blume JD, Bemreuter WK, et al. Locally advanced breast cancer: MR imaging for prediction of response to neoadjuvant chemotherapy – results from ACRIN 6657/I-SPY trial. Radiology 2012;263:663–72.

25. Poplack SP, Tosteson TD, Kogel CA, et al. Digital breast tomosynthesis: initial experience in 98 women with abnormal digital screening mammography. AJR Am J Roentgenol 2007;189(3):616–23.

26. Dromain C, Thibault F, Muller S, et al. Dual-energy contrast-enhanced digital mammography: initial clinical results. Eur Radiol 2011;21:565–74.

27. Hruska CB, Boughey JC, Phillips SW, et al. Scientific Impact Recognition Award: molecular breast imaging: a review of the Mayo Clinic experience. Am J Surg 2008;196:470–6.

28. Brem RF, Floerke AC, Rapelyea JA, et al. Breast-specific gamma imaging as an adjunct imaging modality for the diagnosis of breast cancer. Radiology 2008;247: 651–7.

29. Brem RF, Shahan C, Rapelyea JA, et al. Detection of occult foci of breast cancer using breast-specific gamma imaging in women with one mammographic or clinically suspicious breast lesion. Acad Radiol 2010;17:735–43.

30. Berg WA, Weinberg IN, Narayannan D, et al. High-resolution fluorodeoxyglucose positron emissions tomography with compression ("positron emission mammography") is highly accurate in depicting primary breast cancer. Breast J 2006;12: 309–23.

31. Berg WA, Madsen KS, Schilling K, et al. Breast cancer: comparative effectiveness of positron emission mammography and MR imaging in presurgical planning for the ipsilateral breast. Radiology 2011;258:59–72.

32. Hellquist BN, Duffy SW, Abdsaleh S, et al. Effective of population-based service screening with mammography for women ages 40 to 49 years: evaluation of the Swedish Mammography Screening in Young Women (SCRY) cohort. Cancer 2011;117(4):714–22.

33. Tabar L, Yen MF, Vitak B, et al. Mammography service screening and mortality in breast cancer patients: 20-year follow-up before and after introduction of screening. Lancet 2003;361:1405–10.

34. Gotzsche PC, Olsen O. Is screening for breast cancer with mammography justifiable? Lancet 2000;355:129–34.

35. U.S. Preventive Services Task Force. Screening for breast cancer: U.S. Preventive Services Task Force recommendation statement. Ann Intern Med 2009;151: 716–26.

36. Coldman A, Philips N, Warren L, et al. Breast cancer mortality after screening in British Columbia women. Int J Cancer 2007;120:1076–80.

37. Hendrick RE, Helvie MA. Mammography screening: a new estimate of number needed to screen to prevent one breast cancer. AJR Am J Roentgenol 2012; 198(3):723–8.

38. Wang A, van Houten H, Fan J, et al. Impact of the United States Preventive Services Task Force Update for breast cancer screening on utilization of mammography in women under 50. Academy Health Annual Research Meeting. Orlando, June 24–26, 2012.

39. Harvey JA, Fajardo LL, Innis CA. Previous mammograms in patients with impalpable breast carcinoma: retrospective vs. blinded interpretation. AJR Am J Roentgenol 1993;161:1167–72.

40. Feig SA, Shaber GS, Patchefsky A, et al. Analysis of clinically occult and mammographic occult breast tumors. AJR Am J Roentgenol 1977;128:403–8.

41. Wallis MG, Walsh MT, Lee JR. Review of false negative mammography in a symptomatic population. Clin Radiol 1991;44:13–5.

42. Martin JE, Moskowtiz M, Milbrath JR. Breast cancer missed by mammography. AJR Am J Roentgenol 1979;132:737–9.

43. Cahill CJ, Boulter PS, Gibbs NM, et al. Features of mammographically negative breast tumours. Br J Surg 1981;68:883–4.

44. Mann BD, Giuliano AE, Bassett LW, et al. Delayed diagnosis of breast cancer as a result of normal mammograms. Arch Surg 1983;118:23–4.

45. Bird RE, Wallace TW, Yankaskas BC. Analysis of cancers missed at screening mammography. Radiology 1992;184:613–7.

46. Kalisher L. Factors influencing false negative rates in xeromammography. Radiology 1979;133:297–301.

47. Goerge SK, Evans J, Cohen GP, et al. Characteristics of breast carcinomas missed by screening radiologists. Radiology 1997;204:131–5.

48. Holland R, Hendriks JH, Mravunac M. Mammographically occult breast cancer: a pathologic and radiologic study. Cancer 1983;52:1810–9.

49. Boyd NF, Martin LJ, Bronskill M, et al. Breast tissue composition and susceptibility to breast cancer. J Natl Cancer Inst 2010;102(16):1224–37.

50. Carney PA, Miglioretti DL, Yankaskas BC, et al. Individual and combined effects of age, breast density, and hormone replacement therapy use on the accuracy of screening mammography. Ann Intern Med 2003;138(3):168–75.

51. Rosenberg RD, Hunt WC, Williamson MR, et al. Effects of age, breast density, ethnicity, and estrogen replacement therapy on screening mammographic sensitivity and cancer stage at diagnosis: review of 183,134 screening mammograms in Albuquerque, New Mexico. Radiology 1998;209(2):511–8.

52. Kerlikowske K, Grady D, Barclay J, et al. Likelihood ratios for modern screening mammography. Risk of breast cancer based on age and mammographic interpretation. JAMA 1996;276(1):39–43.

53. Berg WA, Blume JD, Cormack JB, et al, ACRIN 6666 Investigators. Combined screening with ultrasound and mammography vs mammography alone in women at elevated risk of breast cancer. JAMA 2008;299(18):2151–63.

54. Berg WA, Zheng Z, Lehrer D, et al. Detection of breast cancer with addition of annual screening ultrasound or a single screening MRI to mammography in women with elevated breast cancer risk. JAMA 2012;307(13):1394–404.

55. Saslow D, Boetes C, Burke W, et al. American Cancer Society guidelines for breast screening with MRI as an adjunct to mammography. CA Cancer J Clin 2007;57(2):75–89.

# Surgical Management of High-Risk Breast Lesions

Amy C. Degnim, MD[a], Tari A. King, MD[b],*

## KEYWORDS

- High-risk lesion • Atypical hyperplasia • Lobular carcinoma in situ
- Percutaneous breast biopsy • Breast cancer risk • Papillary lesions • Radial scar

## KEY POINTS

- High-risk breast lesions include 2 large main categories: those lesions that are found on percutaneous biopsy that have a significant risk of demonstrating cancer at excision and lesions that indicate an increased risk of breast cancer over a woman's lifetime.
- In general, the following lesions identified on percutaneous breast biopsy should be excised: atypical ductal hyperplasia (ADH), flat epithelial atypia, papillary lesions with atypia, and radial scar with atypia.
- For papillary lesions and radial scars *without atypia*, observation can be considered in select cases with favorable features and radiologic-pathologic concordance; however, surgical excision is a safe approach with low morbidity. Cases that do not undergo surgical excision must be followed with clinical and imaging surveillance to assure stability.
- For percutaneous biopsies demonstrating atypical lobular hyperplasia (ALH) or lobular carcinoma in situ (LCIS), observation can be considered if there are no other associated high-risk lesions in the specimen and/or there is another histologic finding that is concordant with the original imaging lesion (ie, the ALH or LCIS represents an incidental finding); otherwise, surgical excision is a safe approach with low morbidity. Cases that do not undergo surgical excision must be followed with clinical and imaging surveillance to assure stability.
- ADH, ALH, and LCIS are histologic findings that indicate a significantly increased long-term risk of breast cancer that may affect either breast. Women with these findings should be counseled on risks and benefits of prevention strategies.

Funding sources: None.
Conflict of interest: None.
[a] Department of Surgery, Mayo Clinic, 200 First Street Southwest, Rochester, MN 55905, USA;
[b] Breast Service, Department of Surgery, Memorial Sloan-Kettering Cancer Center, 300 East 66th Street, New York, NY 10065, USA
* Corresponding author.
*E-mail address:* kingt@mskcc.org

surgical.theclinics.com

## INTRODUCTION

The term *high-risk lesion* of the breast refers to any of a group of histologic abnormalities that confer an increased risk of breast cancer. The surgeon's role in the clinical management of these lesions is 2-fold and includes issues related to the method of diagnosis as well as strategies for surveillance and risk reduction.

In the era of widespread mammography and image-guided needle biopsies, the surgeon is often presented with a high-risk lesion as a histologic finding on core needle biopsy. In this setting, the key is in understanding which lesions require a surgical excision of the biopsy site to rule out the possibility of an associated malignancy. In the absence of a concurrent malignancy, a high-risk lesion is simply a histologic finding in breast tissue that is associated with an increased risk of breast cancer in the future.

In general, patients who are found to have high-risk lesions are managed long term with surveillance and prevention strategies; but in some circumstances, surgical risk reduction may be considered. In this article, the authors review issues related to the diagnosis of high-risk lesions and recommendations for clinical management.

## HIGH-RISK LESIONS: HISTOLOGIC ENTITIES

The classic high-risk breast lesions, lobular carcinoma in situ (LCIS), atypical ductal hyperplasia (ADH), and atypical lobular hyperplasia (ALH), are those that were identified many years ago as being associated with an increased future risk of breast cancer. In the 1970s, it was recognized that a diagnosis of LCIS conferred an increased risk of breast cancer of approximately 1% per year and that this risk was conferred equally to both breasts.[1] In 1985, Dupont and Page[2] demonstrated that women with either ADH or ALH had an approximate 4-fold increased risk of breast cancer compared with the general population, a level of risk that was approximately one-half of that conferred by a diagnosis of LCIS. With technical advances, the shift to percutaneous core needle biopsy and increased attention to benign histologic findings frequently identified in breast specimens, several additional lesions are now included in the high-risk lesion category, including papillary lesions, radial scar, and flat epithelial atypia (FEA). Each of these is discussed in further detail.

## RATIONALE FOR SURGICAL EXCISION OF HIGH-RISK LESIONS

Percutaneous core needle biopsy of breast abnormalities is subject to several limitations. First, the targeted lesion can be inadequately sampled or clearly missed; fortunately, this occurs only infrequently. However, it is common that only a portion of the lesion is removed, introducing the possibility of sampling error[3]; and the lesions are often fragmented into multiple smaller pieces by the nature of the procedure, which can increase the difficulty in making a definitive histologic diagnosis.[4]

It is well documented that certain histologic diagnoses, when made on core needle biopsy specimens, will frequently be upgraded to cancer when the remaining biopsy site is surgically excised.[5–7] Multiple studies have also shown that the likelihood of upgrading to a diagnosis of cancer is related to the volume of tissue sampled by the needle biopsy, with higher upgrade rates for smaller-gauge biopsy needles (ie, 14G needle vs 11G vacuum-assisted biopsy devices) and larger mammographic lesions.[8–10]

For all of these reasons, it is important to confirm that there is concordance between the radiologic findings and pathologic findings on the core biopsy and to understand which lesions on the core needle biopsy should be surgically excised. When surgical excision is undertaken, the goal is to remove the biopsy site and the original imaging lesion that led to the core needle biopsy to rule out the presence of an associated malignancy.

## RADIOLOGIC-PATHOLOGIC CONCORDANCE

Radiologic-pathologic concordance is required in current practices that perform percutaneous needle biopsy, whether the biopsy is guided by palpation or by ultrasound or stereotactic imaging.[11,12] The combined assessment of clinical, imaging, and pathologic findings that are all internally consistent is referred to as concordance. As a part of the multidisciplinary team that now characterizes modern breast care, the surgeon must also understand and contribute to the concordance assessment of breast core needle biopsy results.[13–16]

To assess concordance, the surgeon must review the original diagnostic mammograms demonstrating the abnormality and also the postbiopsy imaging to assess whether the biopsy marker is located at the site of the original lesion. The histologic findings as described by the pathologist are then interpreted in the context of the clinical and imaging findings to determine if they are all in agreement. Ideally, concordance determination is performed with input from the radiologist, pathologist, and surgeon.

Surgical excision is always indicated when the findings are discordant or there is concern that the target lesion was not sampled. A core needle biopsy demonstrating atypia, or a papillary lesion in the presence of a palpable or imaging mass lesion, is a classic situation that should lead to surgical excision. Additional recommendations for surgical excision are discussed for each high-risk lesion.

## ATYPICAL HYPERPLASIA (ADH AND ALH)

ADH is an epithelial proliferative lesion of the terminal duct lobular unit that demonstrates both cytologic atypia and architectural changes that are similar to ductal carcinoma in situ (DCIS). In ADH, the size and extent of the lesion is smaller, involving only 1 or 2 ducts and measuring less than 2 mm, so it does not meet the criteria for DCIS.[17] Therefore, fragments of tissue from a core biopsy that seem to be ADH would have the same appearance as a small portion of a DCIS lesion. For this reason, sampling error is very relevant in core biopsies demonstrating ADH. Multiple studies of surgical excision of core biopsy sites demonstrating ADH have reported upgrade rates of 10% to 20% **Table 1**.[5,7,10,18–33]

Despite common use of large-gauge vacuum-assisted biopsy devices in more recent years, upgrade rates following a core biopsy diagnosis of ADH are still high enough (31% in a recent publication)[19] that surgical excision is considered to be the standard of care. Recent studies have attempted to define favorable subgroups with ADH on core needle biopsy that do not require surgical excision, such as cases whereby all or more than 95% of calcifications have been removed and there is no mass lesion; however, caution is advised with this approach because other studies have failed to confirm these findings.[34–38]

ALH is a proliferative lesion in which the epithelial cells grow in a confluent fashion of monomorphic cytology that distends the acini and enlarges the terminal duct lobular unit. ALH is similar in appearance to LCIS, but distinguished from it by its lesser extent. When ALH is found on percutaneous biopsy and surgically excised, published upgrade rates to cancer vary widely and range from less than 5% to approximately 50%. However, the literature has been limited by the fact that not all cases in the older series underwent excision, introducing the possibility of selection bias, and many series included results from cases that would be considered discordant.[27,29–31] As

**Table 1**
**Upgrade rates to cancer for various lesions found on percutaneous breast biopsy**

| Lesions on Core Biopsy | Upgrade Rate | | Article, Year |
|---|---|---|---|
| | % | N | |
| ADH | 13 | 5/40 | Burak et al,[18] 2000 |
| | 17 | 11/65 | Winchester et al,[7] 2003 |
| | 12 | 9/78 | Sohn et al,[10] 2007 |
| | 21 | 22/104 | Jackman et al,[5] 2002 |
| | 31 | 132/422 | Deshaies et al,[19] 2011 |
| Papillary lesions | 10 | 13/125 | Rizzo et al,[20] 2008 |
| | 17 | 15/87 | Gendler et al,[21] 2004 |
| | 24 | 19/80 | Valdes et al,[22] 2006 |
| | 37 | 14/38 | Renshaw et al,[23] 2004 |
| FEA | 8 | 2/24 | Sohn et al,[24] 2011 |
| | 13 | 8/60 | Lavoue et al,[25] 2011 |
| | 14 | 5/35 | Chivikula et al,[26] 2009 |
| ALH | 0 | 0/56 | Subhawong et al,[27] 2010 |
| | 1 | 1/81 pure ALH | Shah-Khan et al,[28] 2012 |
| | 3 | 1/40 | Renshaw et al,[29] 2006 |
| | 8 | 5/63 | Karabakhtsian et al,[30] 2007 |
| | 22 | 21/97 | Brem et al,[31] 2008 |
| LCIS | 4 | 3/68 | Rendi et al,[32] 2012 |
| | 3 | 2/72 | Murray MP et al,[33] 2012 |
| | 4 | 2/52 | Renshaw et al,[29] 2006 |
| | 25 | 17/67 | Brem et al,[31] 2008 |

a result of this variability, routine surgical excision of ALH on needle biopsy is controversial.

Although surgical excision is a safe approach, it may be unnecessary in most cases because ALH is often an incidental histologic finding in the surrounding breast tissue of the originally targeted lesion that often proves to be benign. Some surgeons routinely excise all cases of ALH on percutaneous biopsy, whereas others excise only cases with higher suspicion caused by other coexisting high-risk lesions or in cases of ALH associated with mass lesions (ie, discordance) or larger areas of calcifications. Recent reports support observation for select cases of ALH as long as all findings are concordant and there are no other high-risk lesions in the core biopsy specimen.[27,28,39] In cases of ALH or ADH that are not surgically excised, short-term mammographic follow-up is recommended.

Once a concurrent malignancy has been excluded, women with ADH and ALH should be counseled regarding their increased risk of breast cancer in the future and informed about medical treatment options to reduce their risk (**Table 2**). Multiple studies have demonstrated the risk of breast cancer to be approximately 4-fold higher than the general population risk, and the risk is conferred to both breasts.[2,40–42] In a recent study, the degree of long-term breast cancer risk was associated with the volume of atypia found in the tissue, with risk stratified based on 1, 2, or 3 or more foci of atypia (see **Table 2**).[43] The absolute cumulative risk of breast cancer was approximately 20% at 20 years for the group with atypical hyperplasia, with less risk among those with 1 focus and higher risk among those with 3 or more foci of atypical hyperplasia.[43]

In the National Surgical Adjuvant Breast and Bowel Project (NSABP) P-1 study of tamoxifen chemoprevention, women with atypical hyperplasia who received tamoxifen for 5 years achieved an 86% reduction in breast cancer incidence.[44] More

**Table 2**
**Long-term breast cancer risk associated with histologic findings**

| Histologic Finding | Relative Risk | Absolute Risk |
|---|---|---|
| Normal (general population as reference) | 1 | 12% by 80 y of age |
| FEA | 1.5 (very limited data) | Unknown |
| Papillary lesions | ~2 | ~12%–15% at 20 y |
| Radial scar | ~2 | ~12%–15% at 20 y |
| ADH or ALH | ~4 | ~15%–20% at 20 y |
| LCIS | ~10 | ~1% per y; ~20%–25% at 20 y |

recently, the Study of Tamoxifen and Raloxifene (STAR) trial demonstrated that raloxifene results in similar risk reduction to tamoxifen with less toxicity.[45]

## FEA

FEA is a recently described columnar cell breast lesion characterized by cytologic atypia. Columnar cell lesions demonstrate epithelium with a columnar appearance oriented perpendicular to the basement membrane of the acini within terminal duct lobular units. In FEA, the epithelial layer is 1 to 2 cell layers with cytologic atypia characterized by round to ovoid nuclei with nucleoli and loss of polarity.

FEA is a rare lesion, occurring in approximately 5% of percutaneous breast biopsies. Because it is rare and characterized only recently, data on upgrade rates to cancer with surgical excision are limited. Existing published reports indicate that cancer is found in approximately 10% to 15% of FEA cases at surgical excision,[24–26,46] supporting a recommendation for routine surgical excision.

The Nashville Cohort Study provides the only data regarding the long-term risk of breast cancer in women with FEA, and the sample size is small (only 52 women).[47] The study found that women with columnar cell lesions (n = 1261) had a modest increase in breast cancer risk (relative risk, 1.5), yet this risk was not further increased by the presence of FEA. The small number of women with FEA likely limits the accuracy of risk estimation for this subgroup, and further study is needed to define the long-term risk associated with FEA (see **Table 2**).

## PAPILLARY LESIONS

Papillary breast lesions comprise a range of lesions from completely benign findings (intraductal papilloma) to malignant (intraductal papillary carcinoma or invasive papillary carcinoma). These lesions can be difficult to distinguish based on tissue fragments from percutaneous biopsy.[48] Another feature of papillary lesions is that they can be heterogeneous, such that the entire lesion requires histologic evaluation to rule out atypical hyperplasia or cancer. When a core biopsy diagnosis of a papillary lesion is followed by surgical excision, upgrade rates to cancer range from 10% to 35% across series.[20–23]

Papillary lesions without atypia have a lower risk of being upgraded to cancer, leading some to suggest observation rather than excision for selected papillary lesions without atypia, especially if imaging findings confirm that the lesion has been completely removed.[49,50] Papillary lesions without atypia are classified as proliferative benign breast lesions; these lesions confer a modest increase in the risk of future breast cancer: approximately 2-fold more than the general population risk (see **Table 2**).[2,40–42]

The long-term risk of breast cancer associated with papillary lesions with atypia is the same as that conferred by ADH or ALH alone, and women should be counseled accordingly.[51]

## RADIAL SCAR

A radial scar is a breast lesion that can mimic a malignant breast tumor, presenting with a palpable mass and/or as a spiculated lesion on imaging. A radial scar can also be a purely histologic finding without an imaging or palpable correlate. Histologically, a radial scar appears as a fibroelastotic core with multiple proliferative epithelial breast elements, often with adenosis that can demonstrate areas of trapped epithelium within stroma that can be mistaken for infiltrating epithelial cells and malignancy. If a radial scar is an incidental histologic finding in an otherwise benign breast biopsy, no further treatment is needed; however, when a radial scar is present in a core biopsy specimen, there is a risk for misdiagnosis based on the sometimes limited sampling of the epithelial elements and, until recently, surgical excision was recommended for all mammographically or palpably detected radial scar lesions.

Several factors have now been shown to be associated with a higher risk of upgrading to cancer at surgical excision allowing a more selective approach. If a radial scar demonstrates atypia or was biopsied with a 14G or smaller needle, or less than 12 cores were obtained, the upgrade rates are 8% to 28%; these cases should still undergo complete excision. Conversely, radial scars without atypia or those that are sampled with 12 or more cores by an 11G or larger biopsy have reported upgrade rates of 5% or less and may be suitable for short-term follow-up.[52,53] Radial scars are also considered to be proliferative benign breast lesions with an approximately 2-fold increased risk of breast cancer (see **Table 2**).[2,40,54]

## LCIS

LCIS is characterized by small, bland-appearing monomorphic cells with small nuclei that fill and distend at least half the acini of a lobular unit.[55] As stated earlier, ALH has a microscopic pattern similar to LCIS but is generally less extensive. Because the distinction between LCIS and ALH can be subjective, it has been suggested that they both be referred to in a more general category of *lobular neoplasia* (LN); however, this terminology has not been universally adopted.

The term LCIS was first coined in 1941 by Foote and Stewart[56] when they observed this lesion in 14 out of 300 cancerous mastectomy specimens. They hypothesized that LCIS represented a direct precursor to invasive lobular carcinoma and recommended mastectomy as treatment. Emerging data throughout the 1970s demonstrated that the risk of breast cancer following a diagnosis of LCIS was lower than expected for a direct precursor lesion and was conferred equally to both breasts.[1,57,58] These observations, in combination with the fact that the subsequent cancers that developed in women with LCIS were of both the ductal and lobular phenotype, led to the acceptance of LCIS as a marker of increased risk rather than a true precursor.

Compared with the general population, women with LCIS have an 8- to 10-fold increased risk of breast cancer[59]; several studies have demonstrated this risk to be steady over a woman's lifetime such that the risk is approximately 1% per year.[60] In the series with the longest follow-up, the probability of developing carcinoma in situ or invasive cancer by 10 years after the diagnosis of LCIS was 13%, 26% after 20 years, and 35% by 35 years.[61]

LCIS is typically an incidental finding in a breast biopsy performed for another reason. As such, the true incidence of LCIS in the population has been difficult to ascertain. Historical series suggest it is present in up to 4% of otherwise benign breast biopsies,[1,57,58] whereas population-based data reported to Surveillance, Epidemiology, and End Results from 1978 to 1998 demonstrate an incidence of 3.19 per 100 000 women.[62] In the modern era of widespread screening mammography, it has been suggested that LCIS may be associated with calcifications in 21% to 67% of cases[63]; LCIS has also been reported to enhance on magnetic resonance imaging,[64] although these data are limited.

Histologically, LCIS is often multicentric and bilateral.[1,56–58] A diagnosis of LCIS made by surgical excision does not require further surgical intervention. Similarly, the finding of LCIS in the surrounding breast parenchyma of a lumpectomy specimen containing DCIS or invasive carcinoma does not alter surgical management of the breast primary and does not increase the rate of in-breast recurrence in patients undergoing breast conservation.[65–67]

The scenario that often results in controversy is the management of LCIS diagnosed on core biopsy. Similar to the data regarding upgrade rates following a core biopsy diagnosis of ALH, a recent pooled analysis of studies published from 1999 to 2008 demonstrates that the upgrade rate at surgical excision for a core biopsy diagnosis of LCIS also varies widely (0%–50%).[68] Yet these series are limited in that not all patients with LCIS underwent excision and not all cases with radiographic-pathologic discordance were excluded, creating an inherent selection bias and increasing the likelihood of finding an associated malignancy. In addition, in many cases, LCIS or LN were not the only lesions identified in the core biopsy specimen leading to the indication for surgical excision.

More recently, 2 single-institution series have demonstrated that, with careful exclusion of cases with other high-risk lesions on core biopsy (ie, ADH, papilloma, radial scar) and with exclusion of cases with radiographic-pathologic discordance, the actual rate of upstaging to DCIS or invasive cancer is quite low.[32,33] Rendi and colleagues[32] reported an upgrade rate of 4% following surgical excision of 68 cases of LN on core biopsy; similarly, Murray and colleagues[33] reported an upgrade rate of 3% following surgical excision of 72 cases of LN on core biopsy. In both of these series, the cancers identified were small low-grade malignancies. Although both of these series are also retrospective and subject to selection bias, they represent the most careful reviews of this clinical scenario to date and suggest that routine excision is not warranted for all cases of LCIS on core biopsy.

Once a concurrent malignancy has been excluded, women with LCIS should be counseled regarding their increased risk of breast cancer in the future and informed about medical and/or surgical treatment options to reduce their risk. As stated previously in the context of ADH and ALH, prospective randomized data from the NSABP Breast Cancer Prevention Trial (P-1) demonstrated that among high-risk women, tamoxifen decreased the risk of developing invasive breast cancer.[44] Similarly, the NSABP STAR (P-2) trial demonstrated that raloxifene was just as effective as tamoxifen in reducing the risk of breast cancer in high-risk postmenopausal women.[45] Women with LCIS were well represented in both of these studies, comprising 6.2% of 13 338 participants in the NSABP P-1 trial and 9.2% of 19 747 participants in the STAR trial. In both subsets, chemoprevention reduced the risk of developing breast cancer by more than 50%.

In parallel with the surgical management of invasive breast cancer, trends in the surgical management of LCIS have been toward conservative management; in current practice, only a minority of women with LCIS will pursue bilateral prophylactic mastectomy. The option of surgical risk reduction is often considered more strongly in the subset of women with LCIS and other risk factors, such as a strong family history or extremely dense breasts; however, patients considering surgery for risk reduction need to be fully aware of all the risks and benefits of this approach and should be encouraged to consider the impact that prophylactic surgery may have on their quality of life with respect to body image and sexual functioning. They should also be informed that prophylactic mastectomy *does not* completely eliminate cancer risk. The decision to undergo bilateral prophylactic mastectomy is highly individualized and should not be undertaken without ample time to consider all of the available options for risk management.

## SUMMARY

High-risk breast lesions include LCIS, ADH, ALH, FEA, radial scar, and papillary lesions. When these lesions are identified on core needle biopsy, careful radiologic-pathologic concordance is necessary. In general, excision of high-risk lesions is indicated to rule out coexisting malignancy; however, in carefully selected cases, observation with short-term follow-up may be appropriate. Women with LCIS, ADH, and ALH should be counseled about options for breast cancer risk reduction.

## REFERENCES

1. Haagensen CD, Lane N, Lattes R, et al. Lobular neoplasia (so-called lobular carcinoma in situ) of the breast. Cancer 1978;42(2):737–69.
2. Dupont WD, Page DL. Risk factors for breast cancer in women with proliferative breast disease. N Engl J Med 1985;312(3):146–51.
3. Burbank F. Stereotactic breast biopsy of atypical ductal hyperplasia and ductal carcinoma in situ lesions: improved accuracy with directional, vacuum-assisted biopsy. Radiology 1997;202(3):843–7.
4. Corben AD, Edelweiss M, Brogi E. Challenges in the interpretation of breast core biopsies. Breast J 2010;16(Suppl 1):S5–9.
5. Jackman RJ, Birdwell RL, Ikeda DM. Atypical ductal hyperplasia: can some lesions be defined as probably benign after stereotactic 11-gauge vacuum-assisted biopsy, eliminating the recommendation for surgical excision? Radiology 2002;224(2):548–54.
6. Pandelidis S, Heiland D, Jones D, et al. Accuracy of 11-gauge vacuum-assisted core biopsy of mammographic breast lesions. Ann Surg Oncol 2003;10(1):43–7.
7. Winchester DJ, Bernstein JR, Jeske JM, et al. Upstaging of atypical ductal hyperplasia after vacuum-assisted 11-gauge stereotactic core needle biopsy. Arch Surg 2003;138(6):619–22 [discussion: 622–3].
8. Green S, Khalkhali I, Azizollahi E, et al. Excisional biopsy of borderline lesions after large bore vacuum-assisted core needle biopsy- is it necessary? Am Surg 2011;77(10):1358–60.
9. Houssami N, Ciatto S, Ellis I, et al. Underestimation of malignancy of breast core-needle biopsy: concepts and precise overall and category-specific estimates. Cancer 2007;109(3):487–95.
10. Sohn V, Arthurs Z, Herbert G, et al. Atypical ductal hyperplasia: improved accuracy with the 11-gauge vacuum-assisted versus the 14-gauge core biopsy needle. Ann Surg Oncol 2007;14(9):2497–501.
11. American College of Radiology. Practice guidelines for performance of ultrasound-guided percutaneous breast interventional procedures. 2009. Available at: http://www.acr.org ~ /media/ACR/Documents/PGTS/guidelines/US_Guided_Breast.pdf. Accessed January 24, 2013.

12. American College of Radiology. Practice guidelines for the performance of stereotactically guided breast interventional procedures. Rev. 2009. Available at: http://www.acr.org/SecondaryMainMenuCategories/quality_safety/guidelines/breast/stereotactically_guided_breast.aspx. Accessed June 25, 2011.
13. Johnson NB, Collins LC. Update on percutaneous needle biopsy of nonmalignant breast lesions. Adv Anat Pathol 2009;16(4):183–95.
14. Landercasper J, Linebarger JH. Contemporary breast imaging and concordance assessment: a surgical perspective. Surg Clin North Am 2011;91(1):33–58.
15. Masood S, Rosa M. Borderline breast lesions: diagnostic challenges and clinical implications. Adv Anat Pathol 2011;18(3):190–8.
16. The American Society of Breast Surgeons. Position statement on concordance assessment of image-guided breast biopsies and management of borderline or high-risk lesions. 2011. Available at: https://www.breastsurgeons.org/statements/PDF_Statements/Concordance_Assessment.pdf. Accessed September 30, 2010.
17. Page DL, Dupont WD, Rogers LW, et al. Atypical hyperplastic lesions of the female breast. A long-term follow-up study. Cancer 1985;55(11):2698–708.
18. Burak WE Jr, Owens KE, Tighe MB, et al. Vacuum-assisted stereotactic breast biopsy: histologic underestimation of malignant lesions. Arch Surg 2000;135(6): 700–3.
19. Deshaies I, Provencher L, Jacob S, et al. Factors associated with upgrading to malignancy at surgery of atypical ductal hyperplasia diagnosed on core biopsy. Breast 2011;20(1):50–5.
20. Rizzo M, Lund MJ, Oprea G, et al. Surgical follow-up and clinical presentation of 142 breast papillary lesions diagnosed by ultrasound-guided core-needle biopsy. Ann Surg Oncol 2008;15(4):1040–7.
21. Gendler LS, Feldman SM, Balassanian R, et al. Association of breast cancer with papillary lesions identified at percutaneous image-guided breast biopsy. Am J Surg 2004;188(4):365–70.
22. Valdes EK, Tartter PI, Genelus-Dominique E, et al. Significance of papillary lesions at percutaneous breast biopsy. Ann Surg Oncol 2006;13(4):480–2.
23. Renshaw AA, Derhagopian RP, Tizol-Blanco DM, et al. Papillomas and atypical papillomas in breast core needle biopsy specimens: risk of carcinoma in subsequent excision. Am J Clin Pathol 2004;122(2):217–21.
24. Sohn V, Porta R, Brown T. Flat epithelial atypia of the breast on core needle biopsy: an indication for surgical excision. Mil Med 2011;176(11):1347–50.
25. Lavoue V, Roger CM, Poilblanc M, et al. Pure flat epithelial atypia (DIN 1a) on core needle biopsy: study of 60 biopsies with follow-up surgical excision. Breast Cancer Res Treat 2011;125(1):121–6.
26. Chivukula M, Bhargava R, Tseng G, et al. Clinicopathologic implications of "flat epithelial atypia" in core needle biopsy specimens of the breast. Am J Clin Pathol 2009;131(6):802–8.
27. Subhawong AP, Subhawong TK, Khouri N, et al. Incidental minimal atypical lobular hyperplasia on core needle biopsy: correlation with findings on follow-up excision. Am J Surg Pathol 2010;34(6):822–8.
28. Shah-Khan MG, Geiger XJ, Reynolds C, et al. Long-term follow-up of lobular neoplasia (atypical lobular hyperplasia/lobular carcinoma in situ) diagnosed on core needle biopsy. Ann Surg Oncol 2012;19:3131–8.
29. Renshaw AA, Derhagopian RP, Martinez P, et al. Lobular neoplasia in breast core needle biopsy specimens is associated with a low risk of ductal carcinoma in situ or invasive carcinoma on subsequent excision. Am J Clin Pathol 2006;126(2):310–3.

30. Karabakhtsian RG, Johnson R, Sumkin J, et al. The clinical significance of lobular neoplasia on breast core biopsy. Am J Surg Pathol 2007;31(5):717–23.

31. Brem RF, Lechner MC, Jackman RJ, et al. Lobular neoplasia at percutaneous breast biopsy: variables associated with carcinoma at surgical excision. AJR Am J Roentgenol 2008;190(3):637–41.

32. Rendi MH, Dintzis SM, Lehman CD, et al. Lobular in-situ neoplasia on breast core needle biopsy: imaging indication and pathologic extent can identify which patients require excisional biopsy. Ann Surg Oncol 2012;19(3):914–21.

33. Murray MP, Luedtke C, Liberman L, et al. Classic lobular carcinoma in situ and atypical lobular hyperplasia at percutaneous breast core biopsy: Outcomes of prospective excision. Cancer 2012. [Epub ahead of print].

34. Bendifallah S, Defert S, Chabbert-Buffet N, et al. Scoring to predict the possibility of upgrades to malignancy in atypical ductal hyperplasia diagnosed by an 11-gauge vacuum-assisted biopsy device: an external validation study. Eur J Cancer 2012;48(1):30–6.

35. Forgeard C, Benchaib M, Guerin N, et al. Is surgical biopsy mandatory in case of atypical ductal hyperplasia on 11-gauge core needle biopsy? A retrospective study of 300 patients. Am J Surg 2008;196(3):339–45.

36. Nguyen CV, Albarracin CT, Whitman GJ, et al. Atypical ductal hyperplasia in directional vacuum-assisted biopsy of breast microcalcifications: considerations for surgical excision. Ann Surg Oncol 2011;18(3):752–61.

37. Sneige N, Lim SC, Whitman GJ, et al. Atypical ductal hyperplasia diagnosis by directional vacuum-assisted stereotactic biopsy of breast microcalcifications. Considerations for surgical excision. Am J Clin Pathol 2003;119(2):248–53.

38. Wagoner MJ, Laronga C, Acs G. Extent and histologic pattern of atypical ductal hyperplasia present on core needle biopsy specimens of the breast can predict ductal carcinoma in situ in subsequent excision. Am J Clin Pathol 2009;131(1): 112–21.

39. Nagi CS, O'Donnell JE, Tismenetsky M, et al. Lobular neoplasia on core needle biopsy does not require excision. Cancer 2008;112(10):2152–8.

40. Hartmann LC, Sellers TA, Frost MH, et al. Benign breast disease and the risk of breast cancer. N Engl J Med 2005;353(3):229–37.

41. Carter CL, Corle DK, Micozzi MS, et al. A prospective study of the development of breast cancer in 16,692 women with benign breast disease. Am J Epidemiol 1988;128(3):467–77.

42. London SJ, Connolly JL, Schnitt SJ, et al. A prospective study of benign breast disease and the risk of breast cancer. JAMA 1992;267(7):941–4.

43. Degnim AC, Visscher DW, Berman HK, et al. Stratification of breast cancer risk in women with atypia: a Mayo cohort study. J Clin Oncol 2007;25(19):2671–7.

44. Fisher B, Costantino JP, Wickerham DL, et al. Tamoxifen for prevention of breast cancer: report of the National Surgical Adjuvant Breast and Bowel Project P-1 Study. J Natl Cancer Inst 1998;90(18):1371–88.

45. Vogel VG, Costantino JP, Wickerham DL, et al. Effects of tamoxifen vs raloxifene on the risk of developing invasive breast cancer and other disease outcomes: the NSABP Study of Tamoxifen and Raloxifene (STAR) P-2 trial. JAMA 2006;295(23): 2727–41.

46. Piubello Q, Parisi A, Eccher A, et al. Flat epithelial atypia on core needle biopsy: which is the right management? Am J Surg Pathol 2009;33(7):1078–84.

47. Boulos FI, Dupont WD, Simpson JF, et al. Histologic associations and long-term cancer risk in columnar cell lesions of the breast: a retrospective cohort and a nested case-control study. Cancer 2008;113(9):2415–21.

48. Valdes EK, Feldman SM, Boolbol SK. Papillary lesions: a review of the literature. Ann Surg Oncol 2007;14(3):1009–13.
49. Chang JM, Han W, Moon WK, et al. Papillary lesions initially diagnosed at ultrasound-guided vacuum-assisted breast biopsy: rate of malignancy based on subsequent surgical excision. Ann Surg Oncol 2011;18(9):2506–14.
50. Sohn V, Keylock J, Arthurs Z, et al. Breast papillomas in the era of percutaneous needle biopsy. Ann Surg Oncol 2007;14(10):2979–84.
51. Lewis JT, Hartmann LC, Vierkant RA, et al. An analysis of breast cancer risk in women with single, multiple, and atypical papilloma. Am J Surg Pathol 2006; 30:665–72.
52. Brenner RJ, Jackman RJ, Parker SH, et al. Percutaneous core needle biopsy of radial scars of the breast: when is excision necessary? AJR Am J Roentgenol 2002;179(5):1179–84.
53. Linda A, Zuiani C, Furlan A, et al. Radial scars without atypia diagnosed at imaging-guided needle biopsy: how often is associated malignancy found at subsequent surgical excision, and do mammography and sonography predict which lesions are malignant? AJR Am J Roentgenol 2010;194(4):1146–51.
54. Berg JC, Visscher DW, Vierkant RA, et al. Breast cancer risk in women with radial scars in benign breast biopsies. Breast Cancer Res Treat 2008;108(2):167–74.
55. Haagensen CD, editor. Diseases of the breast. 3rd edition. Philadelphia: WB Saunders; 1986.
56. Foote FW, Stewart FW. Lobular carcinoma in situ: a rare form of mammary cancer. Am J Pathol 1941;17(4):491–496.3.
57. Rosen PP, Kosloff C, Lieberman PH, et al. Lobular carcinoma in situ of the breast. Detailed analysis of 99 patients with average follow-up of 24 years. Am J Surg Pathol 1978;2(3):225–51.
58. Wheeler JE, Enterline HT, Roseman JM, et al. Lobular carcinoma in situ of the breast. Long-term follow-up. Cancer 1974;34(3):554–63.
59. Page DL, Kidd TE Jr, Dupont WD, et al. Lobular neoplasia of the breast: higher risk for subsequent invasive cancer predicted by more extensive disease. Hum Pathol 1991;22(12):1232–9.
60. Kilbride KE, Newman LA. Chapter 25: lobular carcinoma in situ: clinical management. In: Harris JR, Lippman ME, Morrow M, et al, editors. Diseases of the breast. 4th edition. Philadelphia: Lippincott Williams & Wilkins; 2010.
61. Bodian CA, Perzin KH, Lattes R. Lobular neoplasia. Long term risk of breast cancer and relation to other factors. Cancer 1996;78(5):1024–34.
62. Li CI, Anderson BO, Daling JR, et al. Changing incidence of lobular carcinoma in situ of the breast. Breast Cancer Res Treat 2002;75(3):259–68.
63. Li CI, Malone KE, Saltzman BS, et al. Risk of invasive breast carcinoma among women diagnosed with ductal carcinoma in situ and lobular carcinoma in situ, 1988-2001. Cancer 2006;106(10):2104–12.
64. Liberman L, Holland AE, Marjan D, et al. Underestimation of atypical ductal hyperplasia at MRI-guided 9-gauge vacuum-assisted breast biopsy. AJR Am J Roentgenol 2007;188(3):684–90.
65. Abner AL, Connolly JL, Recht A, et al. The relation between the presence and extent of lobular carcinoma in situ and the risk of local recurrence for patients with infiltrating carcinoma of the breast treated with conservative surgery and radiation therapy. Cancer 2000;88(5):1072–7.
66. Ciocca RM, Li T, Freedman GM, et al. Presence of lobular carcinoma in situ does not increase local recurrence in patients treated with breast-conserving therapy. Ann Surg Oncol 2008;15(8):2263–71.

67. Moran M, Haffty BG. Lobular carcinoma in situ as a component of breast cancer: the long-term outcome in patients treated with breast-conservation therapy. Int J Radiat Oncol Biol Phys 1998;40(2):353–8.

68. Hussain M, Cunnick GH. Management of lobular carcinoma in-situ and atypical lobular hyperplasia of the breast–a review. Eur J Surg Oncol 2011;37(4):279–89.

# Genetic Predisposition Syndromes and Their Management

David M. Euhus, MD[a,b,*], Linda Robinson, MS[b]

## KEYWORDS

- Breast neoplasms • Gene mutation • Cancer predisposition syndromes
- Genetic counseling • Risk assessment • Risk management

## KEY POINTS

- Although mutations in BRCA1 and BRCA2 account for nearly 50% of the major inherited breast cancer predisposition syndromes, a variety of other high and moderate penetrance genes have been identified.
- Genetic tests that return any result other than deleterious mutation require special consideration and management.
- Professional genetic counselors serve a vital role in the cancer genetics clinic.
- Mutation carriers have several options for managing breast cancer risk, including lifestyle changes, enhanced surveillance, chemoprevention, and prophylactic surgery.
- Genetic counseling and testing should be considered in the initial evaluation of patients with newly diagnosed breast cancer. Patients need this information to make informed decisions about surgery, radiation therapy, and systemic treatments.

## INTRODUCTION

Soon after the French revolution (1789–1799), modern scientific medicine was developed in Paris. Prominent clinician-scientists working to understand the origins of human cancer collected family histories of cancer and debated whether family clusters of cancer proved that cancer was contagious or, rather, was transmitted from parent to offspring. Writing in 1851, the pioneer of modern diagnostic pathology, Hermann Lebert, suggested that "...children come into the world carrying within them the seeds of a cancerous disease which remains latent for thirty to fifty years, but which, once developed, is fatal in the space of a few years."[1] He recognized the value of identifying individuals with an inherited predisposition to cancer and suggested that these individuals might reduce their cancer risk by relocating to regions

Funding Sources: Nil.

Conflict of Interest: Nil.

[a] Department of Surgery, UT Southwestern Medical Center at Dallas, Dallas, TX, USA; [b] Clinical Cancer Genetics, Simmons Comprehensive Cancer Center, UT Southwestern Medical Center at Dallas, Dallas, TX, USA

* Corresponding author. 5323 Harry Hines Boulevard, NB2.402G, Dallas, TX 75390-8548.

*E-mail address:* David.euhus@utsouthwestern.edu

with a low cancer incidence. This prescient grasp of gene-environment interactions predated Gregor Mendel's articulation of the laws of inheritance in 1865,[2] Friedrich Miescher's isolation of DNA in 1871,[3] and Oswald Avery's showing that DNA is the medium of genetic transmission in 1944.[4]

Although early-onset breast cancer was not linked to the D17S74 locus on chromosome 17q21 (later named BRCA1[5]) until 1990,[6] Paul Broca, a contemporary of Herman Lebert, described an apparent family with BRCA in 1866 (**Fig. 1**).[7] He recognized that familial cancer predisposition was rare, that women were disproportionately affected with cancer compared with men, and that cancer rates in these families were at least 15 times greater than those observed in the general population.

The tenets of clinical cancer genetics articulated by Lebert and Broca in the mid-nineteenth century still hold in the twenty-first century. Specifically, major inherited predisposition syndromes account for only 5% to 10% of cases of breast cancer, women are disproportionately affected with hereditary cancer compared with men, and there is great value in identifying high-risk individuals. Ascertainment and assessment of a 3-generation family history of cancer is still the initial step in genetic risk assessment, but genetic testing provides a powerful tool for determining which individuals in a family cluster of cancer are at high risk. Individuals who are found to "carry within them the seeds of a cancerous disease" must understand the time course and magnitude of their cancer risk, the options for enhanced surveillance, and the measures that they can take to reduce their risk. For those recently diagnosed with a hereditary cancer, specific management options must be considered.

## THE GENES

In healthy cells, tumor suppressor genes function to maintain DNA integrity and buffer proliferation signals. These activities slow the rate of accumulation of DNA alterations. For individuals who have inherited an altered copy of 1 of these genes, the process is accelerated and cancers develop at an increased frequency and often at an early age.

TP53 was among the first genes to be definitively associated with familial breast cancer.[8] This gene is a master regulator of DNA damage repair, cell death pathways, and cell cycle control. BRCA1 was cloned in 1994[9] and BRCA2 in 1996.[10–12] Both genes cooperate to maintain DNA integrity by facilitating error-free DNA double-strand break repair (ie, homologous recombination). BRCA1 serves a variety of other functions as well, including regulation of gene expression, cell cycle control, and regulation of protein recycling. Several genes in the Fanconi anemia pathway[13] that interact with BRCA1 in homologous recombination have also been linked to breast cancer, including BARD1, BRIP1/BACH1, MRE11A, NBN, NBS1, RAD50, RAD51C, ATM, and PALB2.[14–17] Other breast cancer susceptibility genes include the cell cycle

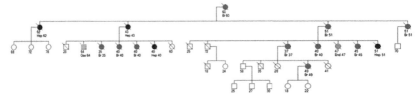

**Fig. 1.** A hereditary breast cancer family described by Paul Broca in 1866.[7] Red circles denote women diagnosed with breast cancer, blue is liver cancer, orange gastric cancer, and green endometrial cancer. Pedigree drawn with CaGene6. (*Data from* Euhus DM. Cancer Gene 2012. Available at: http://www4.utsouthwestern.edu/breasthealth/cagene. Accessed February 1, 2013.)

control proteins CHEK2[18] and p16,[19,20] PTEN, a cytoplasmic protein that buffers proliferation signals (the way a resistor would reduce the current in an electrical circuit),[21,22] CDH1 (E-cadherin), a membrane protein that links cells to other cells,[23,24] and STK11 (LKB1), the Peutz-Jeghers syndrome gene, which regulates how a cell responds to proliferation signals depending on the availability of ATP.[25]

## BASIC GENETICS OF INHERITED PREDISPOSITION

Nearly all of the breast cancer predisposition genes operate in an autosomal-dominant fashion. This expression means that only 1 abnormal copy of the gene needs to be inherited from either the mother or father to significantly increase breast cancer risk. It also means that, on average, about half of the individuals in an affected family are at increased risk for cancer. Some of these genes increase risk of breast cancer more than others (ie, some have a greater penetrance). For example, in some families, a BRCA1 mutation is associated with an 80% lifetime risk of breast cancer, whereas the lifetime risk associated with a CHEK2 mutation is more in the range of 15% to 25%. In addition, mutations are rare for some of the genes, but more common for others. BRCA gene mutations account for about 50% of predisposition to inherited breast cancer, whereas each of the other genes account for fewer than 5% of these cases. The allele frequency for many of these genes varies considerably by ethnicity. For instance, BRCA1 mutations are estimated to occur in 0.06% of non-Jewish individuals, but in up to 2.6% of Ashkenazi Jewish populations.[26,27] The frequency of mutated alleles for most of the other genes is lower than 0.06%. CHEK2 mutations are rare in the United States,[28] but are estimated to occur in up to 1.4% of healthy Finnish individuals.[29] In most cases, a significant family history of cancer is the first clue that there is a mutated gene in the family, but for some genes, such as STK11 and PTEN, new mutations are common (ie, de novo mutation). For these genes, the proband may be the first individual in the family with the syndrome. A working knowledge of mode of inheritance, penetrance, allele frequency, and de novo mutation rates is essential for consistently recognizing heritable cancer predisposition, for precisely identifying the cause, and for managing affected families. **Table 1** lists the major breast cancer predisposition genes in order of penetrance.

## SINGLE-NUCLEOTIDE POLYMORPHISM PANELS

Genome-wide association studies have identified common sequence variants that are associated with a slightly increased risk for breast cancer.[30] One of the most strongly associated variants occurs in FGFR2. This variant is found in 38% of the population and is associated with a 26% increase in risk for breast cancer. This finding means an absolute lifetime risk of about 15%. There is no clinical value for identifying individuals at this risk level, but proponents of these panels assert that there is value in identifying individuals who carry multiple risk-associated single-nucleotide polymorphisms (SNPs). This view is challenged by the observations that more than one-third of women tested would be identified as increased risk, women who are homozygous for all of the risk alleles would have a relative risk for breast cancer of less than 4.0, and more than 1 million women would need to be tested to identify 1 at this risk level.[31] Although these SNP panels are being marketed directly to consumers, it should be recognized that they have no clinical usefulness on an individual basis, but may have some value for population screening. In addition, although many of these SNPs have been shown to modify risk for breast cancer for carriers of the BRCA gene mutation,[32,33] their role in individualized risk assessment has not yet been established.

**Table 1**
**Major breast cancer predisposition genes and syndromes**

| Gene[a] | Lifetime Risk for Breast Cancer (%) | Allele Frequency (%) | Family History and Phenotype Clues |
|---|---|---|---|
| BRCA1[42] | 65–81 | 0.06–1.5 | Hereditary breast ovarian cancer syndrome: early-onset breast cancer, ovarian cancer, modest increase in male breast cancer risk |
| BRCA2[42] | 45–85 | 0.06–1.5 | Hereditary breast ovarian cancer syndrome: early-onset/late-onset breast cancer, ovarian cancer, melanoma, pancreatic cancer, male breast cancer |
| TP53[42] | 50–80 | <0.0005 | Li-Fraumeni syndrome: very-early-onset breast cancer, sarcoma, adrenocortical carcinoma, brain tumors, phyllodes tumor, others (many), ER-positive, PR-positive, human epidermal growth factor receptor 2–positive breast cancer |
| PTEN[42] | 50–85 | 0.0005 | Cowden syndrome: breast cancer, benign and malignant thyroid disease, endometrial cancer, colorectal cancer, macrocephaly, trichilemmomas, palmar-plantar keratoses, oral mucosal papillomatosis, benign breast disease; de novo mutations 11%–48% |
| CDH1[23] | 39–52 | Unknown | Infiltrating lobular cancer, diffuse gastric cancer with signet ring cells |
| STK11[132,133] | 35–50 | 0.004–0.0003 | Peutz-Jeghers syndrome: very-early-onset breast cancer, gastrointestinal cancer, pancreatic cancer, ovarian cancer, hamartomatous polyps of the gastrointestinal tract, oral-labial pigmentation; de novo mutation rate may be as high as 50% |
| PALB2 | 20–30 | 0.2 | Later-onset breast cancer, male breast cancer, pancreatic cancer |
| CHEK2[134] | 15–25 | 0.3–1.7 | Similar cancer spectrum as Li-Fraumeni syndrome but lower penetrance; male breast cancer |
| NF1[135] | 15–25 | 0.02 | Neurofibromatosis: early-onset breast cancer, gliomas, malignant peripheral nerve sheath tumors, café au lait spots; de novo mutations 50% |
| p16[136–138] | 15–25 | Unknown | Familial atypical multiple mole melanoma syndrome: melanoma, pancreatic cancer, dysplastic nevi, breast cancer |

[a] Reference citations point to resources that are useful for clinical management.
*Abbreviations:* ER, estrogen receptor; PR, progesterone receptor.

## THE MUTATIONS

**Fig. 2** shows the basic organization of a gene and some of the most common types of mutations. The most common deleterious mutation is an insertion or deletion of 1 or 2 nucleotides, which creates a frameshift, resulting in early termination of translation

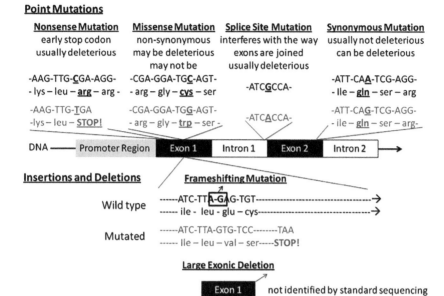

**Fig. 2.** Types of gene mutations observed in breast cancer predisposition genes. Wild-type sequences are shown in black and mutated sequences in red.

and a truncated protein, which can interfere with the normal functions of the full length, wild-type protein produced from the normal sister chromosome. One example is the common Ashkenazi Jewish mutation in BRCA1 known as 185delAG. This nomenclature signifies that at the 185th exonic nucleotide an AG sequence has been deleted.

Although protein-truncating nonsense mutations are nearly always deleterious, other exonic mutations such as point mutations that change 1 amino acid (ie, missense mutations), point mutations that do not change any amino acids (ie, synonymous mutations), and in-frame insertion or deletion of entire triplets may or may not be deleterious. Promoter region and intronic mutations can also be deleterious. This situation is especially true for mutations that occur near the beginning or end of an intron, where they may interfere with subsequent mRNA splicing. An example of 1 such mutation is BRCA1 IVS4+1G>T, which means that the first nucleotide of intervening sequence 4 (ie, the fourth intron) has been changed from a G to a T. Other intronic mutations and promoter region mutations may be deleterious if they affect regulatory regions.

## VARIANTS OF UNCERTAIN CLINICAL SIGNIFICANCE

Although most frameshifting and nonsense mutations generate truncated proteins that interfere with cellular functions and increase cancer risk, disease association is uncertain for many of the single-nucleotide alterations shown in **Fig. 2**. For BRCA1 and BRCA2, it is estimated that 2.9%[34] of identified mutations fall into this latter category. This is a significant improvement over the 7% to 15% rate previously reported.[35,36] Variants of uncertain clinical significance (VUS) rates are higher for non-White populations, but have declined from 22% to 46%[37,38] to 2.6% to 7.8%[34] in recent years. Work is continually ongoing to definitively classify these variants as deleterious or nondeleterious.

From a clinical perspective, patients need to know at the outset that their genetic test may return a VUS. These individuals may need to be managed the same as any individual with a noninformative negative gene test (see later discussion). A record of the genetic test result and patient contact information needs to be maintained so that these individuals can be contacted when the VUS is classified as deleterious or nondeleterious.

## FOUNDER MUTATIONS

Sometimes, during the course of human migration and colonization, small populations of individuals harboring specific mutations become geographically or socially isolated. After many generations of relative isolation, these mutations can become common in the population. The 3 BRCA Ashkenazi founder mutations, BRCA1 185delAG, BRCA1 5382insC, and BRCA2 6174delT, are examples of this situation. It is postulated that mass migration of Spanish Jews to the Americas in 1492 accounts for the high prevalence of Ashkenazi Jewish founder mutations observed in Hispanics.[38] Because these 3 founder mutations account for about 90% of BRCA gene mutations in the Ashkenazi Jewish population,[39] genetic testing usually begins with this 3-gene panel in these individuals.

## GENETIC TESTS

Germline genetic testing is performed on DNA isolated from leukocytes obtained from a venous blood sample or from oral epithelial cells obtained from a saliva sample. If the intent is to test for 1 or a few specific mutations (eg, single-site tests), only limited regions of the gene of interest are assessed. If a more general screen for mutations is desired, DNA sequencing reactions are designed to assess portions of the promoter, some or all of the exons, and sections of the introns that may be involved in messenger RNA (mRNA) splicing. The clinically relevant point is that gene tests are rarely capable of identifying every possible deleterious mutation in a gene. In addition, an idiosyncrasy of the sequencing technology in common use is that it generates a normal read-out if there are rearrangements, duplications, or deletions affecting 1 or more exons. Special testing to identify the 5 most common large rearrangements frequently observed among individuals of European ancestry was added to routine BRCA testing beginning in 2002, but this is a candidate approach that does not identify large rearrangements that are not specifically looked for. Myriad Genetics (Salt Lake City, UT), the primary provider of BRCA gene mutation testing, offers an additional test, called the BRACAnalysis Large Rearrangement Test (BART), which provides a more comprehensive test for rearrangements in BRCA1 and BRCA2. Whether this test is routinely performed or not after a negative BRCA sequencing test is dependent on the personal and family history of cancer (eg, a BRCAPRO mutation probability >30% usually triggers the reflex protocol). For individuals who do not meet the established criteria for BART testing, the test must be ordered and paid for separately. These large rearrangements account for up to 17% of deleterious BRCA gene mutations in individuals of Near-East/Middle-Eastern ancestry and up to 22% for individuals with Latin-American/Caribbean ancestry.[40]

Currently available gene tests are not capable of identifying every deleterious mutation, and testing protocols continue to evolve, making it essential that patients with noninformative negative gene tests remain accessible for retesting as technologies change. The sensitivity of BRCA gene testing is estimated at 80% to 90%. Extended testing may be indicated depending on the family history and ethnic background of the counselee. A negative test must be carefully interpreted in light of all available information.

## THE NONINFORMATIVE NEGATIVE GENE TEST

The positive gene mutation test poses few difficulties in interpretation and should initiate the risk assessment and intervention activities described later. Every negative test requires special consideration and interpretation. Maternal and paternal linage must be considered separately in the interpretation of a negative test. If the cancer predisposition is clearly resident in only 1 lineage, and this predisposition has been adequately explained by the presence of a mutation in 1 or more relatives of that lineage, then a negative gene test is highly informative and the counselee can be reassured that their cancer risk is likely no greater than that of the general population. When all of these criteria are not met, the test result is classified as noninformative negative. Each of the following issues must be addressed for every patient with a noninformative negative test result: could the counselee have inherited an identifiable gene mutation from the other side of the family? Could the gene test have missed a deleterious mutation (ie, is more extensive testing indicated)? Should a different gene be tested? The decision to test other genes can be guided by the family history and phenotype clues listed in **Table 1**. If a noninformative negative gene test cannot be resolved, then the patient must be managed as though they are at increased risk for the cancers associated with the most likely syndrome suggested by the family history.

The best approach for minimizing noninformative negative gene tests is to always test the individual in the family who is most likely to carry a mutation. This is frequently not the individual who is presenting for genetic risk assessment. Every effort should be made to identify and engage the relative with the greatest mutation probability. When family dynamics or early deaths from cancer preclude this strategy, the counselee should be thoroughly educated concerning the likelihood and implications of a noninformative negative test.

## PROFESSIONAL GENETIC COUNSELORS

In 2012, the American College of Surgeons Commission on Cancer accreditation program (http://www.facs.org/cancerprogram/index.html) mandated that cancer risk assessment, genetic counseling, and genetic testing services be provided to patients by a qualified genetic professional either on site or by referral. Practice guidelines for genetic counselors have been well articulated by the National Society of Genetic Counselors.[41] Essential services performed by professional genetic counselors include pretest and posttest counseling and education; interpretation of negative results, which often requires decisions about carrying out more extensive testing, or testing other genes; maintaining patient contact files so that when new gene tests become available or variants of uncertain significance are reclassified the affected patients can be notified; helping newly identified mutation carriers to notify their family members; and aggressively pursuing government, industry, or philanthropic funding to cover the costs of genetic testing for the uninsured or underinsured. These activities are beyond the scope of the average clinical practice. Board-certified professional genetic counselors are essential for the operation of cancer genetics programs.

## IDENTIFYING MUTATION CARRIERS

Genetic testing is expensive and the results can have significant psychosocial impacts; consequently, testing is currently offered selectively. The most pragmatic criteria for offering testing include: (1) the individual is reasonably likely to carry a mutation, (2) the test result would influence health care decisions for the counselee or the counselee's relatives, and (3) there is some mechanism available for paying for the test. The last criterion automatically creates a socioeconomic disparity for the use of cancer genetics services and places third-party payers in the position of defining "reasonably likely to carry a mutation." Guidelines for recommending genetic testing have been published for most of the known hereditary breast cancer syndromes and many, but not all, insurers follow these. The National Comprehensive Cancer Network (NCCN) regularly publishes updated guidelines for several of the syndromes.[42]

Recognizing individuals with a hereditary predisposition to breast cancer usually requires collection and thoughtful evaluation of a 3-generation cancer family history. Early-onset breast cancer is the hallmark of many of the syndromes, but the occurrence of certain combinations of cancers in a family regardless of age at onset may also provide a clue (see **Table 1**). For syndromes with a high de novo mutation rate (eg, Cowden syndrome and Peutz-Jeghers syndrome), the family history may not be helpful, but an astute clinician recognizes the associated phenotypic features on physical examination (see **Table 1**).

Mathematical models such as BRCAPRO,[43] BOADICEA,[26] and Tyrer-Cusick[44] can be used to calculate the probability of a BRCA gene mutation. CancerGene is a widely used desktop program that uses BRCAPRO to estimate mutation probabilities and cancer risks.[45] An online program for calculating the probability of a PTEN mutation is available for patients with suspected Cowden syndrome.[46] Mathematical models are neither sensitive nor specific enough to define a specific mutation probability threshold lower than which genetic testing can be safely avoided,[47] but these models can enhance the accuracy of risk estimations for genetic counselors,[48] and the graphical outputs are useful for risk counseling.

Traditionally, family history screening and referral for genetic counseling have been the responsibility of primary care physicians. These physicians are already overburdened, so it is not surprising that detailed cancer family history screening is not routinely practiced.[49] An alternative approach is to screen large populations of women through mammography departments using brief, validated family history tools.[50,51] In addition, the recognition that 10% to 25% of women diagnosed with triple-negative breast cancer before the age of 50 years carry a BRCA gene mutation[52] provides a way of engaging pathology departments for hereditary breast cancer screening. Ideally, health care providers at all levels would consistently collect detailed cancer family histories and recognize patterns suggesting an inherited predisposition. At a minimum, the single-individual phenotypes listed in **Table 2** should be widely recognized and should prompt cancer genetics referrals.

| Table 2 | |
|---|---|
| **Single-individual phenotypes prompting genetic risk evaluation** | |
| **Phenotype** | **BRCA Mutation Prevalence (%)** |
| Double primary breast-ovarian cancer | 86 |
| Male breast cancer | 8–25 |
| Breast cancer in an Ashkenazi Jewish woman | ~15 |
| Triple-negative breast cancer <60 y of age | 10–25 |
| Ovarian cancer | 10–15 |
| Female breast cancer <45 y of age | ~10 |

## MANAGING RISK FOR PRIMARY BREAST CANCER IN THOSE WHO TEST POSITIVE

A positive gene test permits proactive development and execution of a plan to reduce cancer risk or to diagnose cancer at an early more easily managed stage. Consequently, the initial task after receiving a positive result is to quantify the cancer risk over time. Lifetime breast cancer risk ranges from 65% to 81% for BRCA1 mutation carriers and 45% to 85% for BRCA2 carriers.[53–55] The mean age at diagnosis of breast cancer is about 44 years for BRCA1 mutation carriers and 47 years for BRCA2 carriers, but age at onset varies by family, particularly for BRCA2 families.[56] Some genes, such as TP53 and STK11, are associated with very-early-onset breast cancer, whereas genes like CHEK2 and PALB2 are associated with later-onset breast cancer. In some families, the mutated gene is highly penetrant (ie, most or all of the mutation carriers develop cancer), whereas in other families, gene-gene and gene-environment interactions reduce the cancer risk. A careful assessment of the 3-generation cancer family history in conjunction with the model calculations described in the preceding is helpful at this juncture. Obtaining a sense of the penetrance of the gene mutation in a specific family is particularly helpful for the low or moderate penetrance genes shown in **Table 1**.

## MODIFIERS OF RISK

All BRCA gene mutation carriers are at significantly increased risk for breast cancer, but certain genetic, reproductive, and lifestyle factors can modify this risk. For instance, the Ashkenazi Jewish founder mutation, BRCA2 6174delT, is associated with lower lifetime breast cancer risk (about 55%) compared with other mutations.[39,57] In addition, several SNPs that are known to slightly increase the risk for sporadic breast cancer have been shown to modify risk in BRCA gene mutation carriers.[32,33]

Late age at menarche, early age at first live birth, and increasing numbers of live births have been shown to reduce the risk of sporadic breast cancer. Menarche at or after age 14 years has been associated with a 54% reduction in breast cancer risk for BRCA1 mutation carriers[58,59]; however, early age at first live birth does not seem to reduce risk for breast cancer for BRCA gene mutation carriers.[60] Pregnancy has a minimal effect on risk for breast cancer for BRCA1 mutation carriers, but each pregnancy increases risk by 17% for BRCA2 carriers.[61] Lactation for more than 1 year reduced breast cancer risk by 40% for BRCA1 mutation carriers, but did not seem to have an effect in BRCA2 carriers.[59,62]

Combined hormone replacement therapy (cHRT) is known to increase the risk for sporadic breast cancer. One study[63] has suggested that cHRT does not increase risk in BRCA1 mutation carriers, whereas estrogen-only therapy reduced risk by 49%. Caffeinated coffee is believed to provide antioxidant effects. Consumption of 6 or more cups of caffeinated coffee per day was associated with reduced risk for breast cancer among BRCA1 mutation carriers.[64] Weight gain in adulthood and energy consumption, but not other dietary factors, have been associated with increased risk for breast cancer in BRCA gene mutation carriers.[65] There is evidence that medical radiograph exposure (eg, chest radiographs) before the age of 20 years may increase future breast cancer risk for BRCA gene mutation carriers.[66] The risks of yearly mammography before age 30 years should be carefully considered.

## DEVELOPING AN INDIVIDUALIZED RISK MANAGEMENT STRATEGY

The primary options for managing cancer risk in those who test positive include enhanced surveillance, chemoprevention, and prophylactic surgery. The relative benefits and risks of each of these choices are explained to the patient in detail. Consideration is given to the specific cancer family history, including apparent penetrance and ages at diagnosis, and an understanding is sought of the patient's unique psychosocial perspective, risk tolerance, and family and career goals. Management plans are individualized. There are no hard and fast rules governing what must be done and when. The role of the clinician is to help the well-informed patient develop a personally acceptable plan and then to engage the appropriate multidisciplinary team to execute this plan.

## ENHANCED SURVEILLANCE

The sensitivity of screening magnetic resonance imaging (MRI) for detection of breast cancer in high-risk women ranges from 71% to 94% compared with 33% to 59% for mammography.[67–72] Screening MRI is less specific than mammography, so its use increases the rate of benign breast biopsies (about 10% for the first MRI); but this rate decreases with successive rounds of screening. Screening sonography has a sensitivity of 17% to 65%[69–71] and occasionally identifies a cancer missed by mammography and MRI. Adding modalities to the screening algorithm incrementally increases the cancer detection rate, but also increases the benign biopsy rate. The primary role of sonography is in the further characterization of mammographic or MRI lesions, but the introduction and validation of automated screening sonography platforms may force a reassessment.[73] The combination of clinical breast examination, screening mammography, and screening MRI has a sensitivity of 86% to 94% for detection of breast cancer among BRCA gene mutation carriers.[68,69] The NCCN has recommended that BRCA gene mutation carriers begin practicing breast self-examination at the age of 18 years and twice-yearly clinical breast examination, with yearly screening mammography and MRI beginning at the age of 25 years.[42] Yearly mammography before the age of 30 years may increase risk for breast cancer in BRCA gene mutation carriers, so this recommendation should be reconsidered. The American Cancer Society supports screening MRI for anyone with a lifetime breast cancer risk greater than 20%, making it a reasonable option for most of the syndromes shown in **Table 1**.[74] The age when screening begins may be adjusted according to the earliest age at diagnosis of breast cancer in the family. A common practice is to begin screening 10 years before the earliest age at diagnosis of breast cancer in the family and to stagger the mammography and MRI by 6 months to reduce the screening interval.

## CHEMOPREVENTION

Tamoxifen reduces the risk of breast cancer by nearly 50%, even for women with up to 3 first-degree relatives with breast cancer.[75] Tamoxifen has not been prospectively studied in women with deleterious BRCA gene mutations, but an analysis of 19 mutation carriers included in the NSABP P1 Breast Cancer Prevention Trial suggested a 50% reduction in risk for BRCA2 mutation carriers but no effect for BRCA1 carriers.[76] This finding is not unexpected, because tamoxifen reduces the risk only for estrogen receptor (ER)-positive breast cancer; and, whereas 60% to 75% of BRCA2-associated breast cancers are ER-positive, 70% to 90% of BRCA1-associated breast cancers are ER-negative.[77–79] Tamoxifen is FDA-approved by the US Food and Drug Administration (FDA) for prevention of breast cancer in women aged 35 years or older. Given the early age at onset of breast cancer in BRCA gene mutation carriers, the modern trend for delayed childbirth, and uncertainty concerning the impact of tamoxifen on lifetime risk, tamoxifen is used only infrequently (6%)

among BRCA mutation carriers.[80] Raloxifene, which is FDA-approved for postmenopausal women only, is used even less frequently (3%).

## PROPHYLACTIC BILATERAL SALPINGO-OOPHORECTOMY

Bilateral salpingo-oophorectomy (BSO) reduces the incidence of primary ovarian cancer in BRCA gene mutation carriers by 80% to 96%[81,82]; however, special care must be taken to remove the entire fallopian tube (which is believed to be the origin of many BRCA gene-mutation associated ovarian cancers[83,84]), and systematic protocols should be followed in the operating room and pathology laboratory to identify occult ovarian cancer.[85,86] Premenopausal BSO reduces breast cancer risk by about 50%.[81,87,88] It is not clear whether postmenopausal BSO also reduces breast cancer risk, but its effects on circulating androgen levels are of interest in this regard.[89] Most BRCA2 gene mutation-associated breast cancers are ER-positive, so it is not surprising that BSO reduces breast cancer risk by 64% to 72% in these women.[90,91] Prophylactic BSO also reduces breast cancer risk in BRCA1 gene mutation carriers, but only by 37% to 39%.[90,91] Early, abrupt surgical menopause is associated with disabling quality of life issues in some women.[92] Hormone replacement therapy does not seem to interfere with the risk-reducing effects of BSO[93] and should not be withheld if required. The NCCN guidelines recommend risk-reducing BSO for BRCA gene mutation carriers between the ages of 35 and 40 years.[42] The impact of BSO on risk for breast cancer should not be overestimated for BRCA1 mutation carriers.

## BILATERAL PROPHYLACTIC MASTECTOMY

Bilateral prophylactic mastectomy (BPM) reduces breast cancer risk by more than 90%,[94–96] but 1 year later, 48% of women report feeling more self-conscious and less sexually attractive primarily because of visible scars.[97] Nipple-sparing mastectomy (NSM) provides excellent cosmesis, and the scars can be well hidden by using lateral inframammary incisions (**Fig. 3**). Some have suggested that NSM leaves considerable breast tissue behind and should be avoided in BRCA gene mutation carriers.[98] One of the earliest BPM series (90% of which were NSM) included 214 genetic high-risk women[96] and reported no primary breast cancers among the 26 confirmed BRCA gene mutation carriers after a median follow-up of 13 years.[99] A recent review of NSM supports the oncologic safety of the procedure and suggests that the risk of cancer in the retained nipple is less than 1%.[100] When NSM is performed correctly, the areolar flap is thin relative to the more peripheral flaps. Breast epithelial structures can extend close to the dermis of the breast skin,[101] but terminal duct lobular units are only infrequently identified in excised nipples.[102] Consequently, the volume of residual breast tissue is most related to the area of retained skin and the thickness of the flaps. The nipple-areolar complex accounts for only a tiny fraction of this volume. Patients should be advised that available evidence suggests excellent risk reduction with NSM, but that, theoretically, the risk can be reduced further by taking more skin. Lifetime risk for breast cancer after BPM is estimated at 7% for BRCA gene mutation carriers.[98]

## MANAGING CANCER RISK IN MEN

Lifetime breast cancer risk is estimated at 1.8% for men with BRCA1 mutations and 8.3% for BRCA2.[103] Mutations in CHEK2 PALB2, and PTEN are also associated with an increased risk for male breast cancer. Men who carry BRCA2 gene mutations

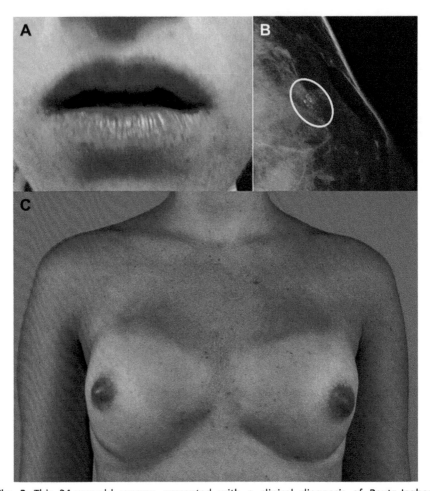

**Fig. 3.** This 24-year-old woman presented with a clinical diagnosis of Peutz-Jeghers syndrome based on a history of intussusception caused by small intestinal hamartomatous polyps at the age of 3 years. Family history was positive for fallopian tube cancer in a maternal aunt (BRCA1/2-negative) and breast cancer in her maternal grandmother. (*A*) Note the lip pigmentation. (*B*) Her first screening mammogram showed a cluster of pleomorphic calcifications (*yellow circle*) diagnosed as ductal carcinoma in situ on core biopsy. (*C*) She underwent bilateral total NSM, and this image shows the postoperative result.

are at increased risk for a variety of other cancers,[104] but the absolute risk for common cancers such as prostate, pancreatic, and melanoma do not seem to justify enhanced surveillance. However, BRCA2 gene mutation carriers are at risk for aggressive, early-onset prostate cancer, which is associated with a higher mortality than sporadic prostate cancer.[105] Screening for breast, prostate, and pancreatic cancer is practiced in some centers.[106] The NCCN guidelines recommend training in breast self-examination, clinical breast examination every 6 months, and consideration of baseline mammography.[42] Our practice is to encourage breast self-examination, begin annual clinical examination and mammography at age 30 years, and annual prostate examination and prostate-specific antigen measurements at age 40 years.

## MANAGING BREAST CANCER IN MUTATION CARRIERS

Breast cancers that arise in the context of a deleterious BRCA1 or BRCA2 gene muta-tion have unique biologic features that directly affect surgical decisions, radiation therapy options, and the choice of systemic agents. Gene mutation testing should be part of the initial evaluation of patients with newly diagnosed breast cancer who are reasonably likely to carry a mutation based on the criteria described in the preceding sections. A thorough review of preoperative genetic testing and the treat-ment implications has been published recently.[107]

## BREAST CANCER OUTCOME

Published data comparing breast cancer–specific and overall survival for BRCA gene mutation-associated and sporadic breast cancer are inconsistent, but generally suggest no difference.[108,109] A recent meta-analysis reported that 5-year progression-free (ipsilateral breast and distant sites) and overall survival are significantly reduced in BRCA1 mutation carriers, but not BRCA2 carriers,[110] whereas a recent international population-based cohort study found that distant recurrence and mortality were higher for BRCA2, but not BRCA1-associated cancers.[111]

## BREAST-CONSERVING SURGERY VERSUS MASTECTOMY

Breast conservation in BRCA gene mutation carriers is associated with the same regional and distant recurrence rates and the same breast cancer–specific and overall survival as mastectomy.[108,109] However, BRCA gene mutation carriers considering breast conservation must understand that ipsilateral breast tumor recurrence (IBTR) rates generally range between 1.7% and 2.7% per year,[109,112] but can be as high as 4% per year for very-early-onset breast cancer (eg, age 42 years or younger).[113] Systemic adjuvant chemotherapy seems to reduce this risk.[109] BRCA gene mutation-associated breast cancer is classified as "Unsuitable for accelerated partial breast irradiation outside of a clinical trial,"[114] but available data suggest that side scatter from whole breast radiation therapy does not increase risk for contralateral breast cancer.[109,113]

Risk for contralateral breast cancer, which ranges from 2.0% to 6.2% per year,[108] should also be considered when making initial surgical decisions. This risk is higher for younger women (eg, <50 years) and for women with 2 or more first-degree relatives with breast cancer.[115] Retrospective data suggest that bilateral mastectomy may be associated with improved breast cancer–specific survival for younger women (eg, <50 years) with hormone receptor negative breast cancer,[116] and for women with family histories of breast cancer.[117]

## BSO

All BRCA gene mutation carriers should consider BSO as an option for reducing ovarian cancer risk, but its value in patients who have newly diagnosed breast cancer is unclear. For example, a recent study that included 302 cases of breast cancer from 9 centers reported that BSO did not significantly reduce the rates of IBTR, contralat-eral breast cancer, or distant recurrence.[109] Conversely, a PROSE (Prevention and Observation of Surgical Endpoints) study that included 1060 patients with BRCA mutation-associated breast cancer reported that, although BSO did not reduce the risk of second primary breast cancers, it was associated with a reduction in breast cancer–specific and all-cause mortality.[90]

## CHEMOTHERAPY DECISIONS

BRCA1 gene mutation carriers treated with anthracycline-based neoadjuvant chemotherapy experience pathologic complete response (pCR) rates that are similar to or greater than those observed among sporadic cases, but responses in BRCA2 patients are more variable.[118–120] Taxanes are among the most commonly used agents for chemotherapy of breast cancer. However, there is evidence that BRCA1-mutated triple-negative breast cancer is highly resistant to docetaxel in the metastatic setting[121] and lower than expected response rates have been observed for both ER-positive and ER-negative BRCA1 mutation-associated breast cancer in the neoadjuvant setting.[122] Until recently, platinum agents were rarely used in breast cancer. Cell-line data suggest that resistance to paclitaxel is directly correlated with sensitivity to cisplatin,[123] and loss of BRCA1 is associated with cisplatin sensitivity.[124] One retrospective study of neoadjuvant chemotherapy that included 102 BRCA1 patients reported a 20% pCR rate for anthracycline-based regimens compared with 83% to 90% for cisplatin.[125,126]

## TARGETED THERAPY

Inhibitors of poly (adenosine diphosphate-ribose) polymerase (PARP) block DNA single-strand break repair. Unrepaired single-strand breaks are converted to double-strand breaks during DNA replication. BRCA-mutated cells are deficient in DNA double-strand break repair, rendering them highly sensitive to PARP inhibitors. An early phase 1 trial of the oral PARP inhibitor, olaparib, in patients with advanced, treatment-refractory cancers observed objective responses in BRCA mutation carriers only, including 1 durable complete clinical response in a patient with breast cancer.[127] A second phase 1 trial restricted to advanced or metastatic breast cancer in BRCA gene mutation carriers recorded a 50% objective response rate for BRCA1 carriers compared with 22% for BRCA2 carriers at the 400-mg twice-daily dose.[128] PARP inhibitors are not approved by the FDA for the treatment of breast cancer, but there are more than a dozen clinical trials open and accruing that target BRCA mutation carriers, many of which include PARP inhibition (ClinicalTrials.gov).

## THE FUTURE OF GENETIC TESTING

The preceding sections describe careful assessment of a 3-generation family history of cancer and attention to phenotypic clues to identify individuals who may have a hereditary predisposition to breast cancer and to determine which gene or genes to test. With the introduction of massive parallel sequencing (ie, next-generation sequencing), it is becoming technically and economically feasible to simultaneously screen large numbers of genes for point mutations, rearrangements, duplications, and deletions.[129,130] These tests are already commercially available (eg, Breast-NextTM[131]), but patent issues exclude BRCA1 and BRCA2. As the cost of these tests diminishes and more genes are added, it is possible that comprehensive genetic testing will become as commonplace as lipid testing for cardiovascular risk assessment. In addition, exome sequencing is increasingly performed for a variety of conditions unrelated to cancer. These screens can surreptitiously identify mutations in breast cancer predisposition genes. Interpreting these test results for patients will impose a heavy burden on cancer genetics professionals because many new variants of uncertain clinical significance will be identified, most of the genes included in these panels have low or moderate penetrance, and there are not enough data to rationally formulate risk management strategies for moderate penetrance mutations.

## REFERENCES

1. Lebert H. Traite pratique des maladies cancereuses. Paris: Librarie de L'Academie Nationale de Medecine; 1851. p. 134–5.
2. Mendel G. Versuche über Pflanzenhybriden Verh. Naturforscher-Verein Brünn 1865;4:3–47.
3. Miescher F. Ueber die chemische Zusammensetzung der Eiterzellen. Medicinisch-Chemische Untersuchungen 1871;4:441–60.
4. Avery OT, MacLeod CM, McCarty M. Studies on the chemical nature of the substance inducing transformation of pneumococcal types: induction of transformation by a desoxyribonucleic acid fraction isolated from pneumococcus type III. J Exp Med 1944;79:137–58.
5. Solomon E, Ledbetter DH. Report of the Committee on the Genetic Constitution of Chromosome 17. Cytogenet Cell Genet 1991;58:686–738.
6. Hall JM, Lee MK, Newman B, et al. Linkage of early-onset familial breast cancer to chromosome 17q21. Science 1990;250:1684–90.
7. Broca P. Traite des tumeurs. Paris: Asselin; 1866. p. 150–2.
8. Malkin D, Li FP, Strong LC, et al. Germ line p53 mutations in a familial syndrome of breast cancer, sarcomas, and other neoplasms. Science 1990;250:1233–8.
9. Miki Y, Swensen J, Shattuck-Eidens D, et al. A strong candidate for the breast and ovarian cancer susceptibility gene BRCA1. Science 1994;266(5182):66–71.
10. Wooster R, Neuhausen SL, Mangion J, et al. Localization of a breast cancer susceptibility gene, BRCA2, to chromosome 13q12-13. Science 1994; 265(5181):2088–90.
11. Wooster R, Bignell G, Lancaster J, et al. Identification of the breast cancer susceptibility gene BRCA2. Nature 1995;378:789–92.
12. Tavtigian SV, Simard J, Rommens J, et al. The complete BRCA2 gene and mutations in chromosome 13q-linked kindreds. Nat Genet 1996;12:333–7.
13. D'Andrea AD, Grompe M. The Fanconi anemia/BRCA pathway. Nat Rev Cancer 2003;3:23–34.
14. Casadei S, Norquist BM, Walsh T, et al. Contribution of inherited mutations in the BRCA2-interacting protein PALB2 to familial breast cancer. Cancer Res 2011; 71:2222–9.
15. Jacquemont C, Taniguchi T. Disruption of the Fanconi anemia pathway in human cancer in the general population. Cancer Biol Ther 2006;5:1637–9.
16. Heikkinen K, Rapakko K, Karppinen SM, et al. RAD50 and NBS1 are breast cancer susceptibility genes associated with genomic instability. Carcinogenesis 2006;27:1593–9.
17. De Nicolo A, Tancredi M, Lombardi G, et al. A novel breast cancer–associated BRIP1 (FANCJ/BACH1) germ-line mutation impairs protein stability and function. Clin Cancer Res 2008;14:4672–80.
18. Bell DW, Varley JM, Szydlo TE, et al. Heterozygous germ line hCHK2 mutations in Li-Fraumeni syndrome. Science 1999;286:2528–31.
19. Borg Å, Sandberg T, Nilsson K, et al. High frequency of multiple melanomas and breast and pancreas carcinomas in CDKN2A mutation-positive melanoma families. J Natl Cancer Inst 2000;92:1260–6.
20. de Snoo FA, Bishop DT, Bergman W, et al. Increased risk of cancer other than melanoma in CDKN2A founder mutation (p16-Leiden)-positive melanoma families. Clin Cancer Res 2008;14:7151–7.
21. Mester J, Eng C. Estimate of de novo mutation frequency in probands with PTEN hamartoma tumor syndrome. Genet Med 2012;14(9):819–22.

22. Marsh DJ, Coulon V, Lunetta KL, et al. Mutation spectrum and genotype-phenotype analyses in Cowden disease and Bannayan-Zonana syndrome, two hamartoma syndromes with germline PTEN mutation. Hum Mol Genet 1998;7: 507–15.

23. Fitzgerald RC, Hardwick R, Huntsman D, et al. Hereditary diffuse gastric cancer: updated consensus guidelines for clinical management and directions for future research. J Med Genet 2010;47:436–44.

24. Schrader KA, Masciari S, Boyd N, et al. Hereditary diffuse gastric cancer: association with lobular breast cancer. Fam Cancer 2008;7:73–82.

25. Hearle N, Schumacher V, Menko FH, et al. Frequency and spectrum of cancers in the Peutz-Jeghers syndrome. Clin Cancer Res 2006;12:3209–15.

26. Antoniou AC, Pharoah PD, McMullan G, et al. A comprehensive model for familial breast cancer incorporating BRCA1, BRCA2 and other genes. Br J Cancer 2002;86:76–83.

27. Janavicius R. Founder BRCA1/2 mutations in Europe: implications for hereditary breast-ovarian cancer prevention and control. EPMA J 2010;1:397–412.

28. Offit K, Pierce H, Kirchhoff T, et al. Frequency of CHEK2*1100delC in New York breast cancer cases and controls. BMC Med Genet 2003;4:1–4.

29. Vahteristo P, Bartkova J, Eerola H, et al. A CHEK2 genetic variant contributing to a substantial fraction of familial breast cancer. Am J Hum Genet 2002;71:432–8.

30. Easton DF, Pooley KA, Dunning AM, et al. Genome-wide association study identifies novel breast cancer susceptibility loci. Nature 2007;447:1087–93.

31. Pharoah PD, Antoniou AC, Easton DF, et al. Polygenes, risk prediction, and targeted prevention of breast cancer. N Engl J Med 2008;358:2796–803.

32. Antoniou AC, Beesley J, McGuffog L, et al. Common breast cancer susceptibility alleles and the risk of breast cancer for BRCA1 and BRCA2 mutation carriers: implications for risk prediction. Cancer Res 2010;70:9742–54.

33. Mulligan AM, Couch FJ, Barrowdale D, et al. Common breast cancer susceptibility alleles are associated with tumour subtypes in BRCA1 and BRCA2 mutation carriers: results from the Consortium of Investigators of Modifiers of BRCA1/2. Breast Cancer Res 2011;13:R110.

34. Eggington JM, Burbridge LA, Roa B, et al. Current variant of uncertain significance rates in BRCA1/2 and Lynch syndrome testing (MLH1, MSH2, MSH6, PMS2, EpCam). American College of Medical Genetics Annual Clinical Genetics Meeting. Charlotte, March 27–31, 2012.

35. Frank TS, Deffenbaugh AM, Reid JE, et al. Clinical characteristics of individuals with germline mutations in BRCA1 and BRCA2: analysis of 10,000 individuals. J Clin Oncol 2002;20:1480–90.

36. Easton DF, Deffenbaugh AM, Pruss D, et al. A systematic genetic assessment of 1,433 sequence variants of unknown clinical significance in the BRCA1 and BRCA2 breast cancer-predisposition genes. Am J Hum Genet 2007;81:873–83.

37. Nanda R, Schumm LP, Cummings S, et al. Genetic testing in an ethnically diverse cohort of high-risk women: a comparative analysis of BRCA1 and BRCA2 mutations in American families of European and African ancestry. JAMA 2005;294:1925–33.

38. Weitzel JN, Lagos V, Blazer KR, et al. Prevalence of BRCA mutations and founder effect in high-risk Hispanic families. Cancer Epidemiol Biomarkers Prev 2005;14:1666–71.

39. Finkelman BS, Rubinstein WS, Friedman S, et al. Breast and ovarian cancer risk and risk reduction in Jewish BRCA1/2 mutation carriers. J Clin Oncol 2012;30: 1321–8.

40. Judkins T, Rosenthal E, Arnell C, et al. Clinical significance of large rearrangements in BRCA1 and BRCA2. Cancer 2012;118(21):5210–6.

41. Riley BD, Culver JO, Skrzynia C, et al. Essential elements of genetic cancer risk assessment, counseling, and testing: updated recommendations of the National Society of Genetic Counselors. J Genet Couns 2012;21:151–61.

42. National Comprehensive Cancer Network. Genetic/familial high-risk assessment: breast and ovarian, NCCN Clinical Practice Guidelines in Oncology v.1.2012. Fort Washington (PA): 2012. Available at: http://www.nccn.org/professionals/physician_gls/PDF/genetics_screening.pdf. Accessed February 1, 2013.

43. Berry DA, Parmigiani G, Sanchez S, et al. Probability of carrying a mutation of breast-ovarian cancer gene BRCA1 based on family history. J Natl Cancer Inst 1997;89:227–38.

44. Tyrer J, Duffy SW, Cuzick J. A breast cancer prediction model incorporating familial and personal risk factors [Erratum appears in Stat Med 2005;24(1):156]. Stat Med 2004;23:1111–30.

45. Euhus DM. Cancer Gene 2012. Available at: http://www4.utsouthwestern.edu/breasthealth/cagene. Accessed February 1, 2013.

46. Cleveland Clinic. Risk calculator for estimating a patient's risk for PTEN mutation. 2012. Available at: http://www.lerner.ccf.org/gmi/ccscore/index.php. Accessed February 1, 2013.

47. Parmigiani G, Chen S, Iversen ES Jr, et al. Validity of models for predicting BRCA1 and BRCA2 mutations [Summary for patients in Ann Intern Med 2007;147(7):I38; PMID: 17909202]. Ann Intern Med 2007;147:441–50.

48. Euhus DM, Smith KC, Robinson L, et al. Pretest prediction of BRCA1 or BRCA2 mutation by risk counselors and the computer model BRCAPRO. J Natl Cancer Inst 2002;94:844–51.

49. Flynn BS, Wood ME, Ashikaga T, et al. Primary care physicians' use of family history for cancer risk assessment. BMC Fam Pract 2010;11:45.

50. Bellcross C. Further development and evaluation of a breast/ovarian cancer genetics referral screening tool. Genet Med 2010;12:240.

51. Bellcross CA, Lemke AA, Pape LS, et al. Evaluation of a breast/ovarian cancer genetics referral screening tool in a mammography population. Genet Med 2009;11:783–9.

52. Kandel MJ, Stadler Z, Masciari S, et al. Prevalence of BRCA1 mutations in triple negative breast cancer [abstract 508]. J Clin Oncol 2006;24:5s.

53. Ford D, Easton DF, Stratton M, et al. Genetic heterogeneity and penetrance analysis of the BRCA1 and BRCA2 genes in breast cancer families: the breast cancer linkage consortium. Am J Hum Genet 1998;62:676–89.

54. Antoniou A, Pharoah PD, Narod S, et al. Average risks of breast and ovarian cancer associated with BRCA1 or BRCA2 mutations detected in series unselected for family history: a combined analysis of 22 studies. Am J Hum Genet 2003;72:1117–30.

55. King MC, Marks JH, Mandell JB. Breast and ovarian cancer risks due to inherited mutations in BRCA1 and BRCA2. Science 2003;302:643–6.

56. Panchal S, Bordeleau L, Poll A, et al. Does family history predict the age at onset of new breast cancers in BRCA1 and BRCA2 mutation-positive families? Clin Genet 2010;77:273–9.

57. Antoniou AC, Pharoah PD, Narod S, et al. Breast and ovarian cancer risks to carriers of the BRCA1 5382insC and 185delAG and BRCA2 6174delT mutations: a combined analysis of 22 population based studies. J Med Genet 2005;42:602–3.

58. Kotsopoulos J, Lubinski J, Lynch HT, et al. Age at menarche and the risk of breast cancer in BRCA1 and BRCA2 mutation carriers. Cancer Causes Control 2005;16:667–74.

59. Gronwald J, Byrski T, Huzarski T, et al. Influence of selected lifestyle factors on breast and ovarian cancer risk in BRCA1 mutation carriers from Poland. Breast Cancer Res Treat 2006;95:105–9.

60. Kotsopoulos J, Lubinski J, Lynch HT, et al. Age at first birth and the risk of breast cancer in BRCA1 and BRCA2 mutation carriers. Breast Cancer Res Treat 2007; 105:221–8.

61. Cullinane CA, Lubinski J, Neuhausen SL, et al. Effect of pregnancy as a risk factor for breast cancer in BRCA1/BRCA2 mutation carriers. Int J Cancer 2005;117:988–91.

62. Jernstrom H, Lubinksi J, Lynch HT, et al. Breast-feeding and the risk of breast cancer in BRCA1 and BRCA2 mutation carriers. J Natl Cancer Inst 2004;96: 209–14.

63. Eisen A, Lubinski J, Gronwald J, et al. Hormone therapy and the risk of breast cancer in BRCA1 mutation carriers. J Natl Cancer Inst 2008;100:1361–7.

64. Nkondjock A, Ghadirian P, Kotsopoulos J, et al. Coffee consumption and breast cancer risk among BRCA1 and BRCA2 mutation carriers. Int J Cancer 2006; 118:103–7.

65. Nkondjock A, Robidoux A, Paredes Y, et al. Diet, lifestyle and BRCA-related breast cancer risk among French-Canadians. Breast Cancer Res Treat 2006; 98:285–94.

66. Gronwald J, Pijpe A, Byrski T, et al. Early radiation exposures and BRCA1-associated breast cancer in young women from Poland. Breast Cancer Res Treat 2008;112:581–4.

67. Kriege M, Brekelmans CT, Boetes C, et al. Efficacy of MRI and mammography for breast-cancer screening in women with a familial or genetic predisposition. N Engl J Med 2004;351:427–37.

68. Leach MO, Boggis CR, Dixon AK, et al. Screening with magnetic resonance imaging and mammography of a UK population at high familial risk of breast cancer: a prospective multicentre cohort study (MARIBS). Lancet 2005;365: 1769–78.

69. Warner E, Plewes DB, Hill KA, et al. Surveillance of BRCA1 and BRCA2 mutation carriers with magnetic resonance imaging, ultrasound, mammography, and clinical breast examination. JAMA 2004;292:1317–25.

70. Sardanelli F, Podo F, D'Agnolo G, et al. Multicenter comparative multimodality surveillance of women at genetic-familial high risk for breast cancer (HIBCRIT study): interim results. Radiology 2007;242:698–715.

71. Weinstein SP, Localio AR, Conant EF, et al. Multimodality screening of high-risk women: a prospective cohort study. J Clin Oncol 2009;27:6124–8.

72. Hagen AI, Kvistad KA, Maehle L, et al. Sensitivity of MRI versus conventional screening in the diagnosis of BRCA-associated breast cancer in a national prospective series. Breast 2007;16:367–74.

73. Kelly K, Dean J, Comulada W, et al. Breast cancer detection using automated whole breast ultrasound and mammography in radiographically dense breasts. Eur Radiol 2010;20:734–42.

74. Saslow D, Boetes C, Burke W, et al. American Cancer Society guidelines for breast screening with MRI as an adjunct to mammography [Erratum appears in CA Cancer J Clin 2007;57(3):185]. CA Cancer J Clin 2010;57: 75–89.

75. Fisher B, Costantino JP, Wickerham DL, et al. Tamoxifen for prevention of breast cancer: report of the National Surgical Adjuvant Breast and Bowel Project P-1 Study. J Natl Cancer Inst 1998;90:1371–88.
76. King MC, Wieand S, Hale K, et al. Tamoxifen and breast cancer incidence among women with inherited mutations in BRCA1 and BRCA2: National Surgical Adjuvant Breast and Bowel Project (NSABP-P1) Breast Cancer Prevention Trial. JAMA 2001;286:2251–6.
77. James PA, Doherty R, Harris M, et al. Optimal selection of individuals for BRCA mutation testing: a comparison of available methods. J Clin Oncol 2006;24: 707–15.
78. Lakhani SR, Van De Vijver MJ, Jacquemier J, et al. The pathology of familial breast cancer: predictive value of immunohistochemical markers estrogen receptor, progesterone receptor, HER-2, and p53 in patients with mutations in BRCA1 and BRCA2. J Clin Oncol 2002;20:2310–8.
79. Robson M, Gilewski T, Haas B, et al. BRCA-associated breast cancer in young women. J Clin Oncol 1998;16:1642–9.
80. Metcalfe KA, Birenbaum-Carmeli D, Lubinski J, et al. International variation in rates of uptake of preventive options in BRCA1 and BRCA2 mutation carriers. Int J Cancer 2008;122:2017–22.
81. Rebbeck TR, Kauff ND, Domchek SM. Meta-analysis of risk reduction estimates associated with risk-reducing salpingo-oophorectomy in BRCA1 or BRCA2 mutation carriers. J Natl Cancer Inst 2009;101:80–7.
82. Finch A, Beiner M, Lubinski J, et al. Salpingo-oophorectomy and the risk of ovarian, fallopian tube, and peritoneal cancers in women with a BRCA1 or BRCA2 mutation. JAMA 2006;296:185–92.
83. Norquist BM, Garcia RL, Allison KH, et al. The molecular pathogenesis of hereditary ovarian carcinoma: alterations in the tubal epithelium of women with BRCA1 and BRCA2 mutations. Cancer 2010;116:5261–71.
84. Crum CP, Drapkin R, Kindelberger D, et al. Lessons from BRCA: the tubal fimbria emerges as an origin for pelvic serous cancer. Clin Med Res 2007;5: 35–44.
85. Powell CB, Kenley E, Chen LM, et al. Risk-reducing salpingo-oophorectomy in BRCA mutation carriers: role of serial sectioning in the detection of occult malignancy. J Clin Oncol 2005;23:127–32.
86. Colgan TJ, Murphy J, Cole DE, et al. Occult carcinoma in prophylactic oophorectomy specimens: prevalence and association with BRCA germline mutation status. Am J Surg Pathol 2001;25:1283–9.
87. Rebbeck TR, Lynch HT, Neuhausen SL, et al. Prophylactic oophorectomy in carriers of BRCA1 or BRCA2 mutations. N Engl J Med 2002;346:1616–22.
88. Kauff ND, Barakat RR. Risk-reducing salpingo-oophorectomy in patients with germline mutations in BRCA1 or BRCA2. J Clin Oncol 2007;25:2921–7.
89. Key TJ, Appleby PN, Reeves GK, et al. Circulating sex hormones and breast cancer risk factors in postmenopausal women: reanalysis of 13 studies. Br J Cancer 2011;105:709–22.
90. Domchek SM, Friebel TM, Singer CF, et al. Association of risk-reducing surgery in BRCA1 or BRCA2 mutation carriers with cancer risk and mortality. JAMA 2010;304:967–75.
91. Kauff ND, Domchek SM, Friebel TM, et al. Risk-reducing salpingo-oophorectomy for the prevention of BRCA1- and BRCA2-associated breast and gynecologic cancer: a multicenter, prospective study. J Clin Oncol 2008; 26:1331–7.

92. Finch A, Metcalfe KA, Chiang JK, et al. The impact of prophylactic salpingo-oophorectomy on menopausal symptoms and sexual function in women who carry a BRCA mutation. Gynecol Oncol 2011;121:163–8.

93. Rebbeck TR, Friebel T, Wagner T, et al. Effect of short-term hormone replacement therapy on breast cancer risk reduction after bilateral prophylactic oophorectomy in BRCA1 and BRCA2 mutation carriers: the PROSE Study Group. J Clin Oncol 2005;23:7804–10.

94. Heemskerk-Gerritsen BA, Brekelmans CT, Menke-Pluymers MB, et al. Prophylactic mastectomy in BRCA1/2 mutation carriers and women at risk of hereditary breast cancer: long-term experiences at the Rotterdam Family Cancer Clinic. Ann Surg Oncol 2007;14:3335–44.

95. Meijers-Heijboer H, van Geel B, van Putten WL, et al. Breast cancer after prophylactic bilateral mastectomy in women with a BRCA1 or BRCA2 mutation. N Engl J Med 2001;345:159–64.

96. Hartmann LC, Schaid DJ, Woods JE, et al. Efficacy of bilateral prophylactic mastectomy in women with a family history of breast cancer. N Engl J Med 1999;340:77–84.

97. Brandberg Y, Sandelin K, Erikson S, et al. Psychological reactions, quality of life, and body image after bilateral prophylactic mastectomy in women at high risk for breast cancer: a prospective 1-year follow-up study. J Clin Oncol 2008;26:3943–9.

98. Rebbeck TR, Friebel T, Lynch HT, et al. Bilateral prophylactic mastectomy reduces breast cancer risk in BRCA1 and BRCA2 mutation carriers: the PROSE Study Group. J Clin Oncol 2004;22:1055–62.

99. Hartmann LC, Sellers TA, Schaid DJ, et al. Efficacy of bilateral prophylactic mastectomy in BRCA1 and BRCA2 gene mutation carriers. J Natl Cancer Inst 2001;93:1633–7.

100. Rusby JE, Smith BL, Gui GP. Nipple-sparing mastectomy. Br J Surg 2010;97:305–16.

101. Dreadin J, Sarode V, Saint-Cyr M, et al. Risk of residual breast tissue after skin-sparing mastectomy. Breast J 2012;18:248–52.

102. Stolier AJ, Wang J. Terminal duct lobular units are scarce in the nipple: implications for prophylactic nipple-sparing mastectomy: terminal duct lobular units in the nipple. Ann Surg Oncol 2008;15:438–42.

103. Tai YC, Domchek S, Parmigiani G, et al. Breast cancer risk among male BRCA1 and BRCA2 mutation carriers. J Natl Cancer Inst 2007;99:1811–4.

104. Mohamad HB, Apffelstaedt JP. Counseling for male BRCA mutation carriers: a review. Breast 2008;17:441–50.

105. Thorne H, Willems AJ, Niedermayr E, et al. Decreased prostate cancer-specific survival of men with BRCA2 mutations from multiple breast cancer families. Cancer Prev Res (Phila) 2011;4:1002–10.

106. Brachot-Simeonova I, Morin G, Gillaux C, et al. What management for the asymptomatic men carriers of BRCA1 or 2 mutation? Results of a survey in the French oncogenetic centers. Bull Cancer 2012;99:417–23 [inFrench].

107. Euhus D, Robinson L. Genetic counseling and genetic testing in the preoperative evaluation of breast cancer patients. Curr Breast Cancer Rep 2012;4:102–9.

108. Liebens FP, Carly B, Pastijn A, et al. Management of BRCA1/2 associated breast cancer: a systematic qualitative review of the state of knowledge in 2006. Eur J Cancer 2007;43:238–57.

109. Pierce LJ, Phillips KA, Griffith KA, et al. Local therapy in BRCA1 and BRCA2 mutation carriers with operable breast cancer: comparison of breast conservation and mastectomy. Breast Cancer Res Treat 2010;121:389–98.

110. Lee EH, Park SK, Park B, et al. Effect of BRCA1/2 mutation on short-term and long-term breast cancer survival: a systematic review and meta-analysis. Breast Cancer Res Treat 2010;122:11–25.
111. Goodwin PJ, Phillips KA, West DW, et al. Breast cancer prognosis in BRCA1 and BRCA2 mutation carriers: an international prospective breast cancer family registry population-based cohort study. J Clin Oncol 2012;30:19–26.
112. Garcia-Etienne CA, Barile M, Gentilini OD, et al. Breast-conserving surgery in BRCA1/2 mutation carriers: are we approaching an answer? Ann Surg Oncol 2009;16:3380–7.
113. Haffty BG, Harrold E, Khan AJ, et al. Outcome of conservatively managed early-onset breast cancer by BRCA1/2 status. Lancet 2002;359:1471–7.
114. Smith BD, Arthur DW, Buchholz TA, et al. Accelerated partial breast irradiation consensus statement from the American Society for Radiation Oncology (ASTRO). Int J Radiat Oncol Biol Phys 2009;74:987–1001.
115. Metcalfe K, Gershman S, Lynch HT, et al. Predictors of contralateral breast cancer in BRCA1 and BRCA2 mutation carriers. Br J Cancer 2011;104:1384–92.
116. Bedrosian I, Hu CY, Chang GJ. Population-based study of contralateral prophylactic mastectomy and survival outcomes of breast cancer patients. J Natl Cancer Inst 2010;102:401–9.
117. Boughey JC, Hoskin TL, Degnim AC, et al. Contralateral prophylactic mastectomy is associated with a survival advantage in high-risk women with a personal history of breast cancer. Ann Surg Oncol 2010;17:2702–9.
118. Chappuis PO, Goffin J, Wong N, et al. A significant response to neoadjuvant chemotherapy in BRCA1/2 related breast cancer. J Med Genet 2002;39:608–10.
119. Delaloge S, Pautier P, Kloos I, et al. BRCA1-linked breast cancer (BC) is highly more chemosensitive than its BRCA2-linked or sporadic counterparts, 27th Congress of the European Society for Medical Oncology. Nice (France): October 18–22, 2002.
120. Hubert A, Mali B, Hamburger T, et al. Response to neo-adjuvant chemotherapy in BRCA1 and BRCA2 related stage III breast cancer. Fam Cancer 2009;8:173–7.
121. Wysocki PJ, Korski K, Lamperska K, et al. Primary resistance to docetaxel-based chemotherapy in metastatic breast cancer patients correlates with a high frequency of BRCA1 mutations. Med Sci Monit 2008;14:SC7–10.
122. Byrski T, Gronwald J, Huzarski T, et al. Response to neo-adjuvant chemotherapy in women with BRCA1-positive breast cancers. Breast Cancer Res Treat 2008;108:289–96.
123. Stordal B, Pavlakis N, Davey R. A systematic review of platinum and taxane resistance from bench to clinic: an inverse relationship. Cancer Treat Rev 2007;33:688–703.
124. Fedier A, Steiner RA, Schwarz VA, et al. The effect of loss of BRCA1 on the sensitivity to anticancer agents in p53-deficient cells. Int J Oncol 2003;22:1169–73.
125. Byrski T, Gronwald J, Huzarski T, et al. Pathologic complete response rates in young women with BRCA1-positive breast cancers after neoadjuvant chemotherapy. J Clin Oncol 2010;28:375–9.
126. Byrski T, Huzarski T, Dent R, et al. Response to neoadjuvant therapy with cisplatin in BRCA1-positive breast cancer patients. Breast Cancer Res Treat 2009;115:359–63.
127. Fong PC, Boss DS, Yap TA, et al. Inhibition of poly(ADP-ribose) polymerase in tumors from BRCA mutation carriers. N Engl J Med 2009;361:123–34.

128. Tutt A, Robson M, Garber JE, et al. Oral poly(ADP-ribose) polymerase inhibitor olaparib in patients with BRCA1 or BRCA2 mutations and advanced breast cancer: a proof-of-concept trial. Lancet 2010;376:235–44.

129. Walsh T, Casadei S, Lee MK, et al. Mutations in 12 genes for inherited ovarian, fallopian tube, and peritoneal carcinoma identified by massively parallel sequencing. Proc Natl Acad Sci U S A 2011;108:18032–7.

130. Walsh T, Lee MK, Casadei S, et al. Detection of inherited mutations for breast and ovarian cancer using genomic capture and massively parallel sequencing. Proc Natl Acad Sci U S A 2010;107:12629–33.

131. Ambry Genetics. BreastNext. 2012. Available at: http://www.ambrygen.com/tests/breastnext. Accessed February 1, 2013.

132. National Comprehensive Cancer Network. Colorectal Cancer Screening, NCCN Clinical Practice Guidelines in Oncology v2.2012. Fort Washington (PA): 2012. Available at: http://www.nccn.org/professionals/physician_gls/pdf/colon.pdf. Accessed February 1, 2013.

133. Beggs AD, Latchford AR, Vasen HF, et al. Peutz-Jeghers syndrome: a systematic review and recommendations for management. Gut 2010;59:975–86.

134. Narod SA. Testing for CHEK2 in the cancer genetics clinic: ready for prime time? Clin Genet 2010;78:1–7.

135. Ferner RE, Huson SM, Thomas N, et al. Guidelines for the diagnosis and management of individuals with neurofibromatosis 1. J Med Genet 2007;44:81–8.

136. Niendorf KB, Tsao H. Cutaneous melanoma: family screening and genetic testing. Dermatol Ther 2006;19:1–8.

137. Kefford RF, Newton Bishop JA, Bergman W, et al. Counseling and DNA testing for individuals perceived to be genetically predisposed to melanoma: a consensus statement of the melanoma genetics consortium. J Clin Oncol 1999;17:3245–51.

138. Lynch HT, Fusaro RM, Lynch JF, et al. Pancreatic cancer and the FAMMM syndrome. Fam Cancer 2008;7:103–12.

# Pathology of Invasive Breast Disease

Adriana D. Corben, MD

## KEYWORDS

- Invasive breast disease • Lesions • Adenocarcinomas

## KEY POINTS

- Invasive breast cancers constitute a heterogeneous group of lesions. Although the most common types are designated ductal and lobular, this distinction is not meant to indicate the site of origin within the mammary ductal system. Most invasive breast cancers arise in the terminal duct-lobular unit regardless of histologic type.
- The main purpose of the identification of specific types of invasive breast carcinoma is to refine the prediction of likely behavior and response to treatment also offered by the other major prognostic factors, which include lymph node stage, histologic grade, tumor size, and lymphovascular invasion. Different histologic types of breast carcinoma have different biologies.

## INTRODUCTION

Invasive breast cancers constitute a heterogeneous group of lesions. Most of them are adenocarcinomas and their histopathologic classification is based on the growth pattern and cytologic features of the tumor. Although the most common types are designated ductal and lobular, this distinction is not meant to indicate the site of origin within the mammary ductal system. Most invasive breast cancers arise in the terminal duct-lobular unit regardless of histologic type.[1]

The main purpose of the identification of specific types of invasive breast carcinoma is to refine the prediction of likely behavior and response to treatment also offered by the other major prognostic factors, which include lymph node stage, histologic grade, tumor size, and lymphovascular invasion. The key clinical aspects are highlighted in **Box 1**.

## MICROINVASIVE CARCINOMA

Microinvasive carcinoma is characterized by the extension of cancer cells beyond the in situ component (ductal carcinoma in situ [DCIS]/lobular carcinoma in situ [LCIS])

Department of Pathology, Memorial Sloan-Kettering Cancer Center, New York, NY 10065, USA
E-mail address: corbena@mskcc.org

Surg Clin N Am 93 (2013) 363–392
http://dx.doi.org/10.1016/j.suc.2013.01.003
0039-6109/13/$ – see front matter © 2013 Elsevier Inc. All rights reserved.

surgical.theclinics.com

---

**Box 1**
**Invasive breast carcinoma**

*Definition:*

- Malignant invasive epithelial lesion of the breast derived from the terminal duct-lobular unit.

*Incidence and location:*

- Common, estimated that 1 in 9 women will develop breast carcinoma in their lifetime.
- Arises anywhere in the breast parenchyma or accessory breast tissue, although most common in the upper outer quadrant.

*Morbidity and mortality:*

- A wide range of clinical behavior is seen with different morphologies.
- Some patients with small grade 1 carcinomas are in essence "cured" by surgical excision; others will die of metastatic disease within a few years.

*Gender, race, and age distribution:*

- A marked female preponderance, although male breast carcinoma may be seen.
- Increasing frequency with increasing patient age; rare in patients in their 20s and 30s without a family history of breast cancer.

*Clinical features:*

- Presents most commonly with an ill-defined mass, sometimes adherent to skin or underlying muscle.
- May also be identified when impalpable by mammographic breast screening programs.

*Radiologic features:*

- Most commonly identified as a mass lesion, often ill-defined on mammography if high grade, or spiculated mass if low grade (grade 1) invasive carcinoma.
- Associated calcifications may be present.
- Ultrasound shows an irregular mass with ill-defined margins and a heterogenous echo texture.

*Prognosis and treatment:*

- Varies widely.
- Depends on pathologic features of the tumor, in particular, the nodal stage, histologic grade, and tumor size.
- Based on these prognostic factors and hormone receptor status, as well as extent of surgery performed, adjuvant treatment may be given and includes hormone manipulation and/or chemotherapy and local radiotherapy.

---

into the adjacent breast tissue with no focus more than 0.1 cm in greatest dimension (**Figs. 1** and **2**). When there are multiple foci of microinvasion, the size of only the largest focus is used by the pathologist to classify the lesion, and the size of the individual foci should not be added together. Lesions that fulfill this definition are staged T1mic.[2]

## INVASIVE DUCTAL CARCINOMA OF NO SPECIFIC TYPE OR NOT OTHERWISE SPECIFIED

Invasive ductal carcinomas (**Fig. 3**) are the most common type of invasive breast cancer, accounting for up to 70% to 75% of the cases in some series. These tumors

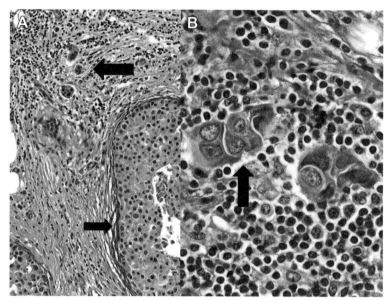

**Fig. 1.** (*A, B*) Microinvasive ductal carcinoma (*large arrow*) near a focus of DCIS (*small arrow*) (hematoxylin and eosin [H&E], ×10 and ×20).

comprise a heterogenous group with regard to pathologic features (**Box 2**) and clinical course.[3]

## INVASIVE LOBULAR CARCINOMA

Invasive lobular carcinomas (**Fig. 4**) account for approximately 5% to 15% of invasive breast carcinomas and are the second most common type.[3] The variation in incidence is related at least in part to differences in diagnostic criteria in different studies. In addition, the increase in frequency of invasive lobular carcinomas in more recent series may be related to the use of postmenopausal hormone replacement therapy.[4]

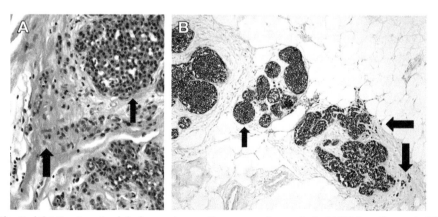

**Fig. 2.** (*A*) Microinvasive lobular carcinoma (*large arrow*) near foci of LCIS (*small arrow*), (*B*) highlighted by the cytokeratin immunostain (H&E, ×10; cytokeratin immunostain, ×20).

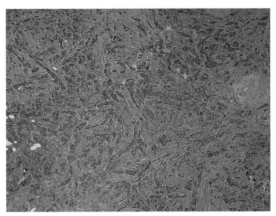

**Fig. 3.** Invasive ductal carcinoma NOS (H&E, ×4).

Invasive lobular carcinomas are characterized by multifocality in the ipsilateral breast and seem to be more often bilateral than other types of invasive breast cancer with a reported range of bilaterality of 6% to 47%. However, some studies have shown the incidence of subsequent contralateral breast cancer among patients with invasive lobular carcinoma to be similar to that of patients with invasive ductal carcinoma.[5–7]

LCIS coexists with invasive lobular carcinoma in 70% to 80% of the cases.[5,8,9] Both in situ and invasive lobular carcinoma typically show loss of expression of E-cadherin, because of either loss of heterozygosity of chromosome 16q22.1, the region of the E-cadherin gene, mutations in the gene encoding this protein, or silencing of gene expression by promoter methylation. This feature distinguishes lobular carcinomas with their loosely cohesive E-cadherin-negative tumor cells from the ductal-type carcinomas (**Fig. 5**), which characteristically exhibit a more

---

**Box 2**
**Invasive ductal carcinoma, not otherwise specified: pathologic features**

*Gross findings:*

- Firm, sometimes rock-hard, well to poorly defined, stellate masses.
- Wide range of sizes at presentation from a few millimeters to many centimeters.

*Microscopic findings:*

- Malignant cells, often forming trabeculae or growing in sheets.
- >50% of tumor shows no special type patterns.

*Immunohistochemical findings:*

- 70%–80% of not otherwise specified (NOS) tumors show estrogen receptor (ER) positivity.
- 15%–30% human epidermal growth factor receptor 2 (HER2) positive.

*Differential diagnosis:*

- Other malignant subtypes of breast carcinomas.
- Rare nonepithelial breast lesions (ie, lymphoma or metastasis).

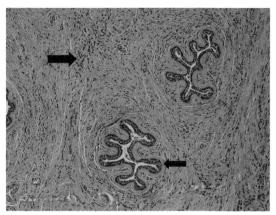

**Fig. 4.** Invasive lobular carcinoma, classical type (*large arrow*), involving benign breast parenchyma (*small arrow*) (H&E, ×10).

cohesive morphology and E-cadherin protein expression, albeit to a variable degree.[10–14]

The pathologic features of invasive lobular carcinomas are highlighted in **Box 3**.

### INVASIVE CARCINOMA WITH DUCTAL AND LOBULAR FEATURES

A small proportion of invasive breast cancers (approximately 5%) are not readily classifiable as either ductal or lobular.[3] They have distinct areas of invasive ductal carcinoma and invasive lobular carcinoma and these are best classified as invasive carcinomas with mixed ductal and lobular features. E-cadherin immunostains may or may not help classifying the lesion.

### INVASIVE TUBULAR CARCINOMA

Tubular carcinoma (**Fig. 7**) is a special type of cancer that is associated with limited metastatic potential and an excellent prognosis. Before the widespread use of

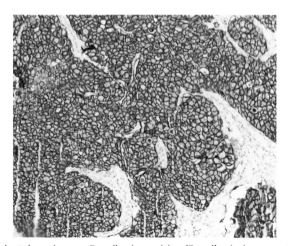

**Fig. 5.** Invasive ductal carcinoma, E-cadherin-positive (E-cadherin immunostain, ×10).

---

**Box 3**
**Invasive lobular carcinoma: pathologic features**

*Gross findings:*

- Some are firm, gritty, gray, and well to poorly defined; indistinguishable from invasive ductal carcinoma.
- In other cases, no mass is grossly evident; the breast tissue may only have a rubbery consistency or be grossly unremarkable and the presence of carcinoma is revealed only on microscopic examination.[15]
- Average size, 2.4 cm.

*Microscopic findings:*

- Subtypes include classical (neoplastic cells in single-file pattern), solid, alveolar, trabecular, mixed, signet ring cell, and pleomorphic.
- Cells show discohesive pattern of infiltration with oval nuclei, small amount of cytoplasm, and intracytoplasmic lumina.
- Usually histologic grade 2; pleomorphic grade 3 (**Fig. 6**).
- LCIS is present in 70% to 80% of the cases.

*Immunohistochemical studies:*

- Negative or reduced staining for E-cadherin.
- Usually positive for ER and progesterone receptor (PR)
- Usually negative for HER2 (except pleomorphic variant).

*Differential diagnosis:*

- Lymphoid population, either benign or lymphomatous infiltrates.
- Pleomorphic variant of invasive lobular carcinoma may be difficult to distinguish from a high-grade invasive ductal carcinoma.

---

screening mammography, tubular carcinomas accounted for less than 4% of all breast cancers.[3] However, these tumors account for a much higher proportion of cancers detected in mammographically screened populations with incidence rates ranging from 7.7% to 27%.[16,17]

The pathologic features of tubular carcinomas are depicted in **Box 4**.

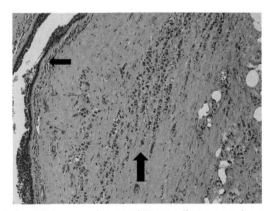

**Fig. 6.** Invasive lobular carcinoma, pleomorphic type (*large arrow*) surrounding a benign duct (*small arrow*) (H&E, ×10).

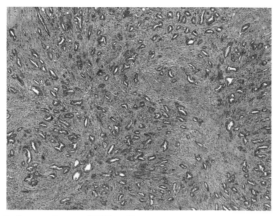

**Fig. 7.** Invasive tubular carcinoma (H&E, ×4).

## INVASIVE CRIBRIFORM CARCINOMA

Invasive cribriform carcinoma (**Fig. 8**) is a well-differentiated cancer associated with a favorable prognosis. It is uncommon, accounting for approximately 1% to 3.5% of invasive breast cancers.[3,18,19]

These carcinomas show pathologic features as listed in **Box 5**.

---

**Box 4**
**Invasive tubular carcinoma: pathologic features**

*Gross findings:*

- Firm, moderately well defined, with stellate/gray cut surface.
- Average size, 1.2–1.6 cm.

*Microscopic findings:*

- Angulated tubules with single layer of epithelial cells.
- Apical snouts often visible.
- Desmoplastic stroma often present.
- 20% multifocal.
- Most associated with low-grade DCIS.
- Often associated with LCIS, atypical ductal hyperplasia, or flat epithelial atypia/columnar cell changes with atypia.

*Immunohistochemical studies:*

- Usually ER and PR positive.
- Usually HER2 negative.
- Markers for myoepithelial cells (ie, p63, calponin) are useful in difficult cases and are negative.

*Differential diagnosis:*

- Radial scar/complex sclerosing lesion.
- Microglandular adenosis.
- Sclerosing adenosis.

---

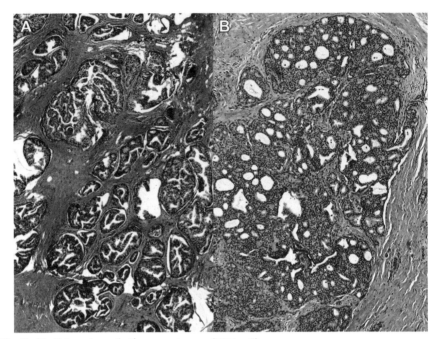

**Fig. 8.** (*A, B*) Invasive cribriform carcinoma (H&E, ×2).

---

**Box 5**
**Invasive cribriform carcinoma: pathologic features**

*Gross findings:*

- Moderately well defined with stellate/gray cut surface.
- Average size, 2.6–3.1 cm.

*Microscopic findings:*

- Islands of tumor cells forming cribriform structures.
- Tumor cells only mildly to moderately pleomorphic.
- Often desmoplastic stromal reaction, occasionally with giant cells.
- 20% of the cases admixed with other histologic patterns, such as tubular carcinoma.
- In about 80% of the cases, there is an associated component of DCIS, usually with a cribriform pattern.

*Immunohistochemical studies:*

- Usually ER and PR positive.
- Usually HER2 negative.

*Differential diagnosis:*

- Adenoid cystic carcinoma.
- Cribriform DCIS.
- Neuroendocrine carcinoma.

## INVASIVE MUCINOUS CARCINOMA

Mucinous carcinoma (also known as colloid carcinoma) **(Fig. 9)** is another special type of cancer that is associated with a relatively favorable prognosis. These tumors are uncommon and in most series account for approximately 2% of invasive breast carcinomas.[3] This tumor type is characterized by a mucinous morphology in greater than 90% of the tumor (pure mucinous carcinoma) with cases composed of 50% to 90% falling into the mixed NOS and mucinous category. Mixed mucinous carcinomas show a less distinct margin, a higher grade, and more mitotically active cytology, and their clinicopathologic features are similar to those of invasive ductal carcinoma, NOS type.

Patients with pure mucinous carcinomas tend to be postmenopausal, with a mean age of 59 to 71 years, but cases in younger patients (<40 y) are also identified who present with a palpable mass. **Box 6** highlights the pathologic features of mucinous carcinomas.

## INVASIVE MEDULLARY CARCINOMA

Medullary carcinomas **(Fig. 10)** are rare and in the author's experience account for less than 1% of all invasive breast cancers. The pathologic diagnosis of this tumor is subject to considerable interobserver variability.[20,21] As a result, its prognostic implications are uncertain. Patients with medullary carcinoma usually present at a younger age than the patients with other breast cancers, and with a palpable mass. Although some patients exhibit axillary lymphadenopathy at the time of presentation, histologic examination of the lymph nodes in such cases typically reveals benign reactive changes rather than metastatic carcinoma. There is an association between mutations in the BRCA1 breast cancer susceptibility gene and the occurrence of medullary carcinomas as well as with invasive ductal carcinomas that have some, but not all, of the features of medullary carcinoma (so-called "atypical medullary carcinoma"). The pathologic features of medullary carcinomas are described in **Box 7**.

## INVASIVE MICROPAPILLARY CARCINOMA

Invasive micropapillary carcinoma **(Fig. 11)** accounts for less than 2% of invasive breast carcinomas in the pure form. It is more common to see foci of invasive micropapillary carcinoma admixed with other histologic types, particularly invasive ductal carcinoma NOS. Up to 75% of patients with this tumor type commonly have axillary

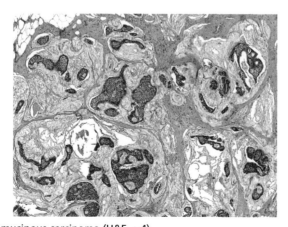

**Fig. 9.** Invasive mucinous carcinoma (H&E, ×4).

---

**Box 6**
**Invasive mucinous carcinoma: pathologic features**

*Gross findings:*

- Well-defined, circumscribed, or bosselated mass with a gelatinous, soft, glistening cut surface.
- Average size, approximately 2 cm.

*Microscopic findings:*

- Nests or trabeculae of tumor cells within large lakes of mucin.
- Tumor cells show most often mild to moderate nuclear pleomorphism.
- Tumor cells have most often a low mitotic count.
- If micropapillary differentiation is present, they become highly angioinvasive carcinomas.

*Immunohistochemical studies:*

- Usually ER and PR positive.
- Usually HER2 negative.
- Neuroendocrine features may be seen.

*Differential diagnosis:*

- Mucocele-like lesion.
- Mucinous cystadenocarcinoma (extremely rare, in elderly women, resembling mucinous cystadenocarcinoma of the ovary and pancreas).
- Metastatic mucinous carcinomas from other sites.

---

lymph node metastases at initial presentation[22–27] and a relatively poor prognosis. The frequency of lymph node involvement is similar for pure invasive micropapillary carcinomas and for those lesions in which the invasive micropapillary growth pattern constitutes only a minor component of the breast cancer. Therefore, it is important that the pathologist recognizes and reports any invasive micropapillary component in an invasive breast cancer, even if present as a minor component. The overall appearance of invasive micropapillary carcinoma may mimic serous papillary

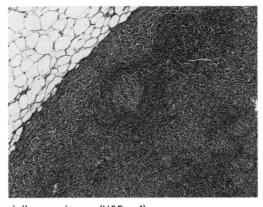

**Fig. 10.** Invasive medullary carcinoma (H&E, ×4).

---

**Box 7**
**Invasive medullary carcinoma: pathologic features**

*Gross findings:*

- Usually well-defined, circumscribed, or multinodular with gray/tan-brown cut surface.
- Areas of hemorrhage, necrosis, or cystic degeneration may be present.
- Average size, 2.5–2.9 cm.

*Microscopic findings:*

- Syncytial growth pattern in >75%.
- Absence of glandular structures.
- Moderate/marked lymphoplasmacytic infiltrate.
- Histologic circumscription.
- Marked (score 3) nuclear pleomorphism.

*Immunohistochemical studies:*

- ER negative.
- HER2 negative.
- p53 positive.

*Differential diagnosis:*

- NOS breast carcinoma.
- Chronic inflammation, lymphoma, or lymph node.

---

carcinoma of the ovary or may simulate lymphovascular invasion (LVI). True LVI has been reported in 33% to 67% of cases and may be extensive. Most tumors (approximately 70%) are associated with a DCIS component with micropapillary and cribriform patterns. Micropapillary carcinomas may occur in the pure form or may be admixed with invasive ductal carcinoma NOS or, in a minority of cases, with mucinous carcinomas.[25] The pathologic features of invasive micropapillary carcinomas are highlighted in **Box 8**.

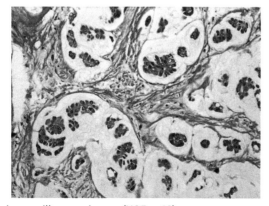

**Fig. 11.** Invasive micropapillary carcinoma (H&E, ×10).

---

**Box 8**
**Invasive micropapillary carcinoma: pathologic features**

*Gross findings:*

- Gray/white, stellate cut surface.
- Average size, 2.4 cm.

*Microscopic findings:*

- Solid/tubular nests within clear spaces.
- Usually a component of mixed tumor.
- Lymphovascular invasion common and a high rate of axillary nodal metastases is seen.

*Immunohistochemical studies:*

- ER positivity in 60%–90%.
- PR positivity in 60%–70%.
- HER2: 45% positive by fluorescence in situ hybridization (FISH) analysis.

*Differential diagnosis:*

- Retraction artifact.
- Ductal NOS carcinoma (ie, missed as a tumor type) or invasive papillary carcinoma.
- Metastatic carcinoma from other primary sites.

---

## INVASIVE METAPLASTIC CARCINOMA

Metaplastic carcinomas (**Fig. 12**) represent a morphologically heterogenous group of invasive breast cancers in which variable portions of the glandular epithelial cells comprising the tumor have undergone transformation into an alternate cell type, either a nonglandular epithelial cell type (ie, squamous cell) or a mesenchymal cell type (ie, spindle cell, chondroid, osseous, myoid, etc).[3] In some cases, particularly in spindle cell and squamous cell carcinomas, the metaplastic elements may occur in pure form without an identifiable component of adenocarcinoma. There is no uniformly agreed on classification scheme or terminology for these tumors.

Metaplastic carcinomas are uncommon, representing less than 1% of all of breast cancers. The prognostic implications of metaplastic carcinomas are difficult to define

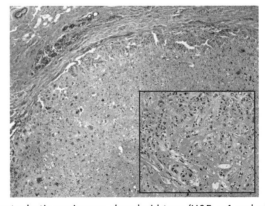

**Fig. 12.** Invasive metaplastic carcinoma, chondroid type (H&E, ×4 and ×20).

> **Box 9**
> **Invasive metaplastic carcinoma: pathologic features**
>
> *Gross findings:*
>
> - Palpable lesion not infrequently associated with rapid growth of short duration.
> - Gray/white, ill-defined cut surface.
> - May have cystic areas of foci of necrosis macroscopically.
> - Wide range of sizes reported, often larger than the other special types.
>
> *Microscopic findings:*
>
> - Squamous or spindle cell (or mixed) infiltrating islands of cells.
> - Spindled component may range from low to high grade and may represent most of the tumor (spindle cell carcinoma).
> - May have heterologous elements (ie, osteocartilagenous differentiation [most common]).
>
> *Immunohistochemical studies:*
>
> - Express cytokeratins, at least focally.
> - Often ER and PR negative.
> - 11%–46% of tumors may demonstrate HER2 overexpression.[3]
>
> *Differential diagnosis:*
>
> - Metastatic carcinoma (squamous) or metastatic or primary sarcoma.
> - Fibromatosis (low-grade variants).
> - Phyllodes tumor.

and are probably related to the type of metaplasia present. Patients with metaplastic carcinoma are similar to patients with invasive ductal carcinoma NOS with regard to their age at presentation, the manner in which their tumors are detected, and the location within the breast in which the tumors arise.[28,29] The pathologic features of the metaplastic carcinoma are described in **Box 9**.

Low-grade adenosquamous carcinoma (**Fig. 13**), an unusual subtype of metaplastic carcinoma, seems to represent a distinct clinicopathologic entity.[30–32] These tumors are typically smaller than other metaplastic carcinomas, with a median size between

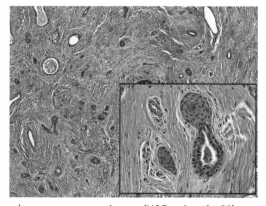

**Fig. 13.** Low-grade adenosquamous carcinoma (H&E, ×4 and ×20).

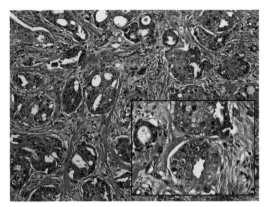

**Fig. 14.** Invasive apocrine carcinoma (H&E, ×4 and ×20).

2 and 2.8 cm (range, 0.5 cm–8.6 cm). They exhibit a firm, yellow cut surface with irregular borders and histologically they are characterized by a stellate morphology composed of infiltrating compressed glands with lumina containing keratin, associated with squamous differentiation (which ranges from 5% to 80%). The differential diagnosis includes syringomatous adenoma of the nipple, reactive squamous metaplasia, and tubular carcinoma. These lesions are locally aggressive, but have a relatively good prognosis when compared with other metaplastic carcinomas.

## INVASIVE APOCRINE CARCINOMA

Although many invasive breast cancers show evidence of apocrine differentiation, less than 1% of invasive breast carcinomas demonstrate pure apocrine features.[3,33–35] Apocrine carcinomas (**Fig. 14**) show the pathologic features listed in **Box 10**.

---

**Box 10**
**Invasive apocrine carcinoma: pathologic features**

*Gross findings:*

- As for tumors of no special type.

*Microscopic findings:*

- Must be 90% apocrine morphology.
- Cells have abundant eosinophilic granular cytoplasm.
- Large nuclei with prominent nucleoli.
- May be admixed with other special types.

*Immunohistochemical studies:*

- Gross cystic disease fluid protein-15 positive.
- ER and PR negative.
- Androgen receptor positive.
- 40%–50% cases show HER2 amplification with FISH.

*Differential diagnosis:*

- Atypical apocrine proliferation in a sclerosing lesion.

---

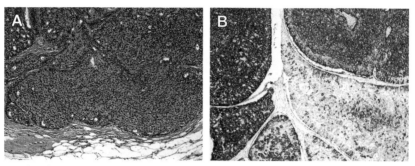

**Fig. 15.** (*A, B*) Invasive neuroendocrine carcinoma. (*A*) H&E, ×4 and (*B*) synaptophysin immu-nostain, ×4.

## INVASIVE NEUROENDOCRINE CARCINOMA

Some invasive breast cancers show evidence of endocrine differentiation (**Fig. 15**) at the morphologic level, histochemical level, immunohistochemical level, or some combination of these.[36–38] With the exception of the rare functioning endocrine tumors, which results in clinical manifestations due to hormone production and secre-tion, these tumors present in a manner similar to other breast cancers without distinc-tive clinical or mammographic findings. The pathologic features of invasive carcinomas with endocrine differentiation (argyrophilic carcinoma) are described in **Box 11**.

## INVASIVE PAPILLARY CARCINOMA

Invasive papillary carcinomas (**Fig. 16**) are rare lesions (up to 2% of all invasive breast cancers) associated with a favorable prognosis and seem to occur more frequently in postmenopausal women. Their pathologic features are highlighted in **Box 12**.

---

**Box 11**
**Invasive neuroendocrine carcinoma: pathologic features**

*Gross findings:*

- Ill-defined mass lesion
- Variable is size, from 1.3 to 5 cm

*Microscopic findings:*

- Infiltrating tumor cells forming nests, trabeculae, or acinar groups.
- Cells may be small and uniform with eosinophilic granular cytoplasm or larger with vesicular nuclei or have a spindle cell morphology.

*Immunohistochemical studies:*

- Chromogranin, synaptophysin, CD56, and NSE positive.
- Cytokeratin 7 positive.
- ER often positive.
- HER2 negative.

*Differential diagnosis:*

- Metastatic neuroendocrine carcinoma (ie, from lung).

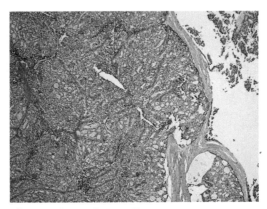

**Fig. 16.** Invasive papillary carcinoma (H&E, ×2).

## ENCAPSULATED (INTRACYSTIC) PAPILLARY CARCINOMA

Traditionally considered to be a variant of DCIS and termed intracystic or encysted papillary carcinoma, the lesion that is now called "encapsulated" papillary carcinoma (**Fig. 17**) is characterized by the presence of papillary carcinoma within an apparent cystically dilated duct. Most frequently encountered in elderly women, these tumors usually present as subareolar mass and/or with nipple discharge. Encapsulated papillary carcinoma may occur alone, but more often the surrounding breast tissue contains foci of low or intermediate nuclear grade DCIS, usually with a cribriform or micropapillary pattern.[39,40] The pathologic features of the encapsulated (intracystic) papillary carcinoma are shown in **Box 13**. Regardless of whether these lesions are in situ or invasive in nature, however, outcome studies have demonstrated

---

**Box 12**
**Invasive papillary carcinoma: pathologic features**

*Gross findings:*

- Well circumscribed.

*Microscopic findings:*

- Invasive cell nests consist of papillae with fibrovascular cores that are covered by malignant epithelial cells.

- Often in association with invasive ductal carcinoma NOS or mucinous carcinoma.

*Immunohistochemical studies:*

- ER and PR positive.

- HER2 negative.

*Differential diagnosis:*

- It may be extremely difficult for the pathologist to distinguish circumscribed nodules of invasive papillary carcinoma from in situ papillary carcinoma.

- At least a subset of lesions reported as "intracystic" and "solid" papillary carcinoma may actually be low-grade invasive carcinomas rather than in situ lesions.

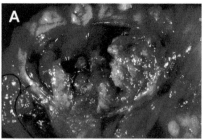
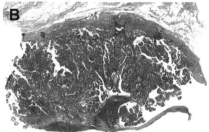

**Fig. 17.** (*A, B*) Encapsulated (intracystic) papillary carcinoma (*A*) gross picture and (*B*) H&E, ×2.

that they are associated with an excellent prognosis with adequate local therapy alone.[41,42]

## INVASIVE SECRETORY CARCINOMA

Invasive secretory carcinoma is a rare tumor that accounts for less than 0.01% of all breast carcinomas, originally described in children, but adult cases are now well recognized. The reported age range is wide, 5 to 87 years. This type of carcinoma has been reported in both female and male patients. Their pathologic features are highlighted in (**Box 14** and **Fig. 18**). Secretory carcinomas in children and young adults (<30 years) are associated with a favorable prognosis. When they occur in older patients, the prognosis may not be as good. Late recurrences (ie, >20 years after diagnosis) have been reported.[44–46]

---

**Box 13**
**Encapsulated (intracystic) papillary carcinoma**

*Gross findings:*

• Friable or bosselated mass with a cystic space.

*Microscopic findings:*

• Characterized by one or occasionally several nodules of papillary carcinoma surrounded by a thick fibrous capsule.

• Myoepithelial cells are not present in the papillae of the tumor.

• In contrast with papillary DCIS (in which myoepithelial cells are present at the periphery of the dilated duct), recent studies failed to demonstrate a peripheral layer of myoepithelial cells, raising the possibility that these lesions may be a form of low-grade invasive carcinoma with an expansile growth pattern or part of a spectrum of progression from in situ to invasive disease.[40,43]

• Areas of unequivocal invasive carcinoma (most often invasive ductal carcinoma NOS) can range from microinvasive (≤0.1 cm) to larger foci.

*Immunohistochemical studies:*

• ER and PR positive.

• HER2 negative.

*Differential diagnosis:*

• Papillary DCIS.

---

> **Box 14**
> **Invasive secretory carcinoma: pathologic features**
>
> *Gross findings:*
>
> - Well-circumscribed, mobile, gray/white/brown masses with a predilection for a subareolar location in prepubertal girls and in men.
> - Resemble fibroadenomas grossly.
> - Mean size, 1.6–2.6 cm.
>
> *Microscopic findings:*
>
> - Often show a central hyalinized area with a cellular periphery.
> - The tumor architecture is solid, papillary, microcystic, cystic, tubular, or a combination thereof.
> - Prominent intracellular and extracellular amphophilic weakly eosinophilic secretion is seen.
> - Associated DCIS may be present.
>
> *Immunohistochemical studies:*
>
> - Most tumors are ER negative.
> - HER2 overexpression has been detected in rare cases.
> - Strong immunoreactivity for S100 protein, alpha-lactalbumin, and polyclonal carcinoembryonic antigen is noted.
>
> *Differential diagnosis:*
>
> - Atypical secretory hyperplasia.

## INVASIVE ADENOID CYSTIC CARCINOMA

Adenoid cystic carcinoma (**Fig. 19**) is a morphologically distinct form of invasive breast carcinoma, analogous to the same morphologic type of carcinoma arising in the salivary glands; it is associated with an excellent prognosis and only rare instances of axillary lymph node metastases have been reported.[47] This rare tumor accounts for only 0.1% of all breast cancers.[3] Median age of presentation is 66 years and 96% of patients are postmenopausal. Often the tumor has a periareolar location. Adenoid cystic carcinoma has peculiar pathologic features (**Box 15**).

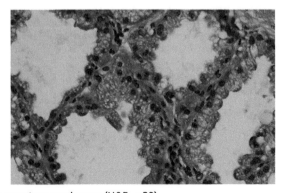

**Fig. 18.** Invasive secretory carcinoma (H&E, ×20).

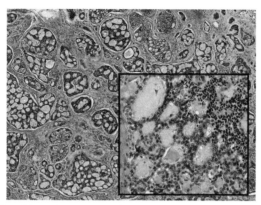

**Fig. 19.** Invasive adenoid cystic carcinoma (H&E, ×4 and ×20).

---

**Box 15**
**Invasive adenoid cystic carcinoma: pathologic features**

*Gross findings:*

- Well-defined nodular mass lesion; however, the microscopic extent of the lesion may be appreciably greater than the grossly evident lesion in 50% to 65% of cases.

- Average, 1.9–2.5 cm.

*Microscopic findings:*

- Infiltrating tumor cells forming solid, trabeculae, or cribriform groups.

- Biphasic with most cells basaloid, small in size, and hyperchromatic lining pseudocysts containing basement membrane material.

- Epithelial cell component lines true acinar structures and are moderate in size with more abundant eosinophilic cytoplasm.

- Epithelial component can assume variable architectural patterns (solid, cribriform, tubular, trabecular, mixed) with the solid variant being the most aggressive clinically.

- Associated DCIS is seen in a minority of cases.

- Perineural invasion is also seen and may be prominent.

- LVI is only rarely identified.

- It may develop in a background of microglandular adenosis.[48]

*Immunohistochemical studies:*

- Basaloid cells express cytokeratin 14, laminin, and collagen IV.

- Glandular cells are positive for cytokeratin 7.

- ER and PR negative.

- HER2 negative.

- Expression of CD117 (c-kit) is a characteristic feature.[49,50]

*Differential diagnosis:*

- Invasive cribriform carcinoma.

- Benign conditions such as collagenous spherulosis.

- High-grade invasive ductal carcinoma, small cell carcinoma, solid papillary carcinoma, and even lymphoma, in the case of a solid variant of adenoid cystic carcinoma.

## INFLAMMATORY CARCINOMA

Inflammatory carcinoma (**Fig. 20**) is a form of locally advanced breast cancer characterized by erythema, edema, induration, and warmth and tenderness of the mammary skin, resulting in a "peau d'orange" appearance.[51] The pathologic correlate of this clinical presentation is the presence of tumor emboli in dermal lymphovascular spaces. The clinical findings are presumed to be due to the lymphatic obstruction by the tumor emboli; the term inflammatory refers to the clinical appearance of the skin.

Skin biopsies from patients with the clinical diagnosis of inflammatory carcinoma do not always demonstrate dermal lymphovascular tumor emboli, possibly because of the limitations of tissue sampling. The pathologist will obtain additional levels through the tissue block in such cases.[3] Conversely, dermal LVI may be seen in the absence of these clinical findings; therefore, this histologic finding in and of itself is insufficient for a diagnosis of inflammatory carcinoma.[52] The invasive component in the breast is most often a high-grade invasive ductal carcinoma NOS, but it may be of any other special types.

## MALE BREAST CANCER

Carcinoma of the male breast is rare (0.6% of all breast cancers) and may be either in situ or invasive. Both lesions tend to occur in a somewhat older age group than in women, with the peak in the sixth decade for the DCIS and the seventh decade for invasive carcinoma. Clinical gynecomastia has not been shown to be a risk factor for carcinoma. However, an increased incidence of breast cancer in men with Klinefelter syndrome has long been recognized.[53] The pathologic features of male breast cancer are highlighted in **Box 16**.

## PROGNOSTIC AND PREDICTIVE FACTORS OF BREAST CANCER

Presently, traditional pathologic factors, such as histologic type, histologic grade, LVI, tumor size, and axillary lymph node status, together with hormone receptor status and HER2 status, represent the principal means for assessing prognosis and determining the likelihood of therapeutic response in patients with breast cancers.

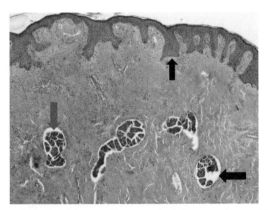

**Fig. 20.** Inflammatory breast carcinoma: Tumor emboli (*large red arrow*) in dermal lymphovascular spaces (*large black arrow;* epidermis: *small arrow*) (H&E, ×4).

---

**Box 16**
**Male breast cancer: pathologic features**

*Gross findings:*

- DCIS tends to be retroareolar in location, nodular, and/or cystic, and often with nipple discharge.
- Invasive carcinomas tend to present with larger, hard irregular stellate tumors and at a higher stage than women with breast cancer, but prognosis is similar to women when matched for stage.

*Microscopic findings:*

- Invasive ductal carcinoma is the most common type, morphologically similar to those seen in women.
- Papillary low-grade and intermediate-grade DCIS is the most frequent histologic pattern.[54]
- High-grade DCIS with comedo necrosis are most seen in association with invasive carcinomas.
- Paget's disease may also be seen.
- Both in situ and invasive lobular carcinoma are extremely uncommon.

*Immunohistochemical studies:*

- ER, PR, and androgen receptor positive.
- HER2 positivity less common than in female breast cancer.

*Differential diagnosis:*

- Metastatic prostate carcinoma: prostate-specific antigen and prostatic acid phosphatase will be helpful in distinguishing it from primary breast carcinoma.
- Myofibroblastoma.
- Fat necrosis, epidermal inclusion cyst.
- Gynecomastia.

---

## HISTOLOGIC TYPE

Some histologic types of breast cancers are associated with a particularly favorable outcome.[55,56] Special types of tumors that have consistently been shown to have an excellent prognosis include tubular, invasive cribriform, mucinous, and adenoid cystic carcinoma. The prognostic significance of medullary carcinoma is controversial. Strict diagnostic criteria for these special types of cancer must be used by the pathologist to observe the favorable outcome reported for these lesions.

## HISTOLOGIC GRADE

The importance of tumor grading as a prognostic factor in patients with breast cancer has been clearly demonstrated in numerous clinical outcome studies.[57,58] In fact, tumor grading has been shown to be of prognostic value even in patients with breast cancers 1 cm and smaller.[59] The grading method in most widespread clinical use presently is the Nottingham combined histologic grading system.[57] In this system, the degree of tubule formation, nuclear grade, and mitotic rate are each assigned a value of 1 to 3; these values are then added together to produce assigned scores from 3 to 9 (**Table 1**). Tumors with total scores of 3 to 5 are categorized as grade 1; those with scores of 6 and 7 are grade 2, and those with scores of 8 and 9 are grade 3.

| Table 1<br>Nottingham system for determining combined histologic grade of invasive breast cancer | | | |
|---|---|---|---|
| Tubules | >75% | 10%–75% | <10% |
| Nuclear grade | Low | Intermediate | High |
| Mitoses | 0–5 | >5–10 | >10 |
| Point value | 1 | 2 | 3 |

### LYMPHOVASCULAR INVASION

The presence of tumor emboli in lymphovascular spaces (**Fig. 21**) has been shown in numerous studies to be an important and independent prognostic factor. The identification of LVI is of particular importance in patients with T1, node-negative breast cancers, because this finding may permit the identification of a subset of patients at increased risk for axillary lymph node involvement and distant metastasis in this otherwise favorable group.[60,61] It has been shown that most small vascular spaces that contain tumor emboli are lymphatic spaces and only a minority are blood vessels.[62]

### TUMOR SIZE

After lymph node status, tumor size represents the next most important prognostic factor for patients with breast cancer. Increasing tumor size is independently associated with a worsening survival. It is important that pathologists measure tumor size as accurately as possible for its prognostic value. If there is a discrepancy between the gross tumor size and the microscopic size, particularly of small breast tumors, it is the microscopic size of the invasive component of the tumor that takes precedence and that should be reported by the pathologist and used for staging.[2]

### AXILLARY LYMPH NODE STATUS

There is uniform agreement that the status of the axillary lymph nodes is the single most important prognostic factor for patients with breast cancer, because the disease-free and overall survival decreases as the number of positive lymph nodes

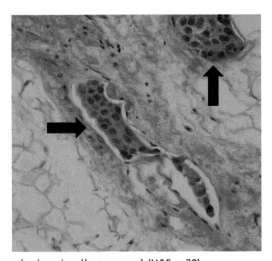

**Fig. 21.** Lymphovascular invasion (*large arrow*) (H&E, ×20).

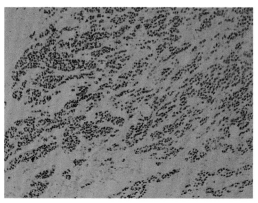

**Fig. 22.** ER-positive invasive ductal carcinoma showing a strong nuclear staining (ER immunostain, ×10).

increases.[63] Axillary lymph node metastases are categorized as macrometastases (>2 mm), micrometastases (≤2 mm but >0.2 mm), and isolated tumor cells (single cells or small clusters of cells not >0.2 mm in size).

## ESTROGEN RECEPTOR AND PROGESTERONE RECEPTOR STATUS

ER and PR represent weak prognostic factors for patients with breast cancer, but these receptors are the strongest predictive factors for response to endocrine therapy. ER and PR assays should be performed on all invasive breast cancers.[63] Both ER and PR are assessed by immunohistochemistry (IHC) on paraffin sections. The cutoff to define positivity is 1% because patients with even 1% ER/PR-positive tumors may benefit from hormonal therapy. About 70% of all breast cancers are ER-positive (**Fig. 22**) and 60% to 65% of all breast cancers are PR-positive (**Fig. 23**).

## HER2 PROTEIN EXPRESSION AND GENE AMPLIFICATION

The analysis of breast cancer specimens for HER2 protein overexpression and/or gene amplification is now standard practice.[64,65] HER2 is a prognostic factor for

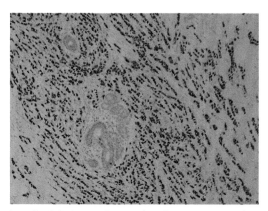

**Fig. 23.** PR-positive invasive lobular carcinoma showing a strong nuclear staining (PR immunostain, ×10).

outcome in both node-negative and node-positive patients and is a predictive factor for response to certain chemotherapeutic and antiendocrine agents. However, the major clinical reason to assess HER2 status is to help select patients for treatment with trastuzumab (Herceptin), a monoclonal antibody targeted to the HER2 protein. HER2/neu is a proto-oncogene that encodes for a transmembrane tyrosine kinase growth receptor, and it is involved in several regulatory pathways in breast, involving proliferation, survival, cell motility, and invasion. HER2 has been mostly measured by IHC, but also by FISH. A positive IHC result is a strong, circumferential (3+) staining in greater than 30% of invasive tumor cells (**Fig. 24**). A positive FISH result using the dual probe system (Pathvysion, Vysion; Abbott Laboratories, Abbott Park, IL) is a HER2/chromosome 17 ratio of greater than 2.2. A 2+ IHC or a HER/chromosome 17 ratio of 1.8 to 2.2 by FISH should be considered equivocal.

Overexpression/amplification is reported in 10% to 34% of invasive breast cancers.

Protein overexpression and gene amplification are concordant in more than 90% of cases.

## OTHER PATHOLOGIC FACTORS

Several other histologic factors have been reported to have prognostic value in patients with invasive breast cancer.

The rate of proliferation, assessed by a variety of methods over the years including mitotic rate, flow cytometric S-phase fraction, and immunostaining for the Ki67 antigen, has been repeatedly demonstrated to be an important prognostic factor.[63]

Blood vessel invasion (ie, invasion of veins and arteries) has been reported to have an adverse effect on clinical outcome. However, there is a broad range in the reported incidence of blood vessel invasion, ranging from less than 5% to almost 50%.[3]

The presence of tumor necrosis has been associated with an adverse effect on clinical outcome.[3] However, it is not clear that this is independent of tumor size and histologic grade.

Perineural invasion is only infrequently observed in invasive breast cancers. This phenomenon is more often seen in association with invasive lobular carcinoma, adenoid cystic carcinoma, and LVI, and it has been shown to be an independent prognostic factor.[3]

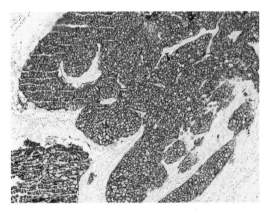

**Fig. 24.** HER2-positive (3+) invasive ductal carcinoma showing a strong and complete membranous staining (HER2 immunostain, ×10).

The extent of DCIS associated with invasive cancers has also been studied as a potential prognostic factor. The presence of an extensive intraductal component ($\geq$25% tumor mass) is a prognostic factor for local recurrence in patients treated with breast-conserving surgery and radiation therapy. In this scenario, it may be more appropriate to obtain a margin of at least 0.2 cm if large amounts of DCIS are

---

**Box 17**
**Major molecular categories of breast cancer determined by gene expression profiling**

*Luminal:*

Gene expression pattern:

• High expression of hormone receptors and associated genes (luminal A > luminal B).

Clinical features:

• Approximately 70% of invasive breast cancers.

• ER-positive and PR-positive.

• Luminal Bs tend to be higher histologic grade than luminal A.

• Some overexpress HER2 (luminal B).

Outcome:

• Favorable prognosis.

*HER2:*

Gene expression pattern:

• High expression of HER2 and other genes in amplicon.

• Low expression of ER and associated genes.

Clinical features:

• Approximately 15% of invasive breast cancers.

• More likely to be high grade and node-negative.

• ER and PR negative.

• HER2 overexpression and gene amplification.

Outcome:

• Poor prognosis.

*Basal:*

Gene expression pattern:

• High expression of basal epithelial genes and basal cytokeratins (EGFR, CK5/6).

• Low expression of ER and associated genes.

• Low expression of HER2.

Clinical features:

• Approximately 15% of invasive breast cancers.

• ER, PR, and HER2 negative.

• BRCA1-associated cancers.

• Particularly common in African American women.

Outcome:

• Poor prognosis.

in proximity to the margin, because it has been shown that 70% of low-grade DCIS, 55% of intermediate-grade DCIS, and 10% of high-grade DCIS may grow discontinuously within the ducts.[66]

## MOLECULAR PROGNOSTIC TESTS

OncotypeDX (Genomic Health, Inc, Redwood City, CA) is a reverse transcription–polymerase chain reaction–based assay that can be performed on paraffin sections. It is based on analysis of the expression of 21 genes and provides a "recurrence score" that correlates with outcome. Although is was initially used to assess prognosis in ER-positive, node-negative patients,[67,68] data have indicated that it is an equally valuable prognostic indicator in ER-positive, node-positive patients.

MammaPrint (Agendia, Netherlands, Amsterdam) is a molecular prognostic test that uses expression array analysis of 70 genes to identify patients with good and poor prognostic signatures.[69,70] This assay requires fresh frozen tumor tissue and is more commonly used in Europe.

## MOLECULAR CLASSIFICATION OF BREAST CANCER

Studies of breast cancers using gene expression profiling have identified several major breast cancer subtypes.[71–73] The best characterized of these have been designated luminal A, luminal B, HER2, and basal-like.[74] These subtypes differ with regard to their patterns of gene expression, clinical features, response to treatment, and outcome. The key features of these breast cancer subtypes are summarized in **Box 17**.

Presently, ER, PR, and HER2 biomarkers can be used as a surrogate for the molecular category of breast cancer as defined by gene expression profiling (**Box 18**),[73] and the basal-like group can be defined more precisely using, in addition, antibodies to

---

**Box 18**
**Immunophenotyping as a surrogate for molecular category using ER, PR, and HER2 status**

*Lumina A:*
- ER positive.
- PR positive.
- HER2 negative.

*Luminal B:*
- ER positive.
- PR positive.
- HER2 positive.

*HER2:*
- ER negative.
- PR negative.
- HER2 positive.

*Basal-like:*
- ER negative.
- PR negative.
- HER2 negative.

CK5/6 and EGFR. Basal-like tumors defined by expression profiling are ER-negative, PR-negative, and HER2-negative and positive for CK5/6 and/or EGFR.[74]

## REFERENCES

1. Wellings SR, Jensen HM, Marcum RG. An atlas of subgross pathology of the human breast with special reference to possible precancerous lesions. J Natl Cancer Inst 1975;55:231–73.
2. AJCC. Cancer staging manual. 7th edition. American joint committe on cancer. Chicago: Springer; 2010.
3. Colditz G, Chia KS. Invasive breast carcinoma: introduction and general features. WHO classification of tumors of the breast. In: Lakhani SR, Ellis IO, Schnitt SJ, et al, editors. 4th edition. 2012. p. 14–31.
4. Chen CL. Hormone replacement therapy in relation to breast cancer. JAMA 2002; 287:734–41.
5. DiCostanzo D. Prognosis in infiltrating lobular carcinoma. An analysis of "classical" and variant tumors. Am J Surg Pathol 1990;14:12–23.
6. Sastre-Garau X. Infiltrating lobular carcinoma of the breast. Clinicopathologic analysis of 975 cases with reference to data on conservatory therapy and metastatic patterns. Cancer 1996;77:113–20.
7. Peiro G. The influence of infiltrating lobular carcinoma on the outcome of patients treated with breast-conserving surgery and radiation therapy. Breast Cancer Res Treat 2000;59:49–54.
8. Wheeler JE. Lobular carcinoma of the breast in situ and infiltrating. Pathol Annu 1976;11:161–88.
9. Azzopardi JG. Problems in breast pathology. Philadelphia: WB Saunders; 1979.
10. Rasbridge SA. Epithelial (E-) and placental (P-) cadherin cell adhesion molecule expression in breast carcinoma. J Pathol 1993;169:245–50.
11. Moll R. Differential loss of E-cadherin expression in infiltrating ductal and lobular carcinomas. Am J Pathol 1993;143:1731–42.
12. Palacios J. Anomalous expression of P-cadherin in breast carcinoma. Correlation with E-cadherin expression and pathologic features. Am J Pathol 1995;146: 605–12.
13. Berx G. E-cadherin is inactivated in a majority of invasive human lobular breast cancers by truncation mutations throughout its extracellular domain. Oncogene 1996;13:1919–25.
14. Nishizaki T. Genetic alterations in lobular breast cancer by comparative genomic hybridization. Int J Cancer 1997;74:513–7.
15. Silverstein MJ. Infiltrating lobular carcinoma. Is it different from infiltrating ductal carcinoma? Cancer 1994;73:1673–7.
16. Rajakariar R. Pathological and biological features of mammographically detected invasive breast carcinomas. Br J Cancer 1995;71:150–4.
17. Cowan WK. The pathological and biological nature of screen-detected breast carcinomas: a morphological and immunohistochemical study. J Pathol 1997; 182:29–35.
18. Page DL. Invasive cribriform carcinoma of the breast. Histopathology 1983;7: 525–36.
19. Venable JG. Infiltrating cribriform carcinoma of the breast: a distinctive clinico-pathologic entity. Hum Pathol 1990;21:333–8.
20. Rubens JR. Medullary carcinoma of the breast. Overdiagnosis of a prognostically favorable neoplasm. Arch Surg 1990;125:601–4.

21. Gaffey MJ. Medullary carcinoma of the breast: interobserver variability in histo-pathologic diagnosis. Mod Pathol 1995;8:31–8.
22. Siriaunkgul S. Invasive micropapillary carcinoma of the breast. Mod Pathol 1993; 6:660–2.
23. Luna-More S. Invasive micropapillary carcinoma of the breast. A new special type of invasive mammary carcinoma. Pathol Res Pract 1994;190:668–74.
24. Paterakos M. Invasive micropapillary carcinoma of the breast: a prognostic study. Hum Pathol 1999;30:1459–63.
25. Walsh MM. Invasive micropapillary carcinoma of the breast: eighty cases of an underrecognized entity. Hum Pathol 2001;32:583–9.
26. Nassar H. Clinicopathologic analysis of invasive micropapillary differentiation in breast carcinoma. Mod Pathol 2001;14:836–41.
27. Zekioglu O. Invasive micropapillary carcinoma of the breast: high incidence of lymph node metastasis with extranodal extension and its immunohistochemical profile compared with invasive ductal carcinoma. Histopathology 2004;44(1):18–23.
28. Kaufman MW. Carcinoma of the breast with pseudosarcomatous metaplasia. Cancer 1984;53:1908–17.
29. Oberman HA. Metaplastic carcinoma of the breast. A clinicopathologic study of 29 patients. Am J Surg Pathol 1987;11:918–29.
30. Rosen PP. Low-grade adenosquamous carcinoma. A variant of metaplastic mammary carcinoma. Am J Surg Pathol 1987;11:351–8.
31. Van Hoeven KH. Low-grade adenosquamous carcinoma of the breast. A clinico-pathologic study of 32 cases with ultrastructural analysis. Am J Surg Pathol 1993; 17:248–58.
32. Drudis T. The pathology of low grade adenosquamous carcinoma of the breast. An immunohistochemical study. Pathol Annu 1994;29(Pt 2):181–97.
33. Mossler JA. Apocrine differentiation in human mammary carcinoma. Cancer 1980;46:2463–71.
34. Eusebi V. Apocrine carcinoma of the breast. A morphologic and immunocyto-chemical study. Am J Pathol 1986;123:532–41.
35. O'Malley FP. The spectrum of apocrine lesions of the breast. Adv Anat Pathol 2004;11:1–9.
36. Bussolati G. Chromogranin-reactive endocrine cells in argyrophilic carcinomas ("carcinoids") and normal tissue of the breast. Am J Pathol 1985;120:186–92.
37. Miremadi A. Neuroendocrine differentiation and prognosis in breast adenocarci-noma. Histopathology 2002;40:215–22.
38. Sapino A. Is detection of endocrine cells in breast adenocarcinoma of diagnostic and clinical significance? Histopathology 2002;40:211–4.
39. Carter D. Intracystic papillary carcinoma of the breast. After mastectomy, radio-therapy or excisional biopsy alone. Cancer 1983;52(1):14–9.
40. Collins LC. Intracystic papillary carcinomas of the breast: a reevaluation using a panel of myoepithelial cell markers. Am J Surg Pathol 2006;30(8):1002–7.
41. Leal C. Intracystic (encysted) papillary carcinoma of the breast: a clinical, path-ological, and immunohistochemical study. Hum Pathol 1998;29(10):1097–104.
42. Harris KP. Treatment and outcome of intracystic papillary carcinoma of the breast. Br J Surg 1999;86(10):1274.
43. Hill CB. Myoepithelial cell staining patterns of papillary breast lesions: from intra-ductal papillomas to invasive papillary carcinomas. Am J Clin Pathol 2005;123(1): 36–44.
44. Krausz T. Secretory carcinoma of the breast in the adults: emphasis on late recur-rence and metastasis. Histopathology 1989;14(1):25–36.

45. Rosen PP. Secretory carcinoma of the breast. Arch Pathol Lab Med 1991;115(2): 141–4.
46. Tavassoli FA. Secretory carcinoma of the breast. Cancer 1980;45(9):2404–13.
47. Page DL. Adenoid cystic carcinoma of breast, a special histopathologic type with excellent prognosis. Breast Cancer Res Treat 2005;93:189–90.
48. Acs G. Microglandular adenosis with transition into adenoid cystic carcinoma of the breast. Am J Surg Pathol 2003;27:1052–60.
49. Mastropasqua MG. Immunoreactivity for c-kit and p63 as an adjunct in the diagnosis of adenoid cystic carcinoma of the breast. Mod Pathol 2005;18:1277–82.
50. Azoulay S. KIT is highly expressed in adenoid cystic carcinoma of the breast, a basal-like carcinoma associated with a favorable outcome. Mod Pathol 2005; 18:1623–31.
51. Lerebours F. Update on inflammatory breast cancer. J Clin Oncol 2005;7:52–8.
52. Guth U. Noninflammatory breast carcinoma with skin involvement. Cancer 2004; 100:470–8.
53. Jackson AW. Carcinoma of male breast in association with the Klinefelter syndrome. Br Med J 1965;1(5429):223–5.
54. Hittmair AP. Ductal carcinoma in situ (DCIS) in the male breast: a morphologic study of 84 cases of pure DCIS and 30 cases of DCIS associated with invasive carcinoma – a preliminary report. Cancer 1998;83(10):2139–49.
55. Ellis IO. Pathological prognostic factors in breast cancer. II. Histological type. Relationship with survival in a large study with long-term follow-up. Histopathology 1992;20:479–89.
56. Rosen PP. Factors influencing prognosis in node-negative breast carcinoma: analysis of 767 T1N0M0/T2N0M0 patients with long-term follow-up. J Clin Oncol 1993;11:2090–100.
57. Elston CW. Pathological prognostic factors in breast cancer. I. The value of histological grade in breast cancer: experience from a large study with long-term follow-up. Histopathology 1991;19:403–10.
58. Page DL. Histologic grading of breast cancer. Let's do it. Am J Clin Pathol 1995; 103:123–4.
59. Chen YY. Prognostic factors for patients with breast cancers 1 cm and smaller. Breast Cancer Res Treat 1998;51:209–25.
60. Leitner SP. Predictors of recurrence for patients with small (one centimeter or less) localized breast cancer (T1a, b N0M0). Cancer 1995;76:2266–74.
61. Lee AK. Lymph node negative invasive breast carcinoma 1 centimeter or less in size (T1a, b N0M0): clinicopathologic features and outcome. Cancer 1997;79: 761–71.
62. Mohammed RA. Improved methods of detection of lymphovascular invasion demonstrate that it is the predominant method of vascular invasion in breast cancer and has important clinical consequences. Am J Surg Pathol 2007;31: 1825–33.
63. Fitzgibbons PL. Prognostic factors in breast cancer. College of American Pathologists Consensus Statement 1999. Arch Pathol Lab Med 2000;124:966–78.
64. Wolf AC. American Society of Clinical Oncology/College of American Pathologists guideline recommendations for human epidermal growth factor receptor 2 testing in breast cancer. J Clin Oncol 2007;25:118–45.
65. Hicks DG. HER2+ breast cancer: review of biologic relevance and optimal use of diagnostic stools. Am J Clin Pathol 2008;129:263–73.
66. Faverly DR. Three dimensional imaging of mammary ductal carcinoma in situ: clinical implications. Semin Diagn Pathol 1994;11(3):193–8.

67. Paik S. A multigene assay to predict recurrence of tamoxifen-treated, node-negative breast cancer. N Engl J Med 2004;351:2817–26.
68. Habel LA. A population-based study of tumor gene expression and risk of breast cancer death among lymph node-negative patients. Breast Cancer Res 2006;8: R25.
69. van de Vijver MJ. A gene-expression signature as a predictor of survival in breast cancer. N Engl J Med 2002;346:1999–2009.
70. Nuyse M. Validation and clinical utility of a 70-gene prognostic signature of women with node-negative breast cancer. J Natl Cancer Inst 2006;98:1183–92.
71. Sorlie T. Gene expression patterns of breast carcinomas distinguish tumor subclasses with clinical implications. Proc Natl Acad Sci U S A 2001;98:10869–74.
72. Sorlie T. Repeated observation of breast tumor subtypes in independent gene expression data sets. Proc Natl Acad Sci U S A 2003;100:8418–23.
73. Brenton JD. Molecular classification and molecular forecasting of breast cancer: ready for clinical application? J Clin Oncol 2005;23:7350–60.
74. Nielsen TO. Immunohistochemical and clinical characterization of the basal-like subtype of invasive breast carcinoma. Clin Cancer Res 2004;10:5367–74.

# Ductal Carcinoma in Situ

Richard J. Bleicher, MD

## KEYWORDS

- Ductal carcinoma in situ • Tamoxifen • Mammography

## KEY POINTS

- Management of ductal carcinoma in situ (DCIS) has evolved from radical surgery to the option of a more minimally invasive approach.
- Although some facets of care for DCIS have not had the benefit of direct prospective trial comparison, data demonstrate that breast conservation surgery performed with administration of radiotherapy, like mastectomy, is feasible and safe, despite the lack of consensus about what constitutes a negative margin.
- Because efforts to find a safe group for elimination of radiotherapy have resulted in data that conflict, radiotherapy still remains standard of care as a part of breast conservation for DCIS.
- Tamoxifen has also shown a significant recurrence benefit, both in the adjuvant treatment setting as well as the prophylactic setting for DCIS, and has become standard in the treatment of receptor-positive disease.

## HISTORY

Ductal carcinoma in situ (DCIS), first termed intraductal, noninvasive, or noninfiltrating carcinoma, was originally treated similarly to invasive breast cancer. Even before mammography was routinely used, DCIS was known to show radiographic calcifications.[1] Mammography was not so critical to the diagnosis of DCIS at that time, because most cases of DCIS presented as a palpable lesion[1] that was most commonly of high-grade comedo histology.[2] The other symptom commonly associated with DCIS (as well as invasive cancer) was bloody nipple discharge, and so this symptom was also considered an indication for diagnostic excision.[1]

DCIS initially accounted for approximately 2% of all breast cancers detected.[3,4] The incidence rates have markedly increased over the past several decades because of widespread implementation of screening mammography in the 1980s and 1990s, with the greatest increase in incidence for women older than 50 years.[5] Although the rate of new cases of DCIS in younger women has continued to increase in the last decade, its incidence in women aged 50 years or older has stabilized since 1999,

Department of Surgical Oncology, Fox Chase Cancer Center, 333 Cottman Avenue, Room C-308, Philadelphia, PA 19111, USA
E-mail address: richard.bleicher@fccc.edu

Surg Clin N Am 93 (2013) 393–410
http://dx.doi.org/10.1016/j.suc.2012.12.001
0039-6109/13/$ – see front matter © 2013 Elsevier Inc. All rights reserved.

and now accounts for 15% to 25% of detected lesions when enumerated by state, and, in 2011, accounted for 57,650 cases, or 20% of all breast cancers detected in the United States.[5]

As with other cancers, the diagnosis of DCIS was achieved by excision before the era of the core needle biopsy. Similarly, for patients having bloody nipple discharge, a central duct excision was standard to establish a diagnosis, because the association with this symptom was recognized as early as the 1950s.[6] Although local excision was standard for diagnosis of DCIS, the treatment of DCIS was more radical, and initially accomplished in a manner identical to that of invasive breast cancers. Although local therapeutic excision was occasionally performed, mastectomy was the primary treatment, via total, modified radical, radical, or extended radical mastectomy in more than 80% of cases[3] with lymph nodes being removed, even although axillary nodal metastases were rarely found.[1] Over the ensuing decades, the surgery varied widely, from bilateral mastectomy to local excision without radiotherapy.[7]

## TERMINOLOGY AND HISTOLOGY
### Histologic Classification

The classification of DCIS has also evolved over the course of several decades as relationships between histologic variants have been clarified. The World Health Organization originally classified malignant breast disease as invasive or noninvasive, and solely divided noninvasive breast cancer into intraductal carcinoma and lobular carcinoma in situ (LCIS).[8] Currently, noninvasive lesions are subclassified under several headings, with LCIS now part of the lobular neoplasia group, DCIS placed under a heading of intraductal proliferative lesions with hyperplasia and atypia, and intraductal papillary carcinomas now occupying a subheading of intraductal papillary neoplasms. DCIS with microscopic ($\leq$1 mm) foci of invasion also occupy a separate classification of microinvasive carcinoma, and male breast lesions have also been separated into 1 category that includes both DCIS and invasive male breast cancer subtypes.[9] Although this method of classifying DCIS lesions seems abstruse, there are fewer clinical management implications to this differentiation than the classification suggests. It is important for the practitioner to know that DCIS of most of these subtypes is treated similarly.

Some of the WHO classification change occurred because DCIS, relative to invasive ductal carcinoma, is not analogous to an LCIS relationship to invasive lobular carcinoma. DCIS and LCIS have similar names because historically LCIS was believed to be the precursor of infiltrating lobular carcinoma. Nonpleomorphic or usual-type LCIS is now known to be a marker for risk and not a cancer itself.

### DCIS and Invasive Cancer

Although DCIS is a malignancy and staged by the American Joint Committee on Cancer as stage 0 breast cancer, the relationship between DCIS and invasive ductal cancer remains a subject of significant controversy, especially because not all DCIS progresses to invasive cancer. The Wellings-Jensen model of evolution of breast cancer, proposed more than 3 decades ago,[10] suggests that there is a progression from normal cells in the terminal duct lobular unit to cells having atypia. These atypical cells then progress to DCIS, which subsequently develops invasive capability. The Sontag-Axelrod theory of progression, proposed in a modeling study in 2005 based on clinical observations,[11] suggests that DCIS is not a progenitor of infiltrating ductal cancer but instead evolves separately in a parallel pathway from a common progenitor.

Genetic alterations in DCIS of differing grades span a spectrum that is similar and analogous to the differences between grades of invasive cancer.[12,13] In a variation on the 2 models of breast cancer pathogenesis, others have more recently suggested that low-grade in situ lesions progress to low-grade invasive cancers, whereas high-grade in situ lesions progress to high-grade invasive lesions, although this has not been uniformly supported in studies of progression of breast cancer.[14] Data from EORTC 10853 (European Organisation for Research and Treatment of Cancer 10853), randomizing patients having DCIS treated with breast conservation to radiotherapy or no radiotherapy, also showed that low-grade, intermediate-grade, and high-grade DCIS recurred as invasive disease at similar rates (9%–13%, $P = .35$) at 10 years.

It is well established that the extent of DCIS correlates with the risk of invasion contained within the in situ lesion. Specifically, DCIS that spans a diameter larger than 5 cm has been found to have a markedly increased risk for the presence of occult invasive disease.[4,15,16] This finding is clinically significant in the workup of patients having what is believed to be pure DCIS, because it suggested that, although DCIS lesion size is not critical for staging, the size of the lesion on diagnostic imaging may have prognostic implications for what is likely to be found on excision, and potentially, operative planning. Other such risk factors for invasion include palpable masses, high-grade histology, and cancerization of lobules,[17,18] which refers to the intraductal spread of DCIS into the lobular unit and not invasion itself.

### Hormone Receptor Expression

DCIS has been extensively characterized histologically, with perhaps the greatest volume of data present for estrogen receptors (ERs) and progesterone receptors (PRs). This area of study is important because of the prominent role that receptor expression plays in current treatment and its association with tumor response. One of the earliest extensive characterizations of ER expression in DCIS estimated the rate to be approximately 45%[19]; however, the threshold to classify expression in this study was that 25% or more of cells had to stain for the receptor, higher than the current 1% threshold for ER (and PR) expression. In this same study, when the presence of any staining was used as the threshold, approximately two-thirds of lesions were considered positive.[19] Subsequent determinations of receptors in DCIS were more consistent with this latter characterization, noting that approximately 65% expressed ERs when 5% to 10% staining is used as the threshold for positivity.[20,21] Other studies note similar or slightly higher rates of ER expression, when 5% or less is used as the definition of ER-positive.[22]

The receptor expression of DCIS also varies by grade, with approximately 75% of low-grade lesions expressing ER, whereas less than half of high-grade lesions do.[20] This finding is consistent with differences seen by histologic subtype[19,21] in which comedo-type DCIS is also more often negative for ERs and PRs than other variants. Although the grade and presence of comedonecrosis are predictors of receptor expression, the correlation is not strong enough to eliminate ER and PR staining in favor of using histology alone to determine whether hormonal therapy is appropriate.[22]

DCIS lesions are also largely PR-positive at a slightly lower rate than for ER expression, at 60% to 70%.[22,23] DCIS lesions, like invasive breast cancers, show a high correlation between ER and PR expression, with few lesions showing PR positivity when tumors are ER-negative, and lesions having 1 or both receptors positive at approximately 80%.[23] Similar to ERs, as grade increases, PR expression declines in DCIS.[22] Nevertheless, both are assayed, because lesions having either ER or PR expression are typically administered endocrine therapy because of the benefit it confers.

## IMAGING EVALUATION OF DCIS
### Mammography

Although several decades ago DCIS was largely diagnosed when found as a palpable abnormality, the routine use of screening mammography has increased the detection of DCIS and the percentage of cases of breast cancer that DCIS accounts for. The routine use of mammography began after dedicated mammography machines were introduced in 1969, and screen-film systems in 1972.[24] This situation led to the Health Insurance Program of Greater New York study, which reported a 30% mortality reduction from mammography and the resulting Breast Cancer Detection Demonstration Project (BCDDP), which also evaluated mammography. The 20-year follow-up from the BCDDP[24] reported a 93.9% to 98.2% 20-year adjusted survival rate for in situ lesions, dependent on age, with younger women having better survival. These studies set the stage for widespread use of mammographic screening for detection of invasive and in situ disease.

DCIS is detected in about 80% of cases by mammography, with more than 80% of those cases showing calcifications.[25,26] Among all mammographically detected non-palpable breast cancers, 68% of calcifications are from DCIS, with these calcifications being associated with necrosis.[27] Meanwhile, although DCIS less frequently presents as a palpable mass compared with several decades ago, 32% of mammographically detected nonpalpable masses with calcifications still represent DCIS, and 5% of masses that have no calcifications do also.[27]

These data about presentation of DCIS are consistent with the notion that mammography is an efficacious screening modality for this disease. In 1 of the largest series of mammographically detected DCIS from the University of California San Francisco,[28] 653,833 mammograms in 540,738 women performed in 1996 and 1997 from the National Cancer Institute's Breast Cancer Surveillance Consortium were reviewed. The study reported that 1 in every 1300 mammograms led to a diagnosis of DCIS and 20.2% of all screen-detected breast cancers were DCIS, with the yield highest among women aged 40 to 49 years (28.2%, 95% confidence interval [CI] 23.9%–32.5%). Meanwhile, the sensitivity for DCIS detection by screening mammography was 86.0% (95% CI 83.2%–88.8%), compared with 75.1% for invasive breast cancers (95% CI 73.5%–76.8%). Sensitivity for DCIS detection did not differ by age, as it did for cases of invasive breast cancer (which increased with age), and the highest sensitivity for detecting DCIS was in women aged 40 to 49 years who had no previous mammogram (97.4%, 95% CI 85%–100%). The rates of nonscreen-detected DCIS were also markedly smaller than the incidence of screen-detected DCIS, supporting the conclusion that mammographic screening is 1 reason why the incidence and proportion of DCIS cases has increased.

### Ultrasonography

Because of the predominance of screen-detected DCIS, with calcifications as the most frequent presentation, ultrasonography has played a minor role in the evaluation of DCIS. Ultrasonography has been investigated for, but has not been shown to be an effective screening modality, and outside its use for palpable abnormalities, does not have a role in either screening or evaluation of DCIS.

### Breast Magnetic Resonance Imaging

Breast magnetic resonance imaging (MRI) is a highly sensitive imaging modality that detects occult foci of breast cancer not seen on mammography in 8% to 40% of cases.[29] The ability of MRI to detect DCIS varies, dependent on the grade of the lesion.

In a large trial of 7319 women from Germany evaluating all women irrespective of risk and not just those presenting with an abnormality, mammography and MRI were both used for screening and compared. MRI showed no difference in sensitivity for low-grade DCIS when compared with mammography, but it had a higher sensitivity for intermediate-grade (31 vs 20%, $P = .013$), and high-grade lesions (87% vs 46%, $P<.0001$). With the approximate 95% 5-year to 10-year survival rate of DCIS detected without the benefit of MRI, and lack of data showing a survival advantage from breast MRI even for invasive cancer[30,31] (with which there is greater room for survival improvement), it remains doubtful that breast MRI would be able to provide any survival benefit if added to routine screening of normal-risk patients for the detection of DCIS.

## NEEDLE BIOPSY
### Fine-Needle Aspiration

Needle biopsy of benign and malignant lesions has been in use since the 1930s,[32] although more widespread use for breast abnormalities did not begin until the 1970s.[33] Fine-needle aspiration (FNA), performed either by palpation or image guidance, allows examination of cells to assess the presence of malignancy as distinguished from hyperplasia and often from atypia.[34] The biopsy technique is convenient because it can be performed with a standard needle and syringe in the office, but it poses difficulty for the pathologist to determine whether a lesion is invasive or in situ even although attempts have been made to distinguish structural features in FNA specimens.[35–37] FNA is consequently less favored than core needle biopsy for establishing a cancer diagnosis, because the need to distinguish DCIS versus invasive breast cancer is critical to determine the proper treatment and operative plan.

### Core Needle Biopsy

In contrast to FNA, core needle biopsy provides accurate assessment, with the benefit of providing architecture for histologic characterization and to distinguish invasive from in situ disease.[38] Core biopsy, whether by palpation, stereotaxis, or sonographic guidance, also frequently provides sufficient tissue for assessment of estrogen and PRs for pretreatment discussion of the role of antiestrogens in DCIS.

   The more germane issue to a surgical practice that surgeons need to be aware of is that the use of core needle biopsy is associated with a low but significant rate of upstaging on final excision. Depending on the number of cores removed and the gauge of the core biopsy needle, complete excision of a lesion diagnosed by core biopsy as DCIS shows invasive cancer in approximately 10% to 20% of cases.[39,40] This finding is clinically most relevant in operative planning, because it relates to management of the axilla, as discussed later.

## SURGICAL AND RADIOTHERAPEUTIC MANAGEMENT OF THE BREAST
### NSABP B-06

The first National Surgical Adjuvant Breast and Bowel Project (NSABP) trial to be performed that had some impact on the surgical management of DCIS was a trial to assess surgical treatment of invasive breast cancer. In NSABP B-06,[41] lumpectomy, lumpectomy with radiotherapy, and mastectomy were compared, and 76 of the 2072 cases were retrospectively found on review to solely have DCIS with no invasive component. This small subset of patients was analyzed,[42] and the lumpectomy group without radiotherapy showed a 43% recurrence rate after an average follow-up of 83 months, with a 7% recurrence rate for lumpectomy with radiation. Although 1 of the 27 patients having mastectomy died of her disease, none of the patients in that group was noted to have local recurrences. The numbers of patients in the 3 groups were all less than 30, and so these recurrence rates must be interpreted with caution, but the investigators concluded that breast conservation was feasible for DCIS, and further investigation was warranted.

### Breast Conservation

Surgical treatment of DCIS dictates that patients undergoing wide excision have negative margins, with larger margins being better, because of a desire to limit recurrence rates. However, there is no consensus on what constitutes an appropriate margin in either DCIS or invasive breast cancer.[43] In light of conflicting data, trials have had widely varying margin criteria, and outcome differences based on margin status have recently been called into question[44] as a result of effective systemic chemotherapy and endocrine agents. The definition of a negative margin is therefore left to the discretion of the practitioner or institution.

Long-standing experience shows that even for patients with low-grade DCIS, elimination of radiotherapy may result in nearly one-third of patients experiencing a local recurrence, and some of these can occur well beyond 10 years postoperatively.[45] Although mastectomy was the standard several decades ago, and although there is no large prospective randomized trial comparing breast conservation therapy (BCT) with mastectomy in DCIS as B-06 did for invasive breast cancer,[46,47] patients have been reported to have low local recurrence and high survival rates with BCT, which includes breast conservation surgery in conjunction with radiotherapy; BCT is a standard treatment option for patients with DCIS.

Although there are innumerable small studies that have confirmed the need for radiotherapy in the setting of breast conservation for DCIS, there are 4 landmark prospective randomized trials that must be mentioned, evaluating radiotherapy for maximizing local control in DCIS. These trials are National Surgical Adjuvant Breast and Bowel Project (NSABP) B-17,[7,48] European Organisation for Research and Treatment of Cancer (EORTC) 10853,[49,50] SweDCIS, and the United Kingdom (UK), Australia, and New Zealand (UK/ANZ) trial.[51] Two large retrospective series, the Collaborative Group Study,[26] which reviewed patients having breast conservation and radiotherapy, and the retrospective series by Kerlikowske and colleagues,[52] which evaluated lumpectomy alone, are of similar size and are also notable. Although each of these large retrospective series is different, they add consistent findings that have made radiotherapy standard of care in the setting of breast conservation for DCIS.

### NSABP B-17

In 1993, the NSABP published results of a trial comparing lumpectomy with lumpectomy with postoperative radiotherapy (50 Gy) for localized DCIS.[7] As breast conservation data started to accumulate for invasive breast cancer, patterns of operation for that disease began to change, leading to a paradox in how breast cancer was treated; invasive disease had local excision with radiotherapy as an option, whereas DCIS lesions still required mastectomy. This paradox prompted further investigation into the value of lumpectomy with or without radiotherapy. NSABP B-17 is considered a landmark trial investigating this paradigm.

There were 818 patients who had DCIS and lumpectomy who were randomized to no breast radiotherapy or radiotherapy at 50 Gy, beginning no later than 8 weeks postoperatively. In a long-term analysis at 207 months, ipsilateral breast recurrences occurred in 35% of the lumpectomy-only group and 19.8% in the group receiving radiotherapy. There was no difference between the arms in the incidence of contralateral breast cancers. This trial, the first results of which were published in 1993, was the first to report the benefit of radiotherapy in this setting. The investigators concluded that lumpectomy and radiotherapy are more appropriate for DCIS than lumpectomy alone.

## EORTC 10853

The EORTC performed a similar trial to evaluate the benefit of radiotherapy for women aged 70 years or younger having completely excised DCIS less than 5 cm without invasion or Paget disease.[49] Axillary dissection was not recommended but, if performed, the axillary lymph nodes needed to be without metastases, and patients having compromised margins were permitted reexcision to negative margins. A total of 1002 patients were randomized to a radiotherapy dose of 50 Gy in 25 fractions within 5 weeks of surgery or no radiotherapy.

At a median follow-up of 10.5 years,[50] the risk of local recurrence was reduced from 26% to 15% with the addition of radiotherapy. Recurrences were nearly evenly split between DCIS (103 patients) and invasive recurrences (106 patients). Contralateral breast cancers were not different in incidence or interval to contralateral breast cancer between the 2 arms. Multivariable model risk factors for recurrence included younger age (specifically, <40 years), detection because of symptoms, intermediately or poorly differentiated DCIS, solid or cribriform growth pattern, positive margins (although n was only 7), and treatment without radiotherapy.

## UK/ANZ Trial

In 2003, the United Kingdom Coordinating Committee on Cancer Research DCIS Working Party began a trial to simultaneously evaluate the benefits of radiotherapy and tamoxifen in the setting of breast conservation for patients having locally excised DCIS.[51] Based on the previously published results of NSABP B-17 and EORTC 10853, and concurrent to NSABP B-24 (later), which began accruing at the time, the trial was designed as a 2 × 2 factorial trial. The 1694 patients who entered the study were permitted to choose how they were randomized. One option was to undergo a complete 2 × 2 randomization to receipt of radiotherapy or not, and receipt of tamoxifen or not. Alternatively, these patients could choose to be randomized solely for the radiotherapy component or solely the tamoxifen component and openly select the other treatment option. There were 912 patients who chose to enter the complete 2 × 2 randomization, whereas 782 chose to be randomized to only 1 of the treatments, with 603 of these latter patients electing not to have radiotherapy (and thus being randomized to either tamoxifen or no tamoxifen).

Patients with unilateral or bilateral DCIS, who were believed to be amenable to breast conservation, were eligible. Two years after the start of the trial, inclusion criteria were amended to allow entry of patients with completely excised microinvasion less than 1 mm. Patients having positive margins and Paget disease were excluded, although reexcision to clear margins was permissible. Radiotherapy was administered as 50 Gy in 25 fractions over 5 weeks with no boost. Tamoxifen was administered at 20 mg daily for 5 years.

There were 1030 patients included in the radiotherapy analysis, with 58 developing a recurrence as DCIS and 60 developing a recurrence as invasive cancer. At a median follow-up of 4.4 years, the rate of recurrence in patients undergoing radiotherapy versus no radiotherapy was 7% versus 16% (P<.0001). Ipsilateral invasive events were reduced by 55% and ipsilateral DCIS by 64%, with contralateral events not affected by radiotherapy. These results again confirmed the findings of the NSABP and EORTC studies, albeit with a lower absolute recurrence rate than occurred in those trials.

### SweDCIS Trial

The Swedish Breast Cancer Group began enrolling patients in a similar trial from 1987 to 1999, in which 1046 women were randomized to radiotherapy or no radiotherapy.[53,54] Patients were eligible if they had DCIS and a clinically negative axilla. Patients having Paget disease, invasive carcinoma, or intracystic carcinoma in situ were excluded. Patients underwent local excision with or without 50 Gy of radiation administered in 25 fractions over 50 weeks, or 54 Gy in 2 series with a gap of 2 weeks, and 11% had microscopically positive margins, with 9% having a margin status unknown.

The absolute risk reduction for radiotherapy was 16% at 10 years, equally decreasing the risk of invasive and in situ events. Consistent with other trials, radiotherapy was more effective with older age, rising from a 6% risk reduction in the youngest to 18% in older patients. The investigators also attempted to find a low-risk group in whom radiotherapy could potentially be spared, but no such group could be found.

### Early Breast Cancer Trialists' Collaborative Group Analysis

In perhaps the most powerful assessment of the benefit afforded by radiotherapy, a meta-analysis by the Early Breast Cancer Trialists' Collaborative Group (EBCTCG) (Oxford Overview)[55] evaluated the 4 major DCIS trials having similar schema for patients having local excision randomized to either radiotherapy or no radiotherapy. These trials included the previously mentioned studies; NSABP B-17, EORTC 10853, SweDCIS, and the UK/ANZ Trial, for a total of 3729 patients evaluated after all exclusions, and a median follow-up of 8.9 woman-years.

Radiotherapy halved the rate of ipsilateral breast events, with a 5-year absolute reduction in risk of 10.5% (7.6% vs 18.1%), and a 10-year reduction of 15.2% (12.9% vs 18.1%). Overall, 24.8% of women had a breast event, and 74% of first events were in the ipsilateral breast. Recurrences were closely split between invasive and noninvasive types irrespective of whether radiotherapy was given, with 92 invasive and 100 noninvasive recurrences in those who had radiotherapy, and 204 invasive and 218 noninvasive recurrences in those who had excision alone. Among a small subset of 291 women within this analysis who did not receive radiotherapy because they were believed to be at low absolute risk of recurrence (negative margins and small low-grade DCIS), the 10-year risk of ipsilateral recurrence was 30.1% and highly significant, again confirming the benefit of radiotherapy, even in a presumably low-risk group.

### Notable Retrospective Series

There are also 2 published studies that, although not prospective randomized trials, are notable because of their large size and focus on DCIS. The first evaluated patients who had lumpectomy and radiotherapy, and the second evaluated lumpectomy alone.

The Collaborative Group Study retrospectively reviewed 1003 women having unilateral mammographically detected DCIS who had BCT at 10 institutions throughout the United States, France, the Netherlands, and Canada.[26] Patients were excluded if they had any physical examination findings, including a breast mass or bloody nipple discharge. This study also required that both breast-conserving surgery and radiotherapy for at least 40 Gy be performed, but margins varied from positive to greater than 2 mm, and no systemic chemotherapy or endocrine treatment was permissible. After a median follow-up of 8.5 years, the overall survival rate at 15 years was 89%, but the disease-specific survival at 15 years was 98% (95% CI 96%–99%). The local failure rate at 15 years was 16%, for invasive cancer and DCIS combined.

The second notable retrospective series is a study of 1036 women from the San Francisco Bay area, aged 40 years and older, treated by lumpectomy alone without radiotherapy.[52] At a median follow-up of 77.9 months, 20.2% of the women experienced a recurrence. Compared with the Collaborative Group Study, which had a true local recurrence rate of invasive recurrences and DCIS recurrences of 3% and 2%, respectively, despite the lack of systemic endocrine therapy, the 5-year recurrence rates in this study for the analogous group (initial DCIS detected by mammography alone) was 6.6% and 14.1% at 5 years, respectively. Data from 2 such separate retrospective studies cannot technically be compared; however, the magnitudes of local failure rates in each of these studies corroborate the randomized trial data and are consistent with smaller series showing a benefit of radiotherapy.

## MANAGEMENT OF THE AXILLA

Historically, patients having DCIS were treated identically to those having invasive breast cancer, with axillary lymph nodes routinely removed.[3] Once sentinel node biopsy was being increasingly used for assessment of the axilla, DCIS was considered an appropriate clinical setting for its use,[56] because of its feasibility and because even although the likelihood of metastatic disease was low, sentinel node biopsy removed fewer nodes, and efforts to incorporate immunohistochemistry to increase the sensitivity of nodal evaluation were ongoing. Studies have now shown that the rate of nodal metastases detected by hematoxylin and eosin staining for pure DCIS is only 1% to 2%.[56,57] This low metastasis rate, controversial significance of immunohistochemically positive nodes, and 5-year survival of 95%[58] even when nodes are not removed have called the value of sentinel node biopsy into question for DCIS. In an extensive review of the data,[59] a panel from the National Cancer Institute found that the benefit did not outweigh the risks of the procedure and therefore did not recommend it for patients having DCIS. The specifics of DCIS with nodal metastases have also recently been investigated in a small series from Finland,[60] which reported that most such metastases are isolated tumor cells or micrometastases, supporting the position that sentinel lymphadenectomy is not necessary in DCIS, because these findings suggest that it is unlikely to affect outcomes.

As noted earlier, patients having high-grade or comedo histology, or having DCIS lesions that span more than 5 cm, are significantly more likely to have invasion identified at complete excision. While sentinel node biopsy was becoming standard of care and indications were being refined, these criteria were considered an indication for sentinel lymphadenectomy in patients with DCIS. Some practitioners still perform sentinel node biopsy when lesions are high grade or more than 5 cm for patients having breast conservation. However, because sentinel lymphadenectomy can be performed accurately after lumpectomy, there is a trend to remove the sentinel nodes only if invasion is found on pathologic examination. Although another procedure may be necessary if invasion is found, it spares the patient the morbidity of nodal removal that may be unnecessary.

When considering DCIS lesions of all grades and sizes, patients having DCIS diagnosed by vacuum-assisted core needle biopsy have an upstaging rate on excision in 10% to 20% of cases.[39,40] depending on the needle gauge and the number of core needle biopsy samples. Because of this risk, although current practice does not routinely prescribe nodal evaluation for evaluation of DCIS, an exception is made for mastectomy patients, because removal of the breast precludes injection of the sentinel node dye, or at best, makes the accuracy of sentinel node biopsy uncertain. Sentinel lymphadenectomy is therefore performed in the setting of mastectomy, in case upstaging is found on pathologic examination of the breast specimen, so that unnecessary axillary dissection need not be performed.

## EFFORTS TO ELIMINATE RADIOTHERAPY FOR DCIS
### Van Nuys Prognostic Index

In 1995, Silverstein and colleagues[61] created the Van Nuys classification, dividing DCIS by nuclear grade, and then those that were not high grade into lesions having or not having comedonecrosis. Thereafter, this classification was used in the Van Nuys Prognostic Index (VNPI),[62] which was created to assist in determining which patients would have an unacceptable risk of local recurrence with BCT whether they received radiotherapy or not. The VNPI added tumor size and margin width to this classification to create a score of 1 to 3 (low risk to high risk) for each variable. The sum of these 3 variables created the overall score.

This classification was then modified to become the University of Southern California/Van Nuys Prognostic Index (USC/VNPI),[63] by adding age to the other 3 variables in the model, because younger patients had been previously noted to have a higher risk for recurrence. This index now created a score ranging from 4 to 12, which was then stratified to predict who could undergo excision alone, who should undergo radiotherapy with local excision, and who required mastectomy. Recurrence in those with scores of 4, 5, and 6 did not benefit from the addition of radiotherapy, those with scores of 7, 8 or 9 received a 12% to 15% local control benefit from radiotherapy, and those having scores of 10, 11, or 12 had 5-year local recurrence rates of nearly 50%, and were believed to require mastectomy.

Despite its apparent practical value, the application of the VNPI and USC/VNPI in clinical practice has remained controversial because of difficulties in reproducing the study results by other investigators.[64–67] The validity also remains in question because the EBCTCG overview of the 4 large prospective DCIS radiotherapy trials showed that radiotherapy was effective in reducing ipsilateral recurrence irrespective of histologic or nuclear grade, the presence of comedonecrosis, or pathologic tumor size.[55]

### Eastern Cooperative Oncology Group 5194

A major prospective trial was launched by the Eastern Cooperative Oncology Group (ECOG) to determine if patients having low-grade or intermediate-grade DCIS could undergo local excision without irradiation.[68] Patients having DCIS 2.5 cm or smaller of low or intermediate grade or DCIS 1 cm or smaller of high grade were eligible. Margins of at least 3 mm were required, and no residual calcifications on postoperative mammogram were permissible. At median follow-up of 6.2 years, the low-grade/ intermediate-grade group comprising 565 patients had a 5-year rate of ipsilateral recurrence of 6.1%, whereas at median follow-up of 6.7 years, the high-grade stratum, consisting of 105 patients, had a rate of 15.3%. The investigators concluded that the low-grade/intermediate-grade group's event rate was acceptable for omission of radiotherapy, unlike the high-grade group, but that additional follow-up is required to determine the long-term outcomes.

### Twenty-One Gene Recurrence Score for DCIS

More recently, genome-directed efforts to determine who may eliminate radiotherapy after breast conservation for DCIS have been pursued. In 2011, data were presented[69] from a trial to evaluate a modification of the 21-gene recurrence score used for determining risk of recurrence in the setting of invasive breast cancer. This study assessed whether this recurrence score, modified for DCIS to range from 0 to 100, might provide better assessment of who may be spared because of a low recurrence risk. This study evaluated 327 patients from ECOG 5194 having either low-grade or intermediate-grade DCIS 2.5 cm or smaller, or high-grade DCIS 1.0 cm or smaller. The DCIS averaged 0.7 cm in size, and median follow-up was 8.8 years. The patients were arbitrarily divided into 3 groups based on their recurrence scores: less than 39 (low), 39 to 54 (intermediate), and 55 or more (high), and although the log rank ($P = .02$) showed that the overall curves differed between the groups, the confidence intervals for in-breast recurrence risk between adjacent groups overlapped at 10 years (low 12.0% [95% CI 8.1%–17.6%], intermediate 24.5% [95% CI 13.8%–41.1%], high 27.3% [95% CI 15.2%–45.9%]). It therefore remains to be seen if the curves are becoming similar or whether the number of patients at 10 years is too few to prevent widening confidence intervals that suggest no statistical difference between the groups.

The study also evaluated 2 multivariable models for risk of in-breast recurrence. Both models used tumor size and postmenopausal status, but 1 added the DCIS score. Tumor size and postmenopausal status were significant in both models, with the DCIS score also noted to be significant when added in ($P = .02$). The results suggest that the recurrence score may have some prognostic ability in determining which patients may be able to be spared radiotherapy, although the study has not yet been published and validation is required.

Although there may be promise in this gene profiling test, it is not known whether this is more or less effective than the VNPI[62] or the Memorial Sloan Kettering DCIS nomogram.[70] This subject is of particular importance in the era of cost containment, because these latter 2 methods of assessment are free, in contrast to the expense of running the 21-gene recurrence score for this purpose. It is hoped that further studies will clarify its value and may allow radiotherapy to be omitted in patients who will not benefit from its use.

## TAMOXIFEN
### NSABP B-24

After NSABP B-17, which established the benefit of radiotherapy with breast conservation for DCIS, NSABP B-24 was designed to investigate tamoxifen in that setting. Previous data had shown that tamoxifen reduced the risk of ipsilateral and contralateral recurrences in patients with invasive breast cancer.[71,72] NSABP B-24 was thus created to randomize patients having breast-conserving surgery with radiotherapy to subsequent tamoxifen or placebo.[73]

There were 1804 patients randomized who had DCIS and a life expectancy of at least 10 years. Patients were excluded if their tumors showed invasion, although LCIS could be seen along with the DCIS, and although axillary dissection was not recommended, patients having an axillary lymphadenectomy were excluded only if the lymph nodes showed metastatic disease, indicating occult invasion. Radiotherapy was standardized at 50 Gy, to be started no later than 8 weeks after surgery, even although patients whose margins were microscopically positive were also not excluded. Tamoxifen was administered in the treatment group at 10 mg twice daily for 5 years, beginning within 56 days of surgery.

At a median follow-up of 74 months, the tamoxifen arm showed 37% fewer breast cancer events overall, with 43% fewer invasive and 31% fewer noninvasive events.[73] The results were further broken down to show that tamoxifen conferred a 38% reduction in ipsilateral breast tumors in women younger than 50 years, and a 22% reduction in those older than 50 years. Patients who were of younger age, had positive margins, or had comedonecrosis were at significantly increased risk for recurrence. A more recent analysis of the B-24 results[74] noted a 15-year rate of invasive ipsilateral tumor recurrence of 10% in the placebo arm and 8.5% in the tamoxifen arm, with 15-year contralateral breast cancer incidence of 10.8% in the placebo arm and 7.3% in the tamoxifen arm.

NSABP B-24 therefore effectively established that tamoxifen provided both ipsilateral and contralateral benefit in patients undergoing breast conservation for DCIS. A retrospective subset analysis of patients from B-24, stratifying by receptor status, reported the benefit to be confined to receptor-positive DCIS,[23] with a 10-year reduction of subsequent breast cancer events of 51% in ER-positive patients and no benefit from tamoxifen for ipsilateral or contralateral events in women with ER-negative DCIS. Because most DCIS lesions do show substantial ER and PR expression,[20] tamoxifen has become a mainstay of treatment in this disease.

### UK/ANZ Trial

As noted earlier, further suggestion of the benefit of tamoxifen was provided in the UK/ANZ trial, which evaluated the effects of radiotherapy and tamoxifen on DCIS undergoing local excision in a 2 × 2 design. Among 1576 patients randomly assigned to receive or not receive tamoxifen, ipsilateral events were 7% in the tamoxifen group and 10% in the no-tamoxifen group, which approached but did not reach significance ($P = .08$). Although there was no difference in rates of contralateral disease, when both ipsilateral and contralateral breast cancer events were combined, there was a significant difference in favor of the tamoxifen group (7% vs 11%, $P = .03$) having fewer events. When the patients with DCIS were subdivided further into those who received radiotherapy and those who did not, tamoxifen conferred no additional benefit in ipsilateral risk reduction in patients who received radiotherapy, but significantly lowered the risk of all events (ipsilateral and contralateral) from 10% to 6% ($P = .03$). This study did not include a subset analysis by ER status.

### NSABP B-35

A trial is under way to assess the role of anastrazole compared with tamoxifen, among patients with ER-positive DCIS. The NSABP B-35 trial[75] randomized women undergoing lumpectomy and radiotherapy to anastrazole or tamoxifen. This study is based on similar data suggesting a benefit for aromatase inhibitors in ER-positive invasive breast cancer[76] and may provide another standard agent for use in DCIS. Analysis is expected in 2014.

## HUMAN EPIDERMAL GROWTH FACTOR 2 (HER2/NEU)
### HER2/neu Expression and Trastuzumab

One of the most clinically relevant histologic assessments performed for invasive breast cancer is assessment of HER2/neu expression. Amplification or overexpression of this gene has been correlated with poor prognosis in invasive breast cancer.[77] In studies of pure DCIS, 66% of lesions are found to overexpress HER2, and although more frequently found in ER-negative or PR-negative DCIS than in ER-positive or PR-positive DCIS, overexpression of HER2 does not correlate with a difference in response to endocrine treatment among receptor-positive lesions.[78]

Trastuzumab is a monoclonal antibody that binds to the HER2/neu receptor. Because adjuvant trastuzumab with chemotherapy results in a survival benefit for women with HER2-positive invasive breast cancer,[79] and because it has been shown to act as a radiosensitizer in other malignancies,[80] its use is being investigated in DCIS.

### NSABP B-43

The NSABP B-43 trial will investigate the potential for trastuzumab to decrease local recurrence rates in DCIS.[81] This is a phase III trial, which randomizes women with HER2-positive DCIS undergoing lumpectomy and radiotherapy to administration or no administration of 2 doses of trastuzumab 3 weeks apart. Patients who are ER-positive or PR-positive will also receive endocrine therapy.

## PREVENTION
### NSABP P-1

The definitive trial for prevention of both DCIS and invasive breast cancer is the NSABP P-1 trial,[82] in which 13,388 women were randomized to receive a placebo or 20 mg of tamoxifen daily for 5 years. Patients were eligible for the trial if they were older than 60 years, or between 35 and 59 years with a 1.66% or greater 5-year risk of breast cancer as calculated by the Gail model,[83] or a had a history of LCIS. The results showed that in addition to the reduction in the risk of invasive cancer, there was a 50% reduction in the annual risk of in situ disease from 2.68 to 1.35 per 1000 women. It was concluded that tamoxifen was an effective preventative agent for women of increased risk, lowering the risk of DCIS and invasive cancer, and that women with DCIS specifically should receive tamoxifen because they have at least as high a risk of developing invasive breast cancer as women with a history of LCIS, for whom the agent showed efficacy in preventing breast cancer.

### STAR Trial

The other landmark prevention trial, known as NSABP P-2, or the STAR (Study of Tamoxifen and Raloxifene) trial assessed the relative preventative value and safety of raloxifene and tamoxifen for developing invasive and noninvasive breast cancer, uterine cancer, bone fractures, and thromboembolic events.[84] There were 19,747 postmenopausal women with an increased 5-year risk of breast cancer similar to the P-1 trial, who were randomized to either 20 mg of daily oral tamoxifen or 60 mg of daily oral raloxifene over 5 years. The trial reported an equal effect between tamoxifen and raloxifene on invasive breast cancer and none of the high-risk subsets (eg, those with atypia, a history of LCIS, increased risk according to the Gail model) were found to have differences between tamoxifen and raloxifene. However, the DCIS findings reported fewer noninvasive lesions, including both LCIS and DCIS in the tamoxifen subgroup relative to raloxifene. This finding did not reach statistical significance, but an update of the trial has found persistence of this trend.[85,86] In the updated results after 81 months of median follow-up, raloxifene was found to be only 78% as effective as tamoxifen in preventing all noninvasive lesions, with the difference between the agents confined to DCIS or cases of mixed DCIS and LCIS. It was also 76% as effective for prevention of invasive cancer; however, raloxifene does have an advantage of a significantly lower risk of endometrial cancer, and no difference for other invasive cancers, events related to ischemic heart disease, or stroke.[84]

## SUMMARY

Management of DCIS has evolved from radical surgery to the option of a more minimally invasive approach. Although some facets of care for DCIS have not had the benefit of direct prospective trial comparison, data show that breast conservation surgery performed with administration of radiotherapy, like mastectomy, is feasible and safe, despite the lack of consensus about what constitutes a negative margin. As efforts to find a safe group for elimination of radiotherapy have resulted in data that conflict, radiotherapy still remains standard of care as a part of breast conservation for DCIS. Tamoxifen has also shown a significant recurrence benefit, both in the adjuvant treatment setting as well as in the prophylactic setting for DCIS, and has become standard in the treatment of receptor-positive disease. Investigation of other agents that are of benefit for invasive breast cancer and show preliminary promise in DCIS, such as anastrazole and trastuzumab, is ongoing.

## REFERENCES

1. Ashikari R, Hajdu SI, Robbins GF. Intraductal carcinoma of the breast. (1960-1969). Cancer 1971;28:1182–7.
2. Winchester DP, Jeske JM, Goldschmidt RA. The diagnosis and management of ductal carcinoma in-situ of the breast. CA Cancer J Clin 2000;50:184–200.
3. Rosner D, Bedwani RN, Vana J, et al. Noninvasive breast carcinoma: results of a national survey by the American College of Surgeons. Ann Surg 1980;192: 139–47.
4. Lagios MD. Duct carcinoma in situ. Pathology and treatment. Surg Clin North Am 1990;70:853–71.
5. Desantis C, Siegel R, Bandi P, et al. Breast cancer statistics, 2011. CA Cancer J Clin 2011;61:409–18.
6. Urban JA. Excision of the major duct system of the breast. Cancer 1963;16:516–20.
7. Fisher B, Costantino J, Redmond C, et al. Lumpectomy compared with lumpectomy and radiation therapy for the treatment of intraductal breast cancer. N Engl J Med 1993;328:1581–6.
8. The world Health Organization Histological Typing of Breast Tumors–Second Edition. The World Organization. Am J Clin Pathol 1982;78:806–16.
9. Tavassoli FA, Devilee P. International Agency for Research on Cancer. World Health Organization. Pathology and genetics of tumours of the breast and female genital organs. Lyon (France): IAPS Press; 2003.
10. Wellings SR, Jensen HM, Marcum RG. An atlas of subgross pathology of the human breast with special reference to possible precancerous lesions. J Natl Cancer Inst 1975;55:231–73.
11. Sontag L, Axelrod DE. Evaluation of pathways for progression of heterogeneous breast tumors. J Theor Biol 2005;232:179–89.
12. Ellsworth RE, Ellsworth DL, Love B, et al. Correlation of levels and patterns of genomic instability with histological grading of DCIS. Ann Surg Oncol 2007;14: 3070–7.
13. Ellsworth RE, Hooke JA, Love B, et al. Correlation of levels and patterns of genomic instability with histological grading of invasive breast tumors. Breast Cancer Res Treat 2008;107:259–65.
14. King TA, Sakr RA, Muhsen S, et al. Is there a low-grade precursor pathway in breast cancer? Ann Surg Oncol 2012;19:1115–21.
15. Yi M, Krishnamurthy S, Kuerer HM, et al. Role of primary tumor characteristics in predicting positive sentinel lymph nodes in patients with ductal carcinoma in situ or microinvasive breast cancer. Am J Surg 2008;196:81–7.
16. Lagios MD, Westdahl PR, Margolin FR, et al. Duct carcinoma in situ. Relationship of extent of noninvasive disease to the frequency of occult invasion, multicentricity, lymph node metastases, and short-term treatment failures. Cancer 1982;50: 1309–14.
17. King TA, Farr GH Jr, Cederbom GJ, et al. A mass on breast imaging predicts co-existing invasive carcinoma in patients with a core biopsy diagnosis of ductal carcinoma in situ. Am Surg 2001;67:907–12.
18. Huo L, Sneige N, Hunt KK, et al. Predictors of invasion in patients with core-needle biopsy-diagnosed ductal carcinoma in situ and recommendations for

a selective approach to sentinel lymph node biopsy in ductal carcinoma in situ. Cancer 2006;107:1760–8.

19. Giri DD, Dundas SA, Nottingham JF, et al. Oestrogen receptors in benign epithelial lesions and intraduct carcinomas of the breast: an immunohistological study. Histopathology 1989;15:575–84.

20. Leal CB, Schmitt FC, Bento MJ, et al. Ductal carcinoma in situ of the breast. Histologic categorization and its relationship to ploidy and immunohistochemical expression of hormone receptors, p53, and c-erbB-2 protein. Cancer 1995;75: 2123–31.

21. Bose S, Lesser ML, Norton L, et al. Immunophenotype of intraductal carcinoma. Arch Pathol Lab Med 1996;120:81–5.

22. Barnes NL, Boland GP, Davenport A, et al. Relationship between hormone receptor status and tumour size, grade and comedo necrosis in ductal carcinoma in situ. Br J Surg 2005;92:429–34.

23. Allred DC, Anderson SJ, Paik S, et al. Adjuvant tamoxifen reduces subsequent breast cancer in women with estrogen receptor-positive ductal carcinoma in situ: a study based on NSABP Protocol B-24. J Clin Oncol 2012;30:1268–73.

24. Smart CR, Byrne C, Smith RA, et al. Twenty-year follow-up of the breast cancers diagnosed during the Breast Cancer Detection Demonstration Project. CA Cancer J Clin 1997;47:134–49.

25. Schouten van der Velden AP, Peeters PH, Koot VC, et al. Clinical presentation and surgical quality in treatment of ductal carcinoma in situ of the breast. Acta Oncol 2006;45:544–9.

26. Solin LJ, Fourquet A, Vicini FA, et al. Long-term outcome after breast-conservation treatment with radiation for mammographically detected ductal carcinoma in situ of the breast. Cancer 2005;103:1137–46.

27. Gajdos C, Tartter PI, Bleiweiss IJ, et al. Mammographic appearance of nonpalpable breast cancer reflects pathologic characteristics. Ann Surg 2002;235: 246–51.

28. Ernster VL, Ballard-Barbash R, Barlow WE, et al. Detection of ductal carcinoma in situ in women undergoing screening mammography. J Natl Cancer Inst 2002;94: 1546–54.

29. Houssami N, Hayes DF. Review of preoperative magnetic resonance imaging (MRI) in breast cancer: should MRI be performed on all women with newly diagnosed, early stage breast cancer? CA Cancer J Clin 2009;59:290–302.

30. Solin LJ, Orel SG, Hwang WT, et al. Relationship of breast magnetic resonance imaging to outcome after breast-conservation treatment with radiation for women with early-stage invasive breast carcinoma or ductal carcinoma in situ. J Clin Oncol 2008;26:386–91.

31. Turnbull LW, Brown SR, Olivier C, et al. Multicentre randomised controlled trial examining the cost-effectiveness of contrast-enhanced high field magnetic resonance imaging in women with primary breast cancer scheduled for wide local excision (COMICE). Health Technol Assess 2010;14:1–182.

32. Martin HE, Ellis EB. Biopsy by needle puncture and aspiration. Ann Surg 1930;92: 169–81.

33. Rimsten A, Stenkvist B, Johanson H, et al. The diagnostic accuracy of palpation and fine-needle biopsy and an evaluation of their combined use in the diagnosis of breast lesions: report on a prospective study in 1244 women with symptoms. Ann Surg 1975;182:1–8.

34. Sneige N, Staerkel GA. Fine-needle aspiration cytology of ductal hyperplasia with and without atypia and ductal carcinoma in situ. Hum Pathol 1994;25:485–92.

35. Pijnappel RM, van den Donk M, Holland R, et al. Diagnostic accuracy for different strategies of image-guided breast intervention in cases of nonpalpable breast lesions. Br J Cancer 2004;90:595–600.

36. Shin HJ, Sneige N. Is a diagnosis of infiltrating versus in situ ductal carcinoma of the breast possible in fine-needle aspiration specimens? Cancer 1998;84: 186–91.

37. Somani A, Hwang JS, Chaiwun B, et al. Fine needle aspiration cytology in young women with breast cancer: diagnostic difficulties. Pathology (Phila) 2008;40: 359–64.

38. Fajardo LL, Pisano ED, Caudry DJ, et al. Stereotactic and sonographic large-core biopsy of nonpalpable breast lesions: results of the Radiologic Diagnostic Oncology Group V study. Acad Radiol 2004;11:293–308.

39. Jackman RJ, Burbank F, Parker SH, et al. Stereotactic breast biopsy of nonpalpable lesions: determinants of ductal carcinoma in situ underestimation rates. Radiology 2001;218:497–502.

40. Burak WE Jr, Owens KE, Tighe MB, et al. Vacuum-assisted stereotactic breast biopsy: histologic underestimation of malignant lesions. Arch Surg 2000;135: 700–3.

41. Fisher B, Redmond C, Poisson R, et al. Eight-year results of a randomized clinical trial comparing total mastectomy and lumpectomy with or without irradiation in the treatment of breast cancer. N Engl J Med 1989;320:822–8.

42. Fisher ER, Leeming R, Anderson S, et al. Conservative management of intraductal carcinoma (DCIS) of the breast. Collaborating NSABP investigators. J Surg Oncol 1991;47:139–47.

43. Taghian A, Mohiuddin M, Jagsi R, et al. Current perceptions regarding surgical margin status after breast-conserving therapy: results of a survey. Ann Surg 2005;241:629–39.

44. Houssami N, Macaskill P, Marinovich ML, et al. Meta-analysis of the impact of surgical margins on local recurrence in women with early-stage invasive breast cancer treated with breast-conserving therapy. Eur J Cancer 2010;46(18):3219–32.

45. Page DL, Dupont WD, Rogers LW, et al. Continued local recurrence of carcinoma 15-25 years after a diagnosis of low grade ductal carcinoma in situ of the breast treated only by biopsy. Cancer 1995;76:1197–200.

46. Fisher B, Anderson S, Bryant J, et al. Twenty-year follow-up of a randomized trial comparing total mastectomy, lumpectomy, and lumpectomy plus irradiation for the treatment of invasive breast cancer. N Engl J Med 2002;347:1233–41.

47. Veronesi U, Cascinelli N, Mariani L, et al. Twenty-year follow-up of a randomized study comparing breast-conserving surgery with radical mastectomy for early breast cancer. N Engl J Med 2002;347:1227–32.

48. Fisher B, Dignam J, Wolmark N, et al. Lumpectomy and radiation therapy for the treatment of intraductal breast cancer: findings from National Surgical Adjuvant Breast and Bowel Project B-17. J Clin Oncol 1998;16:441–52.

49. Julien JP, Bijker N, Fentiman IS, et al. Radiotherapy in breast-conserving treatment for ductal carcinoma in situ: first results of the EORTC randomised phase III trial 10853. EORTC Breast Cancer Cooperative Group and EORTC Radiotherapy Group. Lancet 2000;355:528–33.

50. Bijker N, Meijnen P, Peterse JL, et al. Breast-conserving treatment with or without radiotherapy in ductal carcinoma-in-situ: ten-year results of European Organisation for Research and Treatment of Cancer randomized phase III trial 10853–a study by the EORTC Breast Cancer Cooperative Group and EORTC Radiotherapy Group. J Clin Oncol 2006;24:3381–7.

51. Houghton J, George WD, Cuzick J, et al. Radiotherapy and tamoxifen in women with completely excised ductal carcinoma in situ of the breast in the UK, Australia, and New Zealand: randomised controlled trial. Lancet 2003;362:95–102.

52. Kerlikowske K, Molinaro A, Cha I, et al. Characteristics associated with recurrence among women with ductal carcinoma in situ treated by lumpectomy. J Natl Cancer Inst 2003;95:1692–702.

53. Emdin SO, Granstrand B, Ringberg A, et al. SweDCIS: radiotherapy after sector resection for ductal carcinoma in situ of the breast. Results of a randomised trial in a population offered mammography screening. Acta Oncol 2006;45:536–43.

54. Holmberg L, Garmo H, Granstrand B, et al. Absolute risk reductions for local recurrence after postoperative radiotherapy after sector resection for ductal carcinoma in situ of the breast. J Clin Oncol 2008;26:1247–52.

55. Early Breast Cancer Trialists' Collaborative Group, Correa C, McGale P, et al. Overview of the randomized trials of radiotherapy in ductal carcinoma in situ of the breast. J Natl Cancer Inst Monogr 2010;2010:162–77.

56. Pendas S, Dauway E, Giuliano R, et al. Sentinel node biopsy in ductal carcinoma in situ patients. Ann Surg Oncol 2000;7:15–20.

57. Intra M, Veronesi P, Mazzarol G, et al. Axillary sentinel lymph node biopsy in patients with pure ductal carcinoma in situ of the breast. Arch Surg 2003;138:309–13.

58. Joslyn SA. Ductal carcinoma in situ: trends in geographic, temporal, and demographic patterns of care and survival. Breast J 2006;12:20–7.

59. Zujewski J, Eng-Wong J. Sentinel lymph node biopsy in the management of ductal carcinoma in situ. Clin Breast Cancer 2005;6:216–22.

60. Meretoja TJ, Heikkila PS, Salmenkivi K, et al. Outcome of patients with ductal carcinoma in situ and sentinel node biopsy. Ann Surg Oncol 2012;19:2345–51.

61. Silverstein MJ, Poller DN, Waisman JR, et al. Prognostic classification of breast ductal carcinoma-in-situ. Lancet 1995;345:1154–7.

62. Silverstein MJ, Lagios MD, Craig PH, et al. A prognostic index for ductal carcinoma in situ of the breast. Cancer 1996;77:2267–74.

63. Silverstein MJ. The University of Southern California/Van Nuys prognostic index for ductal carcinoma in situ of the breast. Am J Surg 2003;186:337–43.

64. de Mascarel I, Bonichon F, MacGrogan G, et al. Application of the Van Nuys Prognostic Index in a retrospective series of 367 ductal carcinomas in situ of the breast examined by serial macroscopic sectioning: practical considerations. Breast Cancer Res Treat 2000;61:151–9.

65. Boland GP, Chan KC, Knox WF, et al. Value of the Van Nuys Prognostic Index in prediction of recurrence of ductal carcinoma in situ after breast-conserving surgery. Br J Surg 2003;90:426–32.

66. Asjoe FT, Altintas S, Huizing MT, et al. The value of the Van Nuys Prognostic Index in ductal carcinoma in situ of the breast: a retrospective analysis. Breast J 2007; 13:359–67.

67. MacAusland SG, Hepel JT, Chong FK, et al. An attempt to independently verify the utility of the Van Nuys Prognostic Index for ductal carcinoma in situ. Cancer 2007;110:2648–53.

68. Hughes LL, Wang M, Page DL, et al. Local excision alone without irradiation for ductal carcinoma in situ of the breast: a trial of the Eastern Cooperative Oncology Group. J Clin Oncol 2009;27:5319–24.

69. Solin LJ, Gray R, Baehner FL, et al. A quantitative multigene RT-PCR assay for predicting recurrence risk after surgical excision alone without irradiation for ductal carcinoma in situ (DCIS): a prospective validation study of the DCIS score from ECOG E5194. Cancer Res 2011;71:108s.

70. Rudloff U, Jacks LM, Goldberg JI, et al. Nomogram for predicting the risk of local recurrence after breast-conserving surgery for ductal carcinoma in situ. J Clin Oncol 2010;28:3762–9.
71. Fisher B, Costantino J, Redmond C, et al. A randomized clinical trial evaluating tamoxifen in the treatment of patients with node-negative breast cancer who have estrogen-receptor-positive tumors. N Engl J Med 1989;320:479–84.
72. Fisher B, Redmond C. New perspective on cancer of the contralateral breast: a marker for assessing tamoxifen as a preventive agent. J Natl Cancer Inst 1991;83:1278–80.
73. Fisher B, Dignam J, Wolmark N, et al. Tamoxifen in treatment of intraductal breast cancer: National Surgical Adjuvant Breast and Bowel Project B-24 randomised controlled trial. Lancet 1999;353:1993–2000.
74. Wapnir IL, Dignam JJ, Fisher B, et al. Long-term outcomes of invasive ipsilateral breast tumor recurrences after lumpectomy in NSABP B-17 and B-24 randomized clinical trials for DCIS. J Natl Cancer Inst 2011;103:478–88.
75. U.S. National Institutes of Health. Anastrozole or tamoxifen in treating postmenopausal women with ductal carcinoma in situ who are undergoing lumpectomy and radiation therapy. Available at: http://www.clinicaltrials.gov/ct2/show/NCT00053898?term=B-35&rank=1. Accessed July 25, 2012.
76. Howell A, Cuzick J, Baum M, et al. Results of the ATAC (Arimidex, Tamoxifen, Alone or in Combination) trial after completion of 5 years' adjuvant treatment for breast cancer. Lancet 2005;365:60–2.
77. Pritchard KI, Shepherd LE, O'Malley FP, et al. HER2 and responsiveness of breast cancer to adjuvant chemotherapy. N Engl J Med 2006;354:2103–11.
78. Boland GP, McKeown A, Chan KC, et al. Biological response to hormonal manipulation in oestrogen receptor positive ductal carcinoma in situ of the breast. Br J Cancer 2003;89:277–83.
79. Romond EH, Perez EA, Bryant J, et al. Trastuzumab plus adjuvant chemotherapy for operable HER2-positive breast cancer. N Engl J Med 2005;353:1673–84.
80. Liang K, Lu Y, Jin W, et al. Sensitization of breast cancer cells to radiation by trastuzumab. Mol Cancer Ther 2003;2:1113–20.
81. National Surgical Adjuvant Breast and Bowel Project. NSABP Clinical Trials Overview: Protocol B-43. Available at: http://www.nsabp.pitt.edu/B-43.asp. Accessed July 24.
82. Fisher B, Costantino JP, Wickerham DL, et al. Tamoxifen for prevention of breast cancer: report of the National Surgical Adjuvant Breast and Bowel Project P-1 Study. J Natl Cancer Inst 1998;90:1371–88.
83. Gail MH, Brinton LA, Byar DP, et al. Projecting individualized probabilities of developing breast cancer for white females who are being examined annually. J Natl Cancer Inst 1989;81:1879–86.
84. Vogel VG, Costantino JP, Wickerham DL, et al. Effects of tamoxifen vs raloxifene on the risk of developing invasive breast cancer and other disease outcomes: the NSABP Study of Tamoxifen and Raloxifene (STAR) P-2 trial. JAMA 2006;295:2727–41.
85. Vogel VG, Costantino JP, Wickerham DL, et al. Update of the National Surgical Adjuvant Breast and Bowel Project Study of Tamoxifen and Raloxifene (STAR) P-2 Trial: preventing breast cancer. Cancer Prev Res (Phila) 2010;3:696–706.
86. Bevers TB. Breast cancer prevention: an update of the STAR trial. Curr Treat Options Oncol 2010;11:66–9.

# Surgical Management of the Breast
## Breast Conservation Therapy and Mastectomy

Sarah A. McLaughlin, MD

### KEYWORDS

- Breast conservation • Mastectomy • Breast conservation surgery • Margins
- Surgical trends • Mastectomy • Local recurrence

### KEY POINTS

- Mastectomy and breast conservation offer equivalent survival.
- The surgical goal is complete tumor removal.
- Most women with early stage breast cancers are amenable to breast-conserving surgery.
- Surgical therapy coupled with adjuvant systemic and radiation therapies reduce local recurrence.

The twentieth century witnessed dramatic changes in the surgical management of breast cancer in both the breast and the axilla. Publication of several landmark studies led to the evolution of breast cancer surgery from radical and deforming to breast conserving but also elucidated the systemic nature of the disease. Management of the axilla has mirrored that seen in the breast with movement away from standard axillary node dissection (ALND) toward less radical axillary surgery with the adoption of the sentinel lymph node biopsy. Herein only the surgical management of the breast will be discussed because the management of the axilla is covered elsewhere in this edition.

## FROM RADICAL MASTECTOMY TO BREAST-CONSERVING SURGERY

Several landmark trials with decades of follow-up form the foundation of contemporary breast surgery. The National Surgical Adjuvant Breast and Bowel Project (NSABP) B-04 trial compared radical mastectomy (RM) to total mastectomy (TM) with or without radiation therapy in a prospective randomized fashion. In the TM arm, axillary dissection was performed only if lymph nodes were positive. Enrollment of more than 1600 women began in 1971, and the most recent publication with 25 years of follow-up was published in 2002. The investigators reported no difference in either group with regard

Department of Surgery, Mayo Clinic, 4500 San Pablo Road, Jacksonville, FL 32224, USA
E-mail address: Mclaughlin.sarah@mayo.edu

Surg Clin N Am 93 (2013) 411–428
http://dx.doi.org/10.1016/j.suc.2012.12.006
0039-6109/13/$ – see front matter © 2013 Elsevier Inc. All rights reserved.

to disease-free survival, relapse-free survival, distant-disease-free survival, or overall survival,[1] confirming no advantage to RM.

Subsequently, a total of 6 prospective randomized trials enrolling patients from 1973 to 1989 validated the survival equivalence of mastectomy and breast-conserving surgery. The largest and perhaps most well known is the NSABP B-06 trial. This trial prospectively randomized women with tumors less than 4 cm to mastectomy, lumpectomy, or lumpectomy with radiation. All women had an ALND regardless of treatment assignment or nodal status; negative margins, defined as no tumor at ink, were required. The 20-year follow-up data were published in 2002; the investigators found no difference in disease-free, distant-disease-free, or overall survival[2] between any of the treatment arms. The data did demonstrate, however, a significant reduction in local recurrence (LR) after lumpectomy with the addition of radiation therapy (39.2% vs 14.3%, P<.001) as did the 6 other conservation trials outlined in **Table 1**. Collectively, these trials established breast-conserving therapy (BCT), consisting of margin negative lumpectomy and radiation therapy, as appropriate therapy for women with invasive breast cancer. Based on these trials, the National Institutes of Health (NIH) issued a Consensus Conference statement in 1990 recommending BCT as the preferred surgical treatment of women with early stage breast cancer.[3] Furthermore, they estimated approximately 80% of women with newly diagnosed breast cancer to be eligible for BCT. Not surprisingly, in response to this NIH recommendation, the percentage of women selecting BCT as their therapeutic choice steadily increased.

## PATIENT SELECTION

Long-standing contraindications to BCT exist and are classified as absolute or relative. Absolute contraindications include multicentric disease (tumors in more than one quadrant of the breast), diffuse malignant-appearing calcifications, inflammatory breast cancer, prior radiation to the chest or breast or inability to receive radiation, persistent positive margins despite appropriate attempts for breast-conserving surgery, and the need for radiation during pregnancy.

Relative BCT contraindications may be debated. Surgeons tend to reserve BCT for those women with tumors less than 5 cm in whom negative margins can be achieved while maintaining an acceptable cosmetic outcome. More important, however, than the true size of the tumor is the ratio of the tumor size to the breast size. A 5-cm tumor may be easily excised if located in the upper outer quadrant of a woman with large

**Table 1**
**Prospective randomized trials evaluating mastectomy and breast-conserving surgery**

| Trial | N | Follow-up (y) | Overall Survival Mastectomy (%) | BCT+XRT (%) |
|---|---|---|---|---|
| NSABP B-06[2] | 1851 | 20 | 47.2 | 46.2 |
| National Cancer Institute, United States[68] | 247 | 10 | 75.0 | 77.0 |
| EORTC[69] | 903 | 8 | 64.0 | 66.0 |
| Danish Breast Cancer Group[70] | 793 | 20 | 49.1 | 53.7 |
| Milan[71] | 701 | 20 | 58.8 | 58.3 |
| Institute Gustave-Roussy[72] | 179 | 10 | 80.0 | 79.0 |

*Abbreviations:* BCT, breast-conserving therapy; EORTC, European Organization for Research and Treatment of Cancer; XRT, radiation therapy.

pendulous breasts, whereas excising a 2-cm tumor located in the remote upper inner quadrant or at the 6-o'clock position in a woman with an A-cup breast size may result in an unacceptable cosmetic result. Furthermore the ability to remove multifocal lesions (2 cancers in the same quadrant) must be individualized and made in real time. Active connective tissue disease (especially scleroderma or active systemic lupus erythematosus) involving the skin of the breast precluding radiation is typically considered a contraindication. However, in patients with a connective tissue disorder and no history of involvement of the skin of the breast, radiation may be possible and consultation with a radiation oncologist before surgery may be meaningful in the decision-making process. Having a focally positive margin has long been considered a contraindication for BCT; however, the 2012 National Comprehensive Cancer Network's guidelines permit consideration of BCT in these cases,[4] with the caveat that a higher dose of boost radiation be considered for the tumor bed. Involving a radiation oncologist in this decision would also be helpful. Skin dimpling, nipple and areolar retraction, and tumor location are not contraindications to BCT, yet these should be considered in the preoperative assessment, specifically with respect to the ability to achieve negative margins. Young age is not a contraindication to BCT.

## CURRENT TRENDS IN BREAST SURGERY

Despite the NIH recommendation for BCT, mastectomy rates in the United States have consistently been higher than the anticipated 20% rate estimated by the NIH. In fact, 6 single-institution studies have reported unilateral mastectomy rates ranging between 35% and 52%.[5–10] Reasons for persistent or increasing use of mastectomy are unclear; but many hypothesize this is caused by a variety of clinical factors, such as magnetic resonance imaging (MRI) of the breast,[6,9] young patient age,[10] increased use of genetic testing, patient education and awareness, patient preference,[11] and/or availability and improvements in reconstruction options. Controversy exists as to whether these trends are isolated among individual institutions or reflective of a broader national trend because others find no increase in their mastectomy rates.[5,12] Further, Habermann and colleagues[13] reviewed the breast cancer treatment of 233,754 patients as reported to the Surveillance, Epidemiology, and End Results (SEER) database between 2000 and 2006. They found that mastectomy rates decreased from 40.8% in 2000 to 37.0% in 2006 ($P<.001$). Although this population-based analysis finds contradictory results to the single-institutional series, the SEER data may be slower to identify early trends. Despite this, it still documents mastectomy rates in the United States to be well more than the 20% to 25% rates seen in Europe and elsewhere.[14] Little is known as to why women choose mastectomy when they are eligible for BCT; but one study suggests it may be related to a personal history of contralateral breast cancer, absence of medical comorbidities, or young patient age but does not seem to be influenced by primary tumor characteristics.[11]

Perhaps more significant in recent years than an elevated mastectomy rate has been the profound increase in contralateral prophylactic mastectomies (CPM). Tuttle and colleagues[15] first identified this trend in 2007 noting in a SEER dataset that CPM increased among women undergoing mastectomy from 4.2% in 1998 to 11.0% in 2003. These rates were seen in all stages of cancer and highest in those with young age, lobular histology, and a prior diagnosis of cancer. Memorial Sloan Kettering reviewed their CPM rates and found them to mirror that seen in the SEER database, with rates increasing form 6.7% in 1997 to 24.2% in 2005.[16] Only 13% of patients with CPM had a BRCA mutation or a prior history of mantle radiation, patient groups for whom CPM may be considered routinely; 22% of patients with CPM had ductal carcinoma in situ (DCIS), a noninvasive form of breast cancer without the potential to spread. These trends are difficult to reconcile when one considers that the risk of contralateral breast cancer is estimated to be 0.5% to 0.7% per year and declining in women without a BRCA mutation.[17] However, Abbott and colleagues[18] surveyed 74 women to assess patient perception of contralateral breast cancer risk and found patients estimated their contralateral breast cancer risk to be 31%, well more than the documented rates. Similar to the elevated unilateral mastectomy rates, there is a lack of clarity on the reasons for the increasing rates of CPM, which again seems to be a trend isolated to the United States because a recent European study found only 2.6% of mastectomy patients in Europe choose CPM.[19]

## BCT

The adoption of mammographic screening and improvements in screening techniques has resulted in an increase in the diagnosis of early stage nonpalpable breast cancers amenable to BCT. The term *breast conservation therapy* collectively refers to all surgical definitions for breast preservation procedures with tumor removal, including quadrantectomy, lumpectomy, tumorectomy, partial mastectomy, and others.

Quadrantectomy was popularized by Veronesi and colleagues[20] and refers to an en bloc excision of the skin, breast parenchyma with a 2- to 3-cm margin around the tumor, and pectoralis fascia. Once excised, the remaining breast tissue frequently must be mobilized off the pectoralis muscle and from the skin to allow reapproximation of the tissues with minimal distortion of breast contour and/or the skin. Lumpectomy generally refers to a less generous tissue excision and aims to remove the localized or palpable lesion with about a 1-cm margin. Nonpalpable breast tumors must be localized to aid in removal. Wire localization represents the most widely used technique because the wires may be placed with mammographic, ultrasound, or MRI guidance. Although this has been the standard for years, the process can be inconvenient for patients who must remain with the wire extending through the breast skin risking wire migration during transport. Finally, wire localization requires coordination of both surgery and radiology schedules. Recently, there has been significant interest in other localization options to minimize these concerns, including hematoma-directed ultrasound-guided lumpectomy,[21] radio-guided occult lesion localization,[22] and radioactive seed localization (RSL).[23] All of these options use image-guided localization and can be done intraoperatively or, in the case of seed localization, several days before surgery. Although none of these alternatives have been widely adopted, RSL is gaining favor because the localizing seed is deemed to be safe, does not migrate, and may be associated with lower rates of positive margins.[23,24]

Technically, lumpectomy incisions should be placed directly over the tumor whenever possible to avoid tunneling through the breast, but incision placement should keep in mind the possibility of future mastectomy. The incision is made through the dermis into the subcutaneous tissue, and then flaps are raised in all directions around the tumor to allow for appropriate exposure and mobilization of the breast tissue. Regardless of how the specimen is removed, it should be oriented in some way to ensure margins can be properly inked and identified by the pathologist. Although orientation of the specimen is critical, the precise process of how this is done varies among surgeons, pathologists, and institutions and carries important implications for re-excision surgery. Multiple studies evaluating specimen orientation by surgeon inking, specialized radiopaque margin markers, or shaved oriented cavity margins have been performed without consensus on the best technique. Once the specimen is removed, many surgeons will leave radiopaque clips in the lumpectomy cavity marking the tumor bed to assist with radiation treatment planning and mammographic follow-up. Debate exists as to whether the cavity should be closed after tumor excision given the potential risk of positive margins requiring re-excision; opponents argue that rearranging the breast tissue limits the reidentification of the original positive margin site at re-excision. Finally, the incision is closed in layers, typically with a running monofilament suture for the skin.

## MARGINS

Achieving negative surgical margins is a hallmark of successful BCT because this is associated with a lower rate of LR. However, what constitutes a negative margin remains a matter of significant debate. One particular problem in determining the effect of subtle differences in increasing margin width on local control is the general lack of standardization in specimen processing and microscopic analysis of lumpectomy specimens. It is important to understand how the margin processing is done at one's institution because this can influence interpretation of margin results, rates of positive margins, and the need for re-excision.[25] Both tangential shaved margins and perpendicular inked margins are common techniques for lumpectomy specimen processing. Tangential margin reporting classifies margins as positive or negative, whereas perpendicular margin assessment reports positive or negative and gives a margin distance. This nuance is important because one study found a 49% positive margin rate with tangential shaved margins compared with only 16% if done by the perpendicular margin technique.[26] Further, because the tangential method allows for only a positive or negative result, it limits the surgeon's ability to discriminate among patients with close margins to determine the need for re-excision. As a result, re-excision rates were higher in the tangential arm (75% vs 52%, $P<.001$) despite no difference in residual disease found in the re-excision specimens (27% vs 32%).

The NSABP has long defined a negative margin as no tumor at ink regardless of the proximity of the nearest tumor cell. Historically, other series have argued that margins of more than 1 mm, more than 2 mm, more than 5 mm, or even more than 10 mm provide better local control. A recent meta-analysis reviewed 21 studies and 14 571 patients undergoing BCT.[27] Data demonstrate a significant increase in LR for positive margins with an odds ratio (OR) of 2.42 ($P<.001$) compared with negative margins. Direct comparison between different margin widths found no statistically significant improvement in local control. Although a weak trend was identified suggesting declining LR with increasing margin distance, this trend disappeared after adjustments for radiation boost treatment and endocrine therapy. Also of interest is the lack of standardized practice with respect to re-excision. Wide variation in re-excision patterns exists within and across institutions. McCahill and colleagues[28] reviewed 2206 women undergoing BCT and found only 85% of those with positive margins completed re-excision, whereas 47.9% with margins less than 1 mm, 20.2% of those with 1.0- to 1.9-mm margins, and 6.3% with more than 2.0-mm margins had re-excision. Additionally, re-excision varied from 0% to 70% among surgeons ($P = .003$) and was not affected by surgeon volume. Re-excisions also varied from 1.7% to 20.9% among institutions. These differences underscore the controversies with respect to lumpectomy margins and challenges of using margin status as a quality metric for breast cancer surgery. Regardless, in practice, positive or unknown margins should prompt re-excision because positive margins are associated with significantly increased rates of LR, even with radiotherapy. Diligent margin re-excision can result in successful preservation of the breast in up to 95% of cases,[29] even with multiple re-excisions. Although multiple re-excisions do not affect rates of LR, caution must be used because it may negatively affect cosmetic outcome.

## MRI AND BCT

The use of breast MRI in patients with breast cancer increased dramatically from 10% in 2003 to 27% to 40% by 2007[9,12,30] in part because of its superior sensitivity over mammography in identifying occult malignancies or extensive disease otherwise missed on conventional imaging. Surgeons and patients assumed that better delineation of disease would assist with surgical planning, reduce re-excision rates, and improve local control. However, current data do not validate these perceived benefits. Breast MRI frequently leads to more extensive surgery with wider excision specimens in 3% to 14% of patients and conversion to mastectomy from BCT in 3% to 33%,[31] yet several studies, including the prospective randomized Comparative Effectiveness of MRI in Breast Cancer (COMICE) trial,[30,32,33] found no difference in positive margins or re-excision rates; the prospective randomized MR mammography of nonpalpable breast tumors (MONET) trial[34] found a paradoxically increased rate of positive margins and re-excisions in the MRI group (**Table 2**). Data addressing the effect of MRI on local control are conflicting. One study found a decrease in LR at 40 months in patients having MRI compared with those not having MRI (1.2% vs 6.8%, $P \leq .01$),[35] whereas another found LR rates of 3% at 8 years in MRI patients versus 4% in patients not having MRI ($P = .51$).[36] Further, Solin and colleagues[36] found MRI had no influence on overall survival (86% vs 87%, $P = .51$). Similarly, the COMICE trial has demonstrated no difference in disease-free survival according to MRI usage. Unfortunately, the MONET trial was not designed to address LR or survival.

Incorporation of MRI into the diagnostic algorithm of women with breast cancer varies across the country but may be most appropriate in patients with the following:

- An occult primary breast cancer
- When conventional imaging is suboptimal
- When discordance is present between the physical examination and conventional imaging
- To monitor tumor response after neoadjuvant chemotherapy

Patients undergoing MRI should be counseled regarding the potential need for second-look procedures or additional biopsies and encouraged to complete any additional diagnostic procedures before finalizing the surgical plan because MRI may overestimate the extent of the disease in 33% of patients with unifocal disease and underestimate the extent of disease in 40% of patients with multifocal disease.[37] Finally, it is important to note that the incidence of MRI-only detected additional

**Table 2**
**Trials demonstrating no benefit to MRI in reducing positive-margin rates or additional surgery after BCT**

|  | Study Type | N | Endpoint | No MRI (%) | MRI (%) | P |
|---|---|---|---|---|---|---|
| Pengel[33] | Retrospective | 349 | Positive margins | 19.4 | 13.8 | .17 |
| Bleicher[30] | Retrospective | 577 | Positive margins | 13.8 | 21.6 | .2 |
| COMICE[32] | RCT | 1623 | Reoperation or re-excision | 19.0 | 19.0 | .77 |
| MONET[34] | RCT | 418 | Reoperation or re-excision | 28.0 | 45.0 | .069 |

*Abbreviation:* RCT, prospective randomized controlled trial.

lesions far exceeds contemporary local failure rates of less than 10% with modern adjuvant chemotherapy and radiation regimens.[38]

## NEOADJUVANT CHEMOTHERAPY AND BCT

Neoadjuvant chemotherapy increases eligibility for breast-conserving surgery, especially in patients presenting with locally advanced breast cancer or in borderline cases whereby the tumor-to-breast size ratio will not allow for excision and acceptable cosmetic results. NSABP B-18[39] established the efficacy of neoadjuvant therapy randomizing women with early stage breast cancer to 4 cycles of neoadjuvant or adjuvant doxorubicin plus cyclophosphamide. An updated analysis with more than 16 years of follow-up demonstrates no difference in overall survival, disease-free survival, or event-free survival[40] between the two arms. Further, women receiving neoadjuvant therapy had a higher rate of pathologic negative axillary lymph nodes at surgery and a higher rate of BCT. Overall, 9% of women had a pathologic complete response (pCR). The first-generation trials comparing neoadjuvant with adjuvant chemotherapy are listed in **Table 3**. Second-generation randomized phase III trials incorporating paclitaxel and docetaxel into neoadjuvant regimens as well as those evaluating preoperative targeted therapies like trastuzumab continue to demonstrate improved BCT rates but importantly demonstrate higher pCR rates, 10% to 28% for trials incorporating paclitaxel and docetaxel and 36% to 78% for trials incorporating trastuzumab.[41] Achievement of pCR has been associated with an improved overall survival and disease-free survival.

Surgeons considering neoadjuvant chemotherapy and the possibility of BCT must ensure the tumor is properly marked with a clip before the start of therapy to allow localization and removal of the tumor bed in the event of a pCR. Although imaging regimens for patients undergoing neoadjuvant chemotherapy vary, many clinicians prefer MRI imaging before chemotherapy and then again before surgery to aid in surgical planning. Any imaging abnormalities identified on prechemotherapy imaging should be completely evaluated before the start of treatment.

## ONCOPLASTIC SURGERY

Oncoplastic surgery combines oncologic principles with plastic surgery techniques to enhance the cosmetic outcome. The process includes tumor removal, correction of the tissue defect, reconstruction with rearrangement of the breast parenchyma, and contralateral symmetry procedures. Oncoplastic techniques focus on the following:

- Incision placement
- Nipple location
- Correction of ptosis

**Table 3**
Pathologic complete response and BCT rates among prospective trials comparing neoadjuvant and adjuvant chemotherapy

| | | | BCT Rate (%) | |
| --- | --- | --- | --- | --- |
| Study | N | pCR (%) | Neoadjuvant | Adjuvant |
| Powles[73] | 212 | 10 | 87 | 72 |
| NSABP B-18[39,40] | 1523 | 9 | 68 | 60 |
| EORTC 10902[74] | 698 | 2 | 34 | 23 |

Abbreviation: EORTC, European Organization for Research and Treatment of Cancer.

- A clear understanding of rearrangement techniques based on pedicled breast parenchymal flaps

One particularly rewarding technique associated with high patient satisfaction is the incorporation of tumor excision with a reduction mammoplasty. Perhaps the most important part of the oncoplastic process is the preoperative planning and delineation of the extent of disease as significant rearrangement of breast tissue may preclude the ability to re-excise a positive margin. Marking the tumor bed with clips remains important for future localization.

## RADIATION THERAPY AND BCT

Radiation therapy plays a crucial role in successful BCT and has long been recognized to reduce LR risk by approximately 50%. The 2005 Early Breast Cancer Trialists' Collaborative Group's (EBCTCG) overview analyses demonstrated the influence of local control on long-term survival.[42] The meta-analysis evaluated 42 000 women participating in 78 trials comparing radiotherapy with no radiotherapy, more surgery versus less surgery, and more surgery versus radiotherapy. Specifically with regard to BCT, the EBCTCG collectively analyzed data from 10 trials of 7300 women and found the risk of LR at 5 years to be significantly reduced from 26% after lumpectomy alone to 7% after lumpectomy with radiation therapy, an absolute reduction of 19%. Importantly, however, for the first time, the 2005 meta-analysis demonstrated a significant reduction in the 15 year risk of death from breast cancer from 35.9% among those not having postlumpectomy radiation therapy to 30.5% among those receiving radiation therapy ($P = .0002$ [two-tailed]). The EBCTCG concluded that one breast cancer death at 15 years could be prevented for every 4 LRs avoided.

The EBCTCG recently updated this data in 2011, expanding their analysis to 17 randomized trials of 10 801 women undergoing breast-conserving surgery with and without radiotherapy. This meta-analysis again confirmed that radiation therapy resulted in an overall absolute reduction in LR of 15.7% at 10 years compared with those not receiving radiation (19.3% vs 35.0%, $P<.00001$ [two-tailed])[43]; this translated into an absolute reduction in breast cancer death of 3.8% at 15 years, again reaffirming that preventing 4 LRs at 10 years saves one breast cancer death at 15 years. When the data were analyzed according to nodal status, the absolute reductions in LR and improvements in survival gained from radiation therapy were more profound in those with node-positive disease (**Table 4**). Further review of the node-negative patients according to patient and tumor characteristics was performed in an attempt to identify groups gaining higher benefit from radiation therapy. The investigators found the proportional benefit of radiation to be similar among all groups (about 50% relative reduction in LR), whereas the absolute benefits varied by characteristic, with greater absolute benefit in younger women, higher grade, or larger tumors, and in estrogen receptor (ER)-positive patients not receiving tamoxifen.[43] More importantly,

**Table 4**
EBCTCG local recurrence at 10 years and survival rates at 15 years: meta-analysis of the effects of radiation therapy (XRT) after BCT

|  | N | Any First Recurrence at 10 y | | | Breast Cancer Death At 15 y | | |
|---|---|---|---|---|---|---|---|
|  |  | BCS | BCS+XRT | P | BCS | BCS+XRT | P |
| pN0 | 7287 | 31.0% | 15.6% | P<.00001 (two-tailed) | 20.5% | 17.2% | P = .005 (two-tailed) |
| pN+ | 1050 | 63.7% | 42.5% | P<.00001 (two-tailed) | 51.3% | 42.8% | P = .01 (two-tailed) |

the large sample size of these meta-analyses offered adequate power and long-term follow-up to detect a small but clinically relevant detrimental influence of LR on breast cancer survival. These data validate the importance of local control and demonstrate that optimal local control is achieved through multiple treatment modalities.

Investigations into partial breast irradiation options by external beam, catheter-based, and interstitial-based options are ongoing. Indications vary according to the American Brachytherapy Society and the American Society of Breast Surgeons but generally consider eligibility to be women more than 45 years old, invasive ductal carcinoma or DCIS less than 3 cm, and node negative disease. The NSABP B-39 trial is currently randomizing 4300 women with tumors less than 3 cm and 0 to 3 positive lymph nodes treated with lumpectomy to whole-breast or partial-breast irradiation. The trial is evaluating LR as well as cosmesis and is expected to reach accrual in late 2012.

## LR AFTER BCT

LR after BCT can be described as (1) a true recurrence, one within the primary tumor bed; (2) a marginal miss, one within the same quadrant just outside of the tumor bed; and (3) an elsewhere recurrence, one in a separate quadrant of the breast. Generally, true recurrences and marginal misses account for 46% to 91% of all LRs and tend to occur earlier than elsewhere recurrences.[44] As time lengthens from diagnosis and treatment of the original breast cancer, it becomes more likely that the second tumor is in fact a second primary cancer and not a recurrence. This distinction is made clinically but to date does not affect treatment recommendations. Regardless, the EBCTCG demonstrates that more than 75% of all recurrences occur within 5 years.[42] Risk factors for LR include positive margins, young age, ER-negative receptor status, larger tumor size, positive nodes, and lymphovascular invasion.[45,46] Histologic tumor type and family history are not associated with increased rates of LR. Systemic therapy, especially targeted therapy, reduces the risk of LR. For example, the adjuvant trastuzumab trials demonstrate that patients receiving trastuzumab had a 50% reduction in LR.[47] Similarly, Mamounas and colleagues[48] evaluated LR in estrogen-positive patients enrolled in NSABP B-14 and NSABP B-20 according to the 21-gene recurrence score assay (Oncotype DX, Genomic Health, Redwood City, CA, USA). At 10 years, tamoxifen significantly reduced the risk of LR in the low-risk group from 10.8% to 4.3% ($P<.001$). The addition of chemotherapy further reduced LR to 1.6% in that group ($P = .028$).

Mammography identifies in breast tumor recurrences in 14–47% of patients while physical examination finds 19–60%. Most local recurrences however are found by a combination of both mammography and physical exam. No guidelines exist for the use or MRI for post–breast conservation surgery surveillance, but it should be considered as a problem-solving tool if physical examination findings and mammographic findings are discordant. When tumor recurrence is identified, staging studies should be performed to rule out the presence of synchronous distant disease, which would change the priority for local management. In patients who have previously received radiotherapy, mastectomy is the standard of care surgical treatment option for in breast tumor recurrence. Limited studies have evaluated the potential for repeat BCT but all have demonstrated high rates of second LR ranging from 14% to 48%.[49,50] The disease-free interval from original diagnosis to LR influences long-term survival, with those developing early LR (within 2 years) having significantly worse survival.[51]

## MASTECTOMY

Approximately 30% to 40% of women in the United States are not candidates for BCT or choose mastectomy. Technically, there are many types of mastectomy, including

RM, modified radical, TM, simple, skin-sparing (SSM), nipple-sparing (NSM), subcutaneous, and prophylactic mastectomy (PM). Today, patients commonly undergo a TM or simple-mastectomy in conjunction with sentinel node biopsy for lymph node evaluation. Definitions of mastectomy types are as follows:

- TM or simple mastectomy: removal of the breast, overlying skin, and the nipple and areolar complex
- SSM: same as TM or simple mastectomy but sparing as much skin as possible and the inframammary fold for immediate reconstruction
- NSM: SSM technique also saving the nipple and areolar complex
- Subcutaneous mastectomy: subtotal removal of the breast tissue leaving behind 1 to 2 cm of breast tissue on the mastectomy flaps and the nipple and areolar complex

Although subcutaneous mastectomy is rarely performed in modern breast surgery, understanding that this technique was historically used for prophylaxis in women at elevated risk for breast cancer is important. The term *prophylactic mastectomy* incorporates any of the previously mentioned techniques and implies the procedure is being performed in a healthy breast to reduce the future risk of cancer.

## TECHNIQUE

Incision placement varies on whether or not reconstruction will be performed. In general, however, the incision is performed in an elliptical fashion, incorporating the nipple and areolar complex, and positioned horizontally or obliquely across the chest. Ideally, the incision removes all prior surgical or biopsy scars. Mastectomy flaps are raised to the level of the clavicle superiorly, the sternal edge medially, the inframammary fold or rectus fascia inferiorly, and the latissimus dorsi muscle laterally, leaving behind only a small amount of subcutaneous fat and blood vessels in the subdermal plane on the skin flap. Mastectomy flaps are commonly raised using electrocautery or scalpel dissection. The key to either technique is maintaining adequate retraction of the breast gland with the nondominant hand to identify and maintain the plane of dissection. The flaps are raised in a medial-to-lateral direction as an assistant holds tension on the skin flaps with hook retractors. Some prefer to perform tumescent mastectomy over simple electrocautery or scalpel dissection using a tumescent solution of saline, lidocaine, and epinephrine to infiltrate the subcutaneous fat just below the dermal layer. In this technique, a 60-mL syringe of fluid is injected in the subcutaneous plane across the length of the mastectomy incision to aid in separating the mastectomy plane from the subcutaneous fat. Then with ample retraction of the skin edges toward the operator, the surgeon uses sharp dissection, either with a scalpel or scissors, to create the mastectomy flaps and define the borders of the breast. Regardless of the surgical technique, it is important to recognize that significant interdigitation of the breast tissue and subcutaneous fat exists and the goal is to leave as little breast tissue behind as possible while maintaining viability of the flaps. Of note, not all skin flaps will be of equal thickness because thin women will naturally have thinner mastectomy flaps than obese women. Removal of the breast from the chest wall incorporates the pectoralis major muscle fascia posteriorly and is most easily performed staying parallel to the pectoralis muscle fibers. The mastectomy specimen is oriented by placing a stitch in the axillary tail. In the absence of reconstruction, the cosmetic goal should be to leave the chest wall as flat as possible to allow ease of external prosthesis fitting. Once excess cutaneous deformities (dog-ears) are eliminated, a closed suction drain should be placed and the tissues closed with interrupted dermal sutures followed by a running absorbable suture for the skin.

## SPECIAL CONSIDERATIONS: SSM

Toth and Lappert originally described SSM in 1991.[52] In this initial publication, they defined SSM as the removal of the breast through a smaller incision incorporating the nipple and areolar complex, all biopsy incisions, and allowing access for axillary node dissection. The SSM incision maintains the native skin envelope, limiting skin differences during reconstruction; maintains the natural inframammary fold; and allows for immediate breast reconstruction at the same stage. The investigators concluded SSM offered superior cosmetic results. Using these principles, breast surgeons and plastic surgeons will develop small elliptical or circular incisions around the nipple and areola or even perform mastectomy through a Weiss pattern or reduction mammoplasty incision.

Initial concerns around SSM included oncologic safety and surgical morbidity, both specifically related to the smaller incision, limited exposure, and longer skin flaps. Opponents worried these technical concerns would translate into higher rates of LR and skin flap necrosis. In addition, it was not clear if imaging of the reconstructed breast would be necessary for the residual skin flaps or if the residual skin and reconstructed breast would have to be removed in the event of LR after mastectomy. Although no prospective trials comparing SSM with TM exist, several recent retrospective studies, including a large meta-analysis, have compared SSM with non-SSM, finding no difference in LR (**Table 5**). Given this, contemporary trends, both in the United States and internationally, demonstrate widespread adoption of the SSM technique, with 27% of mastectomy recipients undergoing SSM in 1997 and 75% having SSM by 2001.[53] Further, Kinoshita and colleagues[54] recently reported no difference in disease-free survival (92% and 95%, SSM and non-SSM, respectively) ($P = .75$) or overall survival ($P = .69$) between the two techniques.

## NSM

NSM was originally described in 1962 by Freeman and colleagues[55] and abandoned because of oncologic concerns and cosmetic complications. Interest in this technique, however, increased again in the early twenty-first century. The newer NSM

| Table 5 | | | | | | |
|---------|---|---|---|---|---|---|
| Retrospective studies comparing local recurrence rates after mastectomy, SSM, and NSM | | | | | | |
| Study | N | Follow-up (mo) | LR According to Surgery | | | |
| | | | Mastectomy (%) | SSM (%) | NSM (%) | P |
| Yi[75] | 1810 | 53 | 7.6 | 5.3 | — | .04 |
| Boneti[63] | 293 | NSM 25 SSM 38 | — | 5.0 | 6.0 | .89 |
| Lanitis[65] | 3739 | a | 4.0 | 6.2 | — | OR 1.25 (95% CI 0.81–1.94) |
| Kim[64] | 520 | 63 | 0.9 | 0.8 | 2.0 | .27 |
| Gerber[76] | 246 | 101 | 11.5 | 10.4 | 11.7 | .10 |

*Abbreviation:* CI, confidence interval.
a Meta-analysis with follow-up ranging from 37 to 100 months among 9 studies analyzed.

techniques remove all the breast tissue, similar to SSM or conventional mastectomy, as opposed to the prior descriptions of NSM, which likened the procedure to that of a subcutaneous mastectomy. Furthermore, cosmetically, most plastic surgeons prefer the native nipple to a reconstructed one primarily because reconstructed nipples frequently lose projection over time. Patient satisfaction echoes these opinions; a retrospective study by Jabor and colleagues[56] reported more than 50% of women with reconstructed nipples wish they could improve their nipple projection.

Published series describe a variety of incisions, including inframammary fold, circumareolar, omega (circumareolar with medial and lateral radial extensions), lateral radial, and vertical incisions. The appropriate incision depends on the breast size and shape, the degree of ptosis, presence of prior incisions, type of reconstruction, and surgeon comfort, keeping in mind the ability to reach to anatomic boundaries of the beast (the clavicle, sternum, and inframammary fold) and to perform the same oncologic operation as one would perform in a non-NSM setting. Mastectomy flaps are again raised in the mastectomy plane as previously described. The key difference lies in the removal of tissue behind the nipple and areolar complex. The surgeon should carefully follow the breast parenchyma dissection plane to the areola then dissect it from the nipple and areolar complex sharply, understanding that the ductal tissue converges at the nipple. Although this can be done with electrocautery, sharp dissection with scalpel or scissors allows for careful identification of the planes while minimizing thermal injury to the dermis of the areola. Once the retroareolar breast tissue is separated from the skin, the nipple margin on the specimen should be marked for future orientation. The nipple skin is then inverted, and the remaining ductal tissue is cored from the nipple and sent for frozen section analysis in cancer cases. If tumor cells are identified, the nipple and areola should be removed; if negative, however, it is important to inform patients that the remaining skin of the nipple and areolar complex is functionally similar to a full-thickness skin graft. If tumor cells are identified on the final pathological assessment, the nipple and areolar complex (NAC) should be removed as a second procedure. Frequently, this can be performed without anesthesia given the lack of sensation in the mastectomy skin flap and NAC.

Advances in the NSM technique that allow for removal of the breast parenchyma in a similar fashion to that of SSM or conventional mastectomy have voided some of the oncologic concerns. However, many surgeons still question the safety of leaving the nipple behind, especially for prophylactic indications, arguing that the retained nipple increases the risk of leaving ductal tissue behind and, therefore, decreases the therapeutic benefit of PM. In actuality, this risk is likely low. With an intact breast, the risk of a primary breast cancer originating from the nipple is less than 5%; Paget's disease of the nipple occurs in less than 1% of patients. Available follow-up data suggest that LR rates after NSM are equivalent to SSM or non-SSM, with only a handful of recurrences (about 1%) occurring in the nipple (see **Table 5**).

## PATIENT SELECTION FOR NSM

Patient and tumor factors influence eligibility for NSM. Cosmetically, ideal patients have B- or small C-cup breasts with centrally located nipples. Patients with a large amount of ptosis are not ideal candidates because the position of the nipple can be difficult to correct and the procedure may result in an undesired cosmetic outcome. Patients previously having radiation can have NSM but may have a higher risk for nipple and/or flap necrosis. All patients should be instructed that leaving the NAC intact is purely cosmetic because sensitivity and function is lost in most cases. Oncologically, ideal patients have tumors less than 2 cm located more than 2 cm from the nipple and areolar complex. Tumors more than 4 cm can involve the nipple in 23% to 100% of cases, and careful selection is required if considering an NSM in patients with a larger tumor burden. Attention to patient selection and applying these guidelines will reduce the likelihood of finding occult tumor cells in the nipple. Historic series have reported that tumors located within 2 cm of the nipple will involve the nipple in 36% to 87% of patients, whereas tumors more than 2 cm away from the nipple will involve the nipple in less than 14% of cases.[57–61] To predict nipple involvement, Rusby and colleagues[62] developed a nomogram. Although the nomogram is not widely used, importantly their data identified nipple involvement in 24% of patients, suggesting contingency plans for the nipple and areolar complex should be discussed with all patients before surgery.

## COMPLICATIONS OF NSM

Aside from LR and standard operative risks, nipple necrosis remains the primary risk of NSM, with total nipple necrosis occurring only rarely. Partial nipple necrosis occurs in approximately 10% of cases and is usually managed by conservative means.[63–65] Sometimes healing may take several weeks. Given that patients with NSM tend to have immediate reconstruction, the nipple and areolar complex can be positioned on the native pectoralis muscle in tissue expander reconstruction or on native tissues in autologous flap reconstruction helping to aid in the nipple's recovery.

## PM

Mastectomy performed using any of the previously mentioned techniques without a diagnosis of cancer constitutes a PM. As described earlier, recent trends witness a significant increase in PM despite declining rates of contralateral breast cancer around 0.5% annually or less.[17] PM reduces breast cancer risk by 90% to 95% in all cases and offers the largest absolute risk reduction in those women with BRCA mutations and a lifetime risk of breast cancer ranging from 50% to 80%. In general, patients should be informed that there is no medical indication or survival advantage in favor of PM.

## RECURRENCE AFTER MASTECTOMY

LR after mastectomy occurs in approximately 5% to 8% of early stage breast cancers,[42] with greater than 90% occurring within 3 years of surgery. LR is associated with stage at presentation, lymphovascular invasion, and tumor grade and is reduced by adjuvant therapy. Physical examination identifies most LR as palpable nodules in the skin and soft tissues. Rarely does LR occur in the muscle or behind a breast reconstruction. No surveillance imaging is necessary after mastectomy to evaluate for recurrence. When LR is identified, workup for distant metastatic disease should be performed because 20% to 30% of these women will present with simultaneous distant metastatic disease. Surgical excision to negative margins followed by radiation therapy remains the standard treatment modality in localized recurrences. This sequence achieves local control in 50% to 75% of patients. Occasionally, chemotherapy may be needed to facilitate surgery. Finally, investigators have evaluated the benefit of major chest wall resection (skin, muscle, ribs) in locally recurrent but advanced disease within the chest wall only and found significant morbidity with recurrence as high as 87% and 5-year overall survival of only 18% to 42%.[66,67]

## SUMMARY

- Mastectomy and breast conservation offer equivalent survival.
- The surgical goal is complete tumor removal.
- Most women with early stage breast cancers are amenable to breast-conserving surgery.
- Surgical therapy coupled with adjuvant systemic and radiation therapies reduce LR.

## REFERENCES

1. Fisher B, Jeong JH, Anderson S, et al. Twenty-five-year follow-up of a randomized trial comparing radical mastectomy, total mastectomy, and total mastectomy followed by irradiation. N Engl J Med 2002;347(8):567–75.
2. Fisher B, Anderson S, Bryant J, et al. Twenty-year follow-up of a randomized trial comparing total mastectomy, lumpectomy, and lumpectomy plus irradiation for the treatment of invasive breast cancer. N Engl J Med 2002;347(16):1233–41.
3. NIH Consensus Conference. Treatment of early-stage breast cancer. JAMA 1991; 265(3):391–5.
4. Available at: www.nccn.org.
5. Dang CM, Zaghiyan K, Karlan SR, et al. Increased use of MRI for breast cancer surveillance and staging is not associated with increased rate of mastectomy. Am Surg 2009;75(10):937–40.
6. Pettit K, Swatske ME, Gao F, et al. The impact of breast MRI on surgical decision-making: are patients at risk for mastectomy? J Surg Oncol 2009; 100(7):553–8.
7. McGuire KP, Santillan AA, Kaur P, et al. Are mastectomies on the rise? A 13-year trend analysis of the selection of mastectomy versus breast conservation therapy in 5865 patients. Ann Surg Oncol 2009;16(10):2682–90.
8. Arrington AK, Jarosek SL, Virnig BA, et al. Patient and surgeon characteristics associated with increased use of contralateral prophylactic mastectomy in patients with breast cancer. Ann Surg Oncol 2009;16(10):2697–704.
9. Katipamula R, Degnim AC, Hoskin T, et al. Trends in mastectomy rates at the Mayo Clinic Rochester: effect of surgical year and preoperative magnetic resonance imaging. J Clin Oncol 2009;27(25):4082–8.
10. Adkisson CD, Vallow LA, Kowalchik K, et al. Patient age and preoperative breast MRI in women with breast cancer: biopsy and surgical implications. Ann Surg Oncol 2011;18(6):1678–83.
11. Adkisson CD, Bagaria SP, Parker AS, et al. Which eligible breast conservation patients choose mastectomy in the setting of newly diagnosed breast cancer? Ann Surg Oncol 2012;19(4):1129–36.
12. Carpenter SG, Stucky CC, Dueck AC, et al. Scientific presentation award: the impact of magnetic resonance imaging on surgical treatment of invasive breast cancer. Am J Surg 2009;198(4):475–81.
13. Habermann EB, Abbott A, Parsons HM, et al. Are mastectomy rates really increasing in the United States? J Clin Oncol 2010;28(21):3437–41.
14. Garcia-Etienne CA, Tomatis M, Heil J, et al. Mastectomy trends for early-stage breast cancer: a report from the EUSOMA multi-institutional European database. Eur J Cancer 2012;48(13):1947–56.
15. Tuttle TM, Habermann EB, Grund EH, et al. Increasing use of contralateral prophylactic mastectomy for breast cancer patients: a trend toward more aggressive surgical treatment. J Clin Oncol 2007;25(33):5203–9.

16. King TA, Sakr R, Patil S, et al. Clinical management factors contribute to the decision for contralateral prophylactic mastectomy. J Clin Oncol 2011;29(16): 2158–64.

17. Nichols HB, Berrington de Gonzalez A, Lacey JV Jr, et al. Declining incidence of contralateral breast cancer in the United States from 1975 to 2006. J Clin Oncol 2011;29(12):1564–9.

18. Abbott A, Rueth N, Pappas-Varco S, et al. Perceptions of contralateral breast cancer: an overestimation of risk. Ann Surg Oncol 2011;18(11):3129–36.

19. Guth U, Myrick ME, Viehl CT, et al. Increasing rates of contralateral prophylactic mastectomy - a trend made in USA? Eur J Surg Oncol 2012;38(4):296–301.

20. Veronesi U, Volterrani F, Luini A, et al. Quadrantectomy versus lumpectomy for small size breast cancer. Eur J Cancer 1990;26(6):671–3.

21. Arentz C, Baxter K, Boneti C, et al. Ten-year experience with hematoma-directed ultrasound-guided (HUG) breast lumpectomy. Ann Surg Oncol 2010;17(Suppl 3): 378–83.

22. Van Esser S, Hobbelink M, Van der Ploeg IM, et al. Radio guided occult lesion localization (ROLL) for non-palpable invasive breast cancer. J Surg Oncol 2008;98(7):526–9.

23. Hughes JH, Mason MC, Gray RJ, et al. A multi-site validation trial of radioactive seed localization as an alternative to wire localization. Breast J 2008;14(2): 153–7.

24. McGhan LJ, McKeever SC, Pockaj BA, et al. Radioactive seed localization for nonpalpable breast lesions: review of 1,000 consecutive procedures at a single institution. Ann Surg Oncol 2011;18(11):3096–101.

25. Mendez JE, Lamorte WW, de Las Morenas A, et al. Influence of breast cancer margin assessment method on the rates of positive margins and residual carcinoma. Am J Surg 2006;192(4):538–40.

26. Wright MJ, Park J, Fey JV, et al. Perpendicular inked versus tangential shaved margins in breast-conserving surgery: does the method matter? J Am Coll Surg 2007;204(4):541–9.

27. Houssami N, Macaskill P, Marinovich ML, et al. Meta-analysis of the impact of surgical margins on local recurrence in women with early-stage invasive breast cancer treated with breast-conserving therapy. Eur J Cancer 2010;46(18): 3219–32.

28. McCahill LE, Single RM, Aiello Bowles EJ, et al. Variability in reexcision following breast conservation surgery. JAMA 2012;307(5):467–75.

29. Kearney TJ, Morrow M. Effect of reexcision on the success of breast-conserving surgery. Ann Surg Oncol 1995;2(4):303–7.

30. Bleicher RJ, Ciocca RM, Egleston BL, et al. Association of routine pretreatment magnetic resonance imaging with time to surgery, mastectomy rate, and margin status. J Am Coll Surg 2009;209(2):180–7 [quiz: 294–5].

31. Houssami N, Ciatto S, Macaskill P, et al. Accuracy and surgical impact of magnetic resonance imaging in breast cancer staging: systematic review and meta-analysis in detection of multifocal and multicentric cancer. J Clin Oncol 2008;26(19):3248–58.

32. Turnbull L, Brown S, Harvey I, et al. Comparative effectiveness of MRI in breast cancer (COMICE) trial: a randomised controlled trial. Lancet 2010;375(9714): 563–71.

33. Pengel KE, Loo CE, Teertstra HJ, et al. The impact of preoperative MRI on breast-conserving surgery of invasive cancer: a comparative cohort study. Breast Cancer Res Treat 2009;116(1):161–9.

34. Peters NH, van Esser S, van den Bosch MA, et al. Preoperative MRI and surgical management in patients with nonpalpable breast cancer: the MONET - randomised controlled trial. Eur J Cancer 2011;47(6):879–86.

35. Fischer U, Zachariae O, Baum F, et al. The influence of preoperative MRI of the breasts on recurrence rate in patients with breast cancer. Eur Radiol 2004; 14(10):1725–31.

36. Solin LJ, Orel SG, Hwang WT, et al. Relationship of breast magnetic resonance imaging to outcome after breast-conservation treatment with radiation for women with early-stage invasive breast carcinoma or ductal carcinoma in situ. J Clin Oncol 2008;26(3):386–91.

37. Sardanelli F, Giuseppetti GM, Panizza P, et al. Sensitivity of MRI versus mammography for detecting foci of multifocal, multicentric breast cancer in Fatty and dense breasts using the whole-breast pathologic examination as a gold standard. AJR Am J Roentgenol 2004;183(4):1149–57.

38. Wapnir IL, Anderson SJ, Mamounas EP, et al. Prognosis after ipsilateral breast tumor recurrence and locoregional recurrences in five National Surgical Adjuvant Breast and Bowel Project node-positive adjuvant breast cancer trials. J Clin Oncol 2006;24(13):2028–37.

39. Fisher B, Brown A, Mamounas E, et al. Effect of preoperative chemotherapy on local-regional disease in women with operable breast cancer: findings from National Surgical Adjuvant Breast and Bowel Project B-18. J Clin Oncol 1997; 15(7):2483–93.

40. Rastogi P, Anderson SJ, Bear HD, et al. Preoperative chemotherapy: updates of National Surgical Adjuvant Breast and Bowel Project Protocols B-18 and B-27. J Clin Oncol 2008;26(5):778–85.

41. Mieog JS, van der Hage JA, van de Velde CJ. Preoperative chemotherapy for women with operable breast cancer. Cochrane Database Syst Rev 2007;(2):CD005002.

42. Clarke M, Collins R, Darby S, et al. Effects of radiotherapy and of differences in the extent of surgery for early breast cancer on local recurrence and 15-year survival: an overview of the randomised trials. Lancet 2005;366(9503): 2087–106.

43. Darby S, McGale P, Correa C, et al. Effect of radiotherapy after breast-conserving surgery on 10-year recurrence and 15-year breast cancer death: meta-analysis of individual patient data for 10,801 women in 17 randomised trials. Lancet 2011; 378(9804):1707–16.

44. Dershaw DD, McCormick B, Osborne MP. Detection of local recurrence after conservative therapy for breast carcinoma. Cancer 1992;70(2):493–6.

45. Meyers MO, Klauber-Demore N, Ollila DW, et al. Impact of breast cancer molecular subtypes on locoregional recurrence in patients treated with neoadjuvant chemotherapy for locally advanced breast cancer. Ann Surg Oncol 2011; 18(10):2851–7.

46. Voduc KD, Cheang MC, Tyldesley S, et al. Breast cancer subtypes and the risk of local and regional relapse. J Clin Oncol 2010;28(10):1684–91.

47. Romond EH, Perez EA, Bryant J, et al. Trastuzumab plus adjuvant chemotherapy for operable HER2-positive breast cancer. N Engl J Med 2005; 353(16):1673–84.

48. Mamounas EP, Tang G, Fisher B, et al. Association between the 21-gene recurrence score assay and risk of locoregional recurrence in node-negative, estrogen receptor-positive breast cancer: results from NSABP B-14 and NSABP B-20. J Clin Oncol 2010;28(10):1677–83.

49. Salvadori B, Marubini E, Miceli R, et al. Reoperation for locally recurrent breast cancer in patients previously treated with conservative surgery. Br J Surg 1999; 86(1):84–7.

50. Galper S, Blood E, Gelman R, et al. Prognosis after local recurrence after conservative surgery and radiation for early-stage breast cancer. Int J Radiat Oncol Biol Phys 2005;61(2):348–57.

51. Anderson SJ, Wapnir I, Dignam JJ, et al. Prognosis after ipsilateral breast tumor recurrence and locoregional recurrences in patients treated by breast-conserving therapy in five National Surgical Adjuvant Breast and Bowel Project protocols of node-negative breast cancer. J Clin Oncol 2009;27(15):2466–73.

52. Toth BA, Lappert P. Modified skin incisions for mastectomy: the need for plastic surgical input in preoperative planning. Plast Reconstr Surg 1991;87(6): 1048–53.

53. Sotheran WJ, Rainsbury RM. Skin-sparing mastectomy in the UK–a review of current practice. Ann R Coll Surg Engl 2004;86(2):82–6.

54. Kinoshita S, Nojima K, Takeishi M, et al. Retrospective comparison of non-skin-sparing mastectomy and skin-sparing mastectomy with immediate breast reconstruction. Int J Surg Oncol 2011;2011:876520.

55. Freeman BS. Subcutaneous mastectomy for benign breast lesions with immediate or delayed prosthetic replacement. Plast Reconstr Surg Transplant Bull 1962;30:676–82.

56. Jabor MA, Shayani P, Collins DR, et al. Nipple-areola reconstruction: satisfaction and clinical determinants. Plast Reconstr Surg 2002;110(2):457–63.

57. Lagios MD, Gates EA, Westdahl PR, et al. A guide to the frequency of nipple involvement in breast cancer. A study of 149 consecutive mastectomies using a serial subgross and correlated radiographic technique. Am J Surg 1979; 138(1):135–42.

58. Luttges J, Kalbfleisch H, Prinz P. Nipple involvement and multicentricity in breast cancer. A study on whole organ sections. J Cancer Res Clin Oncol 1987;113(5): 481–7.

59. Morimoto T, Komaki K, Inui K, et al. Involvement of nipple and areola in early breast cancer. Cancer 1985;55(10):2459–63.

60. Simmons RM, Brennan M, Christos P, et al. Analysis of nipple/areolar involvement with mastectomy: can the areola be preserved? Ann Surg Oncol 2002;9(2):165–8.

61. Vyas JJ, Chinoy RF, Vaidya JS. Prediction of nipple and areola involvement in breast cancer. Eur J Surg Oncol 1998;24(1):15–6.

62. Rusby JE, Brachtel EF, Othus M, et al. Development and validation of a model predictive of occult nipple involvement in women undergoing mastectomy. Br J Surg 2008;95(11):1356–61.

63. Boneti C, Yuen J, Santiago C, et al. Oncologic safety of nipple skin-sparing or total skin-sparing mastectomies with immediate reconstruction. J Am Coll Surg 2011;212(4):686–93 [discussion: 93–5].

64. Kim HJ, Park EH, Lim WS, et al. Nipple areola skin-sparing mastectomy with immediate transverse rectus abdominis musculocutaneous flap reconstruction is an oncologically safe procedure: a single center study. Ann Surg 2010; 251(3):493–8.

65. Lanitis S, Tekkis PP, Sgourakis G, et al. Comparison of skin-sparing mastectomy versus non-skin-sparing mastectomy for breast cancer: a meta-analysis of observational studies. Ann Surg 2010;251(4):632–9.

66. Dahlstrom KK, Andersson AP, Andersen M, et al. Wide local excision of recurrent breast cancer in the thoracic wall. Cancer 1993;72(3):774–7.

67. Downey RJ, Rusch V, Hsu FI, et al. Chest wall resection for locally recurrent breast cancer: is it worthwhile? J Thorac Cardiovasc Surg 2000;119(3):420–8.

68. Jacobson JA, Danforth DN, Cowan KH, et al. Ten-year results of a comparison of conservation with mastectomy in the treatment of stage I and II breast cancer. N Engl J Med 1995;332(14):907–11.

69. van Dongen JA, Bartelink H, Fentiman IS, et al. Randomized clinical trial to assess the value of breast-conserving therapy in stage I and II breast cancer, EORTC 10801 trial. J Natl Cancer Inst Monogr 1992;(11):15–8.

70. Blichert-Toft M, Nielsen M, During M, et al. Long-term results of breast conserving surgery vs. mastectomy for early stage invasive breast cancer: 20-year follow-up of the Danish randomized DBCG-82TM protocol. Acta Oncol 2008;47(4):672–81.

71. Veronesi U, Cascinelli N, Mariani L, et al. Twenty-year follow-up of a randomized study comparing breast-conserving surgery with radical mastectomy for early breast cancer. N Engl J Med 2002;347(16):1227–32.

72. Sarrazin D, Le MG, Arriagada R, et al. Ten-year results of a randomized trial comparing a conservative treatment to mastectomy in early breast cancer. Radiother Oncol 1989;14(3):177–84.

73. Powles TJ, Hickish TF, Makris A, et al. Randomized trial of chemoendocrine therapy started before or after surgery for treatment of primary breast cancer. J Clin Oncol 1995;13(3):547–52.

74. van der Hage JA, van de Velde CJ, Julien JP, et al. Preoperative chemotherapy in primary operable breast cancer: results from the European Organization for Research and Treatment of Cancer trial 10902. J Clin Oncol 2001;19(22): 4224–37.

75. Yi M, Kronowitz SJ, Meric-Bernstam F, et al. Local, regional, and systemic recurrence rates in patients undergoing skin-sparing mastectomy compared with conventional mastectomy. Cancer 2011;117(5):916–24.

76. Gerber B, Krause A, Dieterich M, et al. The oncological safety of skin sparing mastectomy with conservation of the nipple-areola complex and autologous reconstruction: an extended follow-up study. Ann Surg 2009;249(3):461–8.

# Management of the Axilla

Barbara Zarebczan Dull, MD, Heather B. Neuman, MD, MS*

## KEYWORDS

- Sentinel lymph node • Axillary lymph node dissection • Breast cancer
- Micrometastases • ACOSOG Z0011

## KEY POINTS

- The disease status of the axilla in breast cancer remains one of the most important factors defining treatment and prognosis.
- The accuracy of SLN biopsy in staging the clinically node-negative axilla has been validated in prospective and randomized controlled trials. SLN should be considered the standard of care for patients without clinically evident axillary disease and patients with negative SLN can be spared the short- and long-term morbidity associated with ALND.
- Although micrometastases or isolated tumor cells may have a statistical association with prognosis, the clinical significance of these is uncertain. Currently, IHC should not be used to evaluate for micrometastases or isolated tumor cells in the SLN. The presence of isolated tumor cells should not be used to direct treatment decision-making.
- Controversies continue to exist regarding the use of SLN biopsies in patients who have undergone previous axillary surgery and those with multicentric breast cancer. Determining the optimal timing of SLN biopsy in patients undergoing neoadjuvant chemotherapy remains challenging.
- ACOSOG Z001 is a practice-changing trial that allows ALND to be avoided in select patients with positive SLNs undergoing breast conservation.

## INTRODUCTION

The status of the axillary lymph nodes is one of the most important factors impacting overall prognosis and treatment decision-making for breast cancer.[1] Axillary surgery has long been an integral part of breast cancer treatment to stage the axilla and provide locoregional control. Traditionally, this has been accomplished by performing a formal axillary lymph node dissection (ALND). However, ALND is now reserved for patients with a clinically positive axilla or positive lymph nodes confirmed on needle biopsy. In patients with a clinically negative axilla, a sentinel lymph node (SLN) biopsy can be performed safely at the time of mastectomy or lumpectomy, sparing patients the morbidity associated with ALND.

No financial disclosures.
Department of Surgery, University of Wisconsin School of Medicine and Public Health, 600 Highland Avenue, H4/726 CSC, Madison, WI 53792-7375, USA
* Corresponding author.
E-mail address: neuman@surgery.wisc.edu

## ADDRESSING THE CLINICALLY NEGATIVE AXILLA

### SLN Biopsy

The sentinel node is based on the concept that breast cancers drain to a single node or nodes, the sentinel nodes, before draining to more distal nodes. It was first described in 1977 by Cabanas[2] in work on penile carcinoma metastases. It was concluded that if the biopsied sentinel node is negative, the likelihood of additional lymph nodes being positive is low and further surgery is therefore not warranted. This concept was first applied to breast cancer in the early 1990s,[3,4] with the first multicenter validation study published in 1998.[5] Since that time, several prospective observational and randomized controlled trials have examined SLN biopsy in breast cancer,[6-9] leading to SLN biopsy being considered standard of care for evaluation of the axilla in patients with clinically node-negative breast cancer.

One of the earliest randomized trials examining the use of SLN biopsy was reported by Veronesi and colleagues[6] in 2003. They randomized 516 patients with breast cancer with tumors less than 2 cm in diameter to receive an SLN biopsy followed by routine ALND or SLN biopsy followed by an ALND only if the SLN contained metastases. The SLN was identified in 98.5% of patients with a sensitivity of 91.2%.[6] After 10 years of follow-up, no difference was observed between the groups for local axillary recurrence (0% in the SLN biopsy group vs 2% in the ALND group) or disease-free survival (89.9% vs 88.8%).[10]

Similar SLN identification, false-negative rates, and disease-free survival have since been demonstrated in several other large prospective and randomized controlled trials.[7-9,11] The largest include the prospective American College of Surgeons Oncology Group (ACOSOG) Z0010 trial[11] and the randomized National Surgical Adjuvant Breast and Bowel Project (NSABP) B-32 trial.[8] ACOSOG Z0010 is a multicenter, prospective observational study designed to examine the clinical significance of SLN micrometastases; this study also identified eligible patients for the randomized ACOSOG Z0011 trial (discussed later). Patients with T1 or T2 clinically node-negative breast cancer underwent SLN biopsy. A total of 198 surgeons participated in this trial. An SLN was identified in 98.7% of patients.[12] At a median follow-up of 3.1 years, the local recurrence rate (ie, the clinical false-negative rate) was 0.3%.[12]

Finally, the NSABP B-32 was a randomized controlled trial of 5611 patients from 80 academic and community centers in the United States and Canada that took place between 1999 and 2004[8]; 187 surgeons participated in the trial.[13] The objective was to compare locoregional recurrence, morbidity, and survival of SLN biopsy alone versus SLN followed by ALND. In this trial the rate of SLN identification was 97.3% and the false-negative rate was 9.8%; tumors in the lateral region of the breast, prior excisional biopsies, and removal of less than two SLN was associated with increased false-negative rates.[13] No difference in locoregional recurrence, overall survival, or disease-free survival was observed between the trial arms.[8]

These multicenter trials involving hundreds of academic and community surgeons demonstrate that SLN mapping can be performed accurately in patients with early stage breast cancer. Based on these data, SLN should be considered standard of care and patients with negative SLNs spared the morbidity of an ALND (**Table 1**).

### Technical Details

#### Blue dye versus radiocolloid tracer

No consensus exists regarding the optimal means of performing lymphoscintigraphy. However, most surgeons who perform lymphatic mapping report using blue dye and radiotracer. In a survey of the Fellows of the American College of Surgeons, 90% of

| Table 1 Accuracy of SLN biopsy | | | | | |
|---|---|---|---|---|---|
| | Veronesi et al[6] | Sentinella/GIVOM[7] | ALMANAC[9] | ACOSOG Z0010[12] | NSABP B-32[13] |
| Study design | RCT | RCT | RCT | Prospective | RCT |
| Year | 2003 | 2007 | 2006 | 2007 | 2010 |
| Patient enrollment | 516 | 697 | 991 | 5327 | 5611 |
| SLN identification | 98.5% | 95% | 98% | 98.7% | 97.3% |
| Sensitivity | 91.2% | 83.3% | 93.3% | NR | 90.2% |
| False-negative rate | 8.8% | 16.7% | 6.7% | 0.3%[a] | 9.8% |

[a] False-negative rate based on a median clinical follow-up of 31 months.

respondents stated that they used both methodologies.[14] Similarly, 79.4% of participating surgeons in the ACOSOG Z0010 Trial reported using both modalities, whereas 14.8% used blue dye and 5.7% only radiotracer.[12] No relationship between lymphoscintigraphy technique and the identification of an SLN has been observed in prospective or randomized trials.[15] Surgeon experience is the most important factor influencing successful SLN mapping.[12] In cases where an SLN cannot be identified, an ALND is the standard of care.

*Injection site*
Injection for lymphoscintigraphy can occur either subdermally around the areola or directly around the tumor. The concordance of the two injections sites was examined in a prospective study of 68 patients, reported in 1999 by Klimberg and colleagues.[16] Patients received an injection of technetium-99 sulfur colloid in the subareolar area of the breast, and an injection of isosulfan blue around the tumor. Four patients did not have an SLN identified; however, the SLNs in 62 of the 64 patients who had successful SLN identification were identified as hot and blue, suggesting that the site of injection has minimal impact on which lymph nodes are identified as the SLNs.[16] This observation was extended in a 2007 multicenter trial of 459 patients where the detection rate of SLNs was significantly higher in the patients undergoing periareolar injection compared with peritumoral injections.[17] Given these findings and the ease of a subareolar injection, this technique is favored by many surgeons.

*Morbidity*
One of the benefits of SLN biopsy is the decreased morbidity compared with ALND. However, complications do occur. Wound infections, seromas, paresthesias, lymphedema, and decreased shoulder abduction have all been reported in the literature after SLN biopsy (**Table 2**).

Wound infection is uncommon after SLN biopsy.[9,19,20,22] Results from ACOSOG Z0010/11 demonstrated a wound infection rate of 1% (only 0.1% requiring readmission for treatment with intravenous antibiotics).[19] Seroma formation after SLN biopsy is similarly uncommon.[19,22–25] Patients in the ACOSOG Z0010 trial had a 7.1% incidence of seroma formation, with only 0.4% necessitating drain placement for treatment.[19] This trial identified increasing age, removal of greater than or equal to five lymph nodes, and use of radiocolloid-only mapping technique to be associated with increased risk of seroma formation.[19]

Another common morbidity is arm paresthesias in the form of numbness and tingling. Although much of the early postoperative paresthesias resolve, some persist

**Table 2**
**Morbidity after SLN biopsy compared with ALND**

| Morbidity | Veronesi et al[6a] | | Sentinella/ GIVOM[18a] | | ALMANAC[9b] | | ACOSOG Z0010/ 11[19,20c] | | NSABP B-32[21a] | |
|---|---|---|---|---|---|---|---|---|---|---|
| | SLN | ALND | SLN | ALND | SLN | ALND | SLN | ALND | SLN | ALND |
| Wound infection | NR | NR | NR | NR | 11% | 15% | 1% | 8% | NR | NR |
| Seroma | NR | NR | NR | NR | NR | NR | 7.1% | 14% | NR | NR |
| Paresthesias | 1% | 68% | 7% | 15% | 11% | 31% | 9% | 44% | 10% | 36% |
| Lymphedema | 0% | 12% | 4% | 8% | 5%[d] | 13%[d] | 7% | 11% | 8% | 14% |

Abbreviation: NR, not reported.
[a] Morbidity data at 24 months.
[b] Morbidity data at 12 months.
[c] Morbidity data at 6 months.
[d] Subjective rate of lymphedema presented.

as long as 24 months.[6,18,21] At 24 months postoperative, 9.9% of patients in the NSABP B-32 trial reported numbness, whereas 9.2% reported residual tingling.[21] This contrasts with the study by Veronesi and colleagues,[6] where only 1% of SLN patients reported persistent paresthesias. The varying rates of paresthesias are likely caused by the subjective nature of patient self-reporting, but demonstrate that for patients this may significantly impact quality of life.

Lymphedema is one of the most feared complications after axillary surgery. Early studies reported a 0% incidence of lymphedema after SLN biopsy.[6,25] However, larger trials including ACOSOG Z0010 and NSABP B-32 (which used objective measurements of arm circumference) have demonstrated rates of lymphedema after SLN biopsy of 7% and 9%, respectively.[19,21] Multivariate analysis performed on the data from ACOSOG Z0010 found that increasing age and body mass index were significantly associated with development of lymphedema.[19]

It is not uncommon for patients to have decreased shoulder range of motion after axillary surgery secondary to postoperative pain. The NSABP B-32 trial found that 41% of patients had deficits in shoulder abduction 1 week postoperatively. However, most resolve and by 6 months only 6% of patients reported decreased shoulder abduction.[21] These results are similar to those reported by the Sentinel Node Biopsy versus Axillary Clearance and the Sentinella-GIVOM trials.[18,26]

Finally, an uncommon, but potentially life-threatening complication that can occur during SLN biopsy is an allergic reaction to isosulfan blue dye. Reactions can range from a mild rash or blue hives to more serious anaphylaxis. The NSABP-32 trial reported an incidence of 0.4% for mild grade I and II allergic reactions and 0.2% of more severe grade III and IV reactions, such as anaphylaxis and cardiac or respiratory arrest.[13]

## Indications

Based on these and other trials, the current recommendations from the American Society of Clinical Oncology state that SLN biopsy is indicated in T1 and T2 tumors without clinical involvement of the axilla.[27] These indications are in accordance with the 2010 American Society of Breast Surgeons guidelines for performing SLN biopsy with the addition that SLN biopsy be performed in patients undergoing a mastectomy for ductal carcinoma in situ (DCIS).[28]

## Contraindications

Although SLN biopsy is a well-established alternative to ALND in T1 and T2 breast cancers, several contraindications to performing the procedure exist. Palpable axillary lymph nodes are an absolute contraindication to SLN biopsy and these patients should be offered an ALND if metastatic disease is confirmed. Large T4 tumors and inflammatory breast cancer are also considered contraindications to SLN biopsy because tumor deposits may decrease the reliability of lymphatic mapping.

Because isosulfan and lymphazurine blue dye have not been proved to be safe in pregnancy, SLN localization using dye is contraindicated in pregnant women.[29] There are also limited data regarding the risk of radiotracer to an unborn fetus. A recent study demonstrated that fetal exposure to radiolabeled colloid during SLN biopsy is less than 0.3% of the Nuclear Regulatory Commission guideline for limitations during pregnancy.[30] Although use of radiotracer is probably safe in pregnancy, data are limited and pregnancy, therefore, is considered a relative contraindication to SLN biopsy.[29,31]

## Areas of Ongoing Controversy

### Ductal carcinoma in situ

Patients with DCIS do not undergo routine examination of the axillary lymph nodes because, by definition, DCIS has little to no metastatic potential. However, studies have demonstrated that certain DCIS patients at high-risk for microinvasive disease may benefit from an SLN biopsy.[32,33] In a 2000 study by Klauber-DeMore and colleagues,[32] it was found that 12% of their 76 patients with high-risk DCIS had metastatic disease in the SLN. Similar findings were reported in 2006 by Goyal and colleagues[33] using the Breast Test Wales database. In their series, 38% of the 587 patients with DCIS were found to have invasive disease on final pathology. Axillary nodal staging was performed in 269 patients, with nodal metastases in 13%. In both studies, presence of a palpable or imaging-identified mass was associated with upstaging to invasive cancer.

Because of the risk of upstaging at the time of surgery, SLN biopsy should be considered in any patient with DCIS undergoing mastectomy. Furthermore, in patients undergoing lumpectomy in whom there is increased suspicion that microinvasive or invasive carcinoma will be identified, consideration of an SLN biopsy at the time of their breast surgery is reasonable.

### Prior axillary surgery

Prior axillary surgery is a relative contraindication to SLN biopsy because lymphatic drainage may be disrupted, theoretically leading to an inability to identify an SLN or an increased false-negative rate. The largest study examining this has been published from the Memorial Sloan-Kettering Cancer Center (MSKCC), looking at their experience with 117 patients with breast cancer undergoing reoperative SLN after either a prior SLN biopsy or an ALND.[34] The SLN was successfully identified in 55% of patients. Likelihood of successful mapping was higher after a previous SLN biopsy (74%) than an ALND (38%). Of the 63 patients with successful mapping, 30% (N = 19) had a nonaxillary drainage site identified; 8 had ipsilateral axillary drainage in addition to a second site, whereas 11 had only nonaxillary drainage. At a median 2.2 years of follow-up, no axillary recurrences were observed. The authors concluded that an SLN can be identified in most patients who have had prior axillary surgery, albeit it at a lower rate than for initial SLN biopsies. However, further research is needed to define the true false-negative rate given the limited follow-up.

### Multicentric breast disease

There has been concern that multiple tumors within the breast may drain to different SLNs, making an SLN biopsy unreliable. Several retrospective studies have addressed this question and found the SLN identification rate to exceed 95%.[35–37] False-negative rate (confirmed by back-up ALND) was 8.8% in a retrospective review of the ALMANAC trial[38] and 8% in a large single institution study.[36] Two other single-institution studies have reported their clinical axillary recurrence for patients with multi-centric cancer and negative SLN's.[35,37] An axillary recurrence rate of 0% was reported in a study of 142 patients at a median follow-up of 28.8 months,[35] and a rate of 2.2% at 5-years in a study of 337 patients.[37] Although these retrospective studies suggest that SLN could be an alternative to ALND in patients with multicentric breast cancer, larger prospective patient studies with longer follow-up are needed to confirm the efficacy of SLN biopsy in this setting.

### T3 or T4 tumors

Limited prospective data exist to support the accuracy of SLN biopsy in patients with large primary tumors. Several retrospective studies examining this question have found the SLN identification rate to be more than 97%.[39–41] The false-negative rate (confirmed in most cases by completion ALND after SLN) was 3%. These favorable findings need to be interpreted in the context of the overall tumor burden for patients with larger breast tumors, where 62.5% to 76.7% of patients have metastases in the SLN.[39–41]

### Management of Positive SLNs

ALND has been the standard of care for patients with a positive SLN. Recent research, however, has questioned whether all patients with a positive SLN require a completion ALND. In patients with clinically node-negative disease, the SLN is the only involved node in 40% to 60% of patients, which raises the question as to whether ALND offers additional therapeutic benefit for all patients.[24,42]

This question was addressed prospectively in the ASOCOG Z0011 trial.[43] Patients with T1 and T2 tumors undergoing lumpectomy who were found to have metastatic disease in the SLNs were randomized to undergo either completion axillary dissection or no further treatment of the axilla.[43] All patients were required to have negative margins in the breast excision, and went on to have whole-breast irradiation. Low-volume nodal disease was required, with all eligible patients having less than three positive nodes and no gross extranodal disease. Adjuvant treatment was per the primary team, with 96% receiving chemotherapy and 47% endocrine therapy. The trial closed early because of low accrual and events rates, reaching only 47% of its accrual goals (891 patients enrolled). Median follow-up for the evaluable patients was 6.3 years. At 5 years, the local recurrence rate was 1.6% in the SLN biopsy group compared with 3.1% in the ALND arm.[44] There was also no difference in 5-year disease-free survival (89.9% vs 88.8%).[43] The authors concluded that for select patients with node-positive breast cancer and low-volume axillary disease, an SLN biopsy alone does not result in inferior survival or inadequate local control.

This trial's eligibility criteria apply to a very select group of patients: women with low-volume breast and axillary disease undergoing lumpectomy with radiation. It is likely that some of the low axillary lymph nodes were covered by the radiation fields and therefore received treatment; this specific question is currently being examined by the study investigators. Additionally, most women received systemic therapy (either chemotherapy, endocrine therapy, or both), which impacts local recurrence and over-all survival. Finally, approximately 40% of patients had only micrometastases in the SLN, emphasizing the low-volume axillary disease that was included in this trial.

Although the data cannot be widely generalized to all patients with breast cancer, this study should be considered a practice-changing trial for the subset of women with positive SLNs undergoing breast conservation.

## Micrometastatic Disease

Controversy also exists regarding the significance of isolated tumor cells and micrometastases found on SLN biopsies. The enhanced pathologic assessment associated with the SLN biopsy has resulted in the identification of increasingly small deposits of metastatic disease and subsequent upstaging of cancer. The American Joint Committee on Cancer staging system has changed to reflect this and includes three categories of nodal metastases: (1) isolated tumor cells (no cluster greater than <0.2 mm, pN0[i+]); (2) micrometastases (0.2–2 mm, pN1mi); and (3) macrometastases (>2 mm).[31] However, the clinical significance of these very small metastatic deposits is uncertain. The Dutch Micrometastases and Isolated Tumor Cells: Relevant and Robust or Rubbish (MIRROR) trial was a retrospective analysis of 2756 patient who underwent an SLN biopsy before 2006 and were found to have isolated tumor cells or micrometastases in the regional lymph nodes.[45] They compared outcomes for 856 patients with node-negative disease and no systemic therapy with patients with isolated tumor cells or micrometastases who did (N = 995) and did not (N = 856) receive systemic therapy. Disease-free survival was poorer in patients with either isolated tumor cells or micrometastases in the SLN (76.5% vs 85.7%; $P<.001$), suggesting these small tumor deposits have some prognostic significance.[45] However, this study included contralateral breast cancer in the definition of a disease "event" (accounting for 29% of events). Because development of contralateral breast cancer is unlikely to be related to the presence of micrometastatic axillary disease, this definition makes these findings difficult to interpret.

ACOSOG Z0010[11] and the NSABP B-032[46] trials examined the significance of occult metastases in the SLN. In ACOSOG Z0010, routine immunohistochemistry was performed on SLN specimens to increase identification of isolated tumor cells and micrometastases. In this study, no difference in 5-year overall (95.7% vs 95.1%) or disease-free (92.2% vs 90.4%) survival was observed between patients with node-negative versus IHC-positive SLNs.[11] Similarly, NSABP-B32 performed IHC staining in all SLNs found to be negative on initial processing.[46] No difference in overall or disease-free survival was observed in patients with IHC-detected metastases versus true-negative SLNs.

Although the Dutch MIRROR study suggests that some prognostic significance may be associated with isolated tumor cells or micrometastatic disease,[45] this has not been confirmed in large prospectively collected data. No role for the routine use of IHC staining for breast cancer SLNs exists and the presence of IHC-detected SLN metastases should not guide treatment decision-making.[47]

## ADDRESSING THE CLINICALLY POSITIVE AXILLA
### Axillary Lymph Node Dissection

### Indications

ALND is indicated in patients with clinically positive axillary lymph nodes and those that are found to be positive on needle biopsy. Completion ALND for positive SLNs, including micrometastases, is also currently recommended by the American Society of Clinical Oncology guidelines.[27] ALND is the first-line surgical treatment in cases in which SLN biopsy is contraindicated, such as large primary tumors and inflammatory breast cancer.

## Complications

Multiple studies have demonstrated that the rate of various immediate- and long-term complications is significantly increased after ALND compared with SLN biopsy (see **Table 2**).[20,21,48] The more extensive dissection required during an ALND leads to increased rates of wound infection, seroma formation, and lymphedema compared with SLN biopsy.[20,49,50]

Wound infection rates from 8% to 15% have been reported in randomized controlled trials.[20,51] Postoperative seromas are also relatively common, identified in a recent meta-analysis as the most common complication after ALND.[52] Seromas were identified in 14% of patients undergoing ALND in ACOSOG Z0011.[20]

In performing a thorough ALND, the surgeon often has to sacrifice sensory nerves that cross the axilla, specifically the intercostobrachial nerve. Subsequently, postoperative paresthesias are common. A report by Roses and colleagues[53] found that 76.5% of their 200 patients who underwent ALND reported paresthesias, with only 22% achieving full resolution after 1 year of follow-up. These rates of sensory deficits are similar to those reported in studies by Purushotham and coworkers and Veronesi and coworkers, which reported 1-year rates of 65% and 68%, respectively.[6,54] More recent trials, such as the ALMANAC, ACOSOG Z0011, and NSABP B-32 trials, have demonstrated a self-reported rate of paresthesias of 31%, 39%, and 44.6% after ALND.[9,20,21,55] These paresthesias may be permanent.

Lymphedema is one of the most commonly recognized lifelong complications following ALND. The rates among studies and trials vary widely (6%–70%) depending on whether the lymphedema is self-reported or objective measurements of the arm are performed.[21,53,56–58] Lymphedema most commonly develops within the first year of surgery, but may develop as long as 20 years after surgery.[56,59] The extent of axillary surgery, postoperative wound infection, and postoperative axillary radiation have all been found to increase risk of lymphedema.[50,56,60–63]

Range of motion deficits can occur as a result of ALND. In the NSABP B-32 trial, 75% of patients reported difficulties with shoulder abduction after ALND in the immediate postoperative period; this decreased to only 9% by 6 months.[21] These findings are similar to those of the ALMANAC trial.[9]

## OVERALL AREAS OF CONTROVERSY
### Neoadjuvant Chemotherapy and Timing of SLN Biopsy

Neoadjuvant chemotherapy is an accepted initial treatment of patients with large breast cancers who wish to undergo breast conservation and for those with locally advanced breast cancer.[64] Down-staging of the tumor occurs in most patients, with 26% to 50% achieving a pathologic complete response to neoadjuvant chemotherapy.[65–69] Because this response occurs in the primary tumor and the nodal basin, it makes the timing of SLN mapping for patients undergoing neoadjuvant chemotherapy controversial.

The pros and cons of preneoadjuvant versus postneoadjuvant chemotherapy SLN biopsy are listed in **Table 3**. The greatest benefit to performing SLN biopsy before neoadjuvant chemotherapy is to allow for accurate staging of the axilla at the time of diagnosis. This information provides not only prognostic information, but can be used to inform decisions for adjuvant radiation. However, this approach requires patients to undergo two separate surgical procedures and, if the pretreatment SLN if found to be positive, commits them to an ALND regardless of their response to neoadjuvant therapy. In contrast, postneoadjuvant SLN biopsy accounts for patients' response to chemotherapy and theoretically can spare patients with a good response

**Table 3**
**Pros and cons of preneoadjuvant and postneoadjuvant chemotherapy SLN biopsy**

| Preneoadjuvant SLN Biopsy | Postneoadjuvant SLN Biopsy |
|---|---|
| *Pros* | |
| Accurate staging of the axilla at initial diagnosis | Direct additional treatment based on response to chemotherapy |
| Provide prognostic information by documenting response to treatment | Identify patients with response to chemotherapy that can be spared an ALND |
| Increase ability to inform adjuvant radiation therapy decisions | |
| *Cons* | |
| Commit patients to ALND regardless of response to neoadjuvant therapy | Uncertainty regarding initial nodal status (loss of prognostic information) |
| Requires two surgical procedures | Higher false-negative rate |
| Complications of SLN biopsy may delay chemotherapy | Increased rates of mapping failure |
| Delayed ALND may be technically more difficult | Chemotherapy may make SLN biopsy technically more difficult |

an ALND. However, lower rates of SLN identification and increased false-negative rates[70] make the accuracy of postneoadjuvant therapy SLN biopsy uncertain.

ACOSOG Z1071, a prospective multi-institution phase II study designed to validate the postneoadjuvant chemotherapy SLN false-negative rate in patients who presented with pathologically confirmed axillary lymph nodes, has completed accrual and results are pending.[71] Until these results are available, the merits of preneoadjuvant and postneoadjuvant chemotherapy SLN biopsy should be considered when making decisions for SLN timing for an individual patient.

## FUTURE DIRECTIONS
### AMAROS Trial

Axillary radiation therapy has been evaluated as an alternative to ALND. Previous small studies have demonstrated low axillary recurrence and no difference in survival in patients with clinically negative lymph nodes.[72–74] The After Mapping of the Axilla: Radiotherapy or Surgery? (AMAROS) study is a prospective, randomized control comparing ALND with axillary radiation therapy in patients with early breast cancer with positive SLNs.[75] The trial began accruing patients in 2001 and completed accrual in April of 2010. The results of this study have not yet been published, but the results may change the management of axillary lymph node metastases.

### Endoscopic Axillary Surgery

To decrease the morbidity of SLN biopsy and ALND, the concept of endoscopic axillary surgery has been introduced. Few studies have demonstrated significant benefits of endoscopic axillary surgery when compared with traditional operative techniques. In one of the first studies to evaluate this technique, Kuehn and colleagues[76] published a study of 53 patients undergoing endoscopic ALND. In this study they found that postoperative seroma formation and lymphedema were not significantly reduced compared with conventional surgery, but operative time was greatly increased. In a similar prospective study by Langer and colleagues,[77] a 15% rate of seroma formation requiring drainage was reported and 4% of patients developed port site metastases. A more recent study reported decreased drainage and operative blood loss with endoscopic axillary dissection, but found that the number of lymph nodes removed was significantly lower than with ALND.[78] Based on these and other studies, the risks of port site metastases and missed axillary lymph nodes outweigh the benefits of endoscopic axillary surgery.

### Axillary Reverse Mapping

The concept of axillary reverse mapping (ARM) is based on the hypothesis that the lymphatic channels draining the breast are different from those draining the upper arm.[79] Therefore, if the upper arm lymphatics can be mapped and visualized during an ALND, they then can be preserved thereby minimizing lymphedema. In one of the first studies describing ARM, Thompson and colleagues[80] successfully identified blue lymphatics draining the upper arm in 61% of patients. They removed the ARM nodes in 64% of patients in which they could be identified and found them to be negative for breast cancer. Similar results were found by Nos and colleagues,[81] with identification of ARM nodes in 71% of their patient population. A 2009 study by Klimberg and colleagues[82] was the first to demonstrate that lymphedema may be reduced by preserving the ARM nodes. This study included 220 patients and found that in 2.8% of patients the SLN shared a common lymphatic channel with the ARM lymphatics and 40.6% of patients had ARM lymphatics adjacent to the SLN, which were at high risk of injury. Overall, at 6-month follow-up, no patients in whom the ARM nodes were preserved had lymphedema. Additional prospective randomized trials need to be performed to validate the true impact of ARM on minimizing the development of lymphedema.

### Use of Axillary Ultrasound

In the absence of clinically palpable lymph nodes, ultrasound of the axilla has been found to be a useful adjunct in determining preoperatively which patients may have axillary metastases. Established criteria for evaluating a lymph node as suspicious for malignancy include cortical thickening greater than 3 mm; absence of the fatty hilum; and presence of nonhilar blood flow (increased vascularity).[83–86] Suspicious lymph nodes can then be biopsied before surgery, facilitating surgical planning. Sensitivity rates of axillary ultrasound with needle biopsy have been reported to range from 20% to 80%[87] and varies based on the population evaluated. Based on these data, the American Society of Breast Surgeons recommends that preoperative axillary ultrasound be performed if the surgeon or radiologist has experience in performing the study, thereby increasing the cost effectiveness of SLN biopsy.[28]

### Nomograms

To determine which patients may benefit from further axillary surgery after the identification of a positive SLN, researchers at several institutions have developed nomograms to calculate the likelihood of additional non-SLNs being positive.[88–90] One of the first nomograms was developed at MSKCC and uses tumor size, type, and grade, number of positive and negative SLNs, method of detection of those SLNs, and estrogen receptor status in determining the risk of additional positive non-SLNs.[88] The most recent nomogram from MD Anderson Cancer Center includes many of the variables in the MSKCC nomogram, but additionally included the size of SLN metastases.[91] Based on this research, nomograms can be used to inform patient discussion as to whether to proceed with completion ALND, but should not be the only determining factor.

**REFERENCES**

1. Fisher B, Bauer M, Wickerham DL, et al. Relation of number of positive axillary nodes to the prognosis of patients with primary breast cancer. An NSABP update. Cancer 1983;52:1551–7.
2. Cabanas RM. An approach for the treatment of penile carcinoma. Cancer 1977; 39:456–66.
3. Giuliano AE, Dale PS, Turner RR, et al. Improved axillary staging of breast cancer with sentinel lymphadenectomy. Ann Surg 1995;222:394–9 [discussion: 399–401].
4. Krag DN, Weaver DL, Alex JC, et al. Surgical resection and radiolocalization of the sentinel lymph node in breast cancer using a gamma probe. Surg Oncol 1993;2:335–9 [discussion: 40].
5. Krag D, Weaver D, Ashikaga T, et al. The sentinel node in breast cancer–a multi-center validation study. N Engl J Med 1998;339:941–6.
6. Veronesi U, Paganelli G, Viale G, et al. A randomized comparison of sentinel-node biopsy with routine axillary dissection in breast cancer. N Engl J Med 2003;349:546–53.
7. Zavagno G, De Salvo GL, Scalco G, et al. A randomized clinical trial on sentinel lymph node biopsy versus axillary lymph node dissection in breast cancer: results of the Sentinella/GIVOM trial. Ann Surg 2008;247:207–13.
8. Krag DN, Anderson SJ, Julian TB, et al. Sentinel-lymph-node resection compared with conventional axillary-lymph-node dissection in clinically node-negative patients with breast cancer: overall survival findings from the NSABP B-32 rand-omised phase 3 trial. Lancet Oncol 2010;11:927–33.
9. Mansel RE, Fallowfield L, Kissin M, et al. Randomized multicenter trial of sentinel node biopsy versus standard axillary treatment in operable breast cancer: the ALMANAC Trial. J Natl Cancer Inst 2006;98:599–609.
10. Veronesi U, Viale G, Paganelli G, et al. Sentinel lymph node biopsy in breast cancer: ten-year results of a randomized controlled study. Ann Surg 2010;251: 595–600.
11. Giuliano AE, Hawes D, Ballman KV, et al. Association of occult metastases in sentinel lymph nodes and bone marrow with survival among women with early-stage invasive breast cancer. JAMA 2011;306:385–93.
12. Posther KE, McCall LM, Blumencranz PW, et al. Sentinel node skills verification and surgeon performance: data from a multicenter clinical trial for early-stage breast cancer. Ann Surg 2005;242:593–9 [discussion: 599–602].
13. Krag DN, Anderson SJ, Julian TB, et al. Technical outcomes of sentinel-lymph-node resection and conventional axillary-lymph-node dissection in patients with clinically node-negative breast cancer: results from the NSABP B-32 randomised phase III trial. Lancet Oncol 2007;8:881–8.
14. Lucci A, Kelemen PR, Miller C, et al. National practice patterns of sentinel lymph node dissection for breast carcinoma. J Am Coll Surg 2001;192:453–8.
15. Morrow M, Rademaker AW, Bethke KP, et al. Learning sentinel node biopsy: results of a prospective randomized trial of two techniques. Surgery 1999;126: 714–20 [discussion: 720–2].
16. Klimberg VS, Rubio IT, Henry R, et al. Subareolar versus peritumoral injection for location of the sentinel lymph node. Ann Surg 1999;229:860–4 [discussion: 4–5].
17. Rodier JF, Velten M, Wilt M, et al. Prospective multicentric randomized study comparing periareolar and peritumoral injection of radiotracer and blue dye for the detection of sentinel lymph node in breast sparing procedures: FRANSENODE trial. J Clin Oncol 2007;25:3664–9.

18. Del Bianco P, Zavagno G, Burelli P, et al. Morbidity comparison of sentinel lymph node biopsy versus conventional axillary lymph node dissection for breast cancer patients: results of the sentinella-GIVOM Italian randomised clinical trial. Eur J Surg Oncol 2008;34:508–13.

19. Wilke LG, McCall LM, Posther KE, et al. Surgical complications associated with sentinel lymph node biopsy: results from a prospective international cooperative group trial. Ann Surg Oncol 2006;13:491–500.

20. Lucci A, McCall LM, Beitsch PD, et al. Surgical complications associated with sentinel lymph node dissection (SLND) plus axillary lymph node dissection compared with SLND alone in the American College of Surgeons Oncology Group Trial Z0011. J Clin Oncol 2007;25:3657–63.

21. Ashikaga T, Krag DN, Land SR, et al. Morbidity results from the NSABP B-32 trial comparing sentinel lymph node dissection versus axillary dissection. J Surg Oncol 2010;102:111–8.

22. Wernicke AG, Shamis M, Sidhu KK, et al. Complication rates in patients with negative axillary nodes 10 years after local breast radiotherapy after either sentinel lymph node dissection or axillary clearance. Am J Clin Oncol 2013;36(1):12–9.

23. Burak WE, Goodman PS, Young DC, et al. Seroma formation following axillary dissection for breast cancer: risk factors and lack of influence of bovine thrombin. J Surg Oncol 1997;64:27–31.

24. Giuliano AE, Haigh PI, Brennan MB, et al. Prospective observational study of sentinel lymphadenectomy without further axillary dissection in patients with sentinel node-negative breast cancer. J Clin Oncol 2000;18:2553–9.

25. Schrenk P, Rieger R, Shamiyeh A, et al. Morbidity following sentinel lymph node biopsy versus axillary lymph node dissection for patients with breast carcinoma. Cancer 2000;88:608–14.

26. Gill G, SNAC Trial Group of the Royal Australasian College of Surgeons (RACS) and NHMRC Clinical Trials Centre. Sentinel-lymph-node-based management or routine axillary clearance? One-year outcomes of sentinel node biopsy versus axillary clearance (SNAC): a randomized controlled surgical trial. Ann Surg Oncol 2009;16:266–75.

27. Lyman GH, Giuliano AE, Somerfield MR, et al. American Society of Clinical Oncology guideline recommendations for sentinel lymph node biopsy in early-stage breast cancer. J Clin Oncol 2005;23:7703–20.

28. American Society of Breast Surgeons guidelines for performing sentinel lymph node biopsy in breast cancer. 2010. Available at: https://www.breastsurgeons.org/statements/2010-Nov-05_Guidelines_on_Performing_SLN.pdf. Accessed July 10, 2012.

29. Krontiras H, Bland KI. When is sentinel node biopsy for breast cancer contraindicated? Surg Oncol 2003;12:207–10.

30. Pandit-Taskar N, Dauer LT, Montgomery L, et al. Organ and fetal absorbed dose estimates from 99mTc-sulfur colloid lymphoscintigraphy and sentinel node localization in breast cancer patients. J Nucl Med 2006;47:1202–8.

31. Wiatrek R, Kruper L. Sentinel lymph node biopsy indications and controversies in breast cancer. Maturitas 2011;69:7–10.

32. Klauber-DeMore N, Tan LK, Liberman L, et al. Sentinel lymph node biopsy: is it indicated in patients with high-risk ductal carcinoma-in-situ and ductal carcinoma-in-situ with microinvasion? Ann Surg Oncol 2000;7:636–42.

33. Goyal A, Douglas-Jones A, Monypenny I, et al. Is there a role of sentinel lymph node biopsy in ductal carcinoma in situ?: analysis of 587 cases. Breast Cancer Res Treat 2006;98:311–4.

34. Port ER, Garcia-Etienne CA, Park J, et al. Reoperative sentinel lymph node biopsy: a new frontier in the management of ipsilateral breast tumor recurrence. Ann Surg Oncol 2007;14:2209–14.
35. Knauer M, Konstantiniuk P, Haid A, et al. Multicentric breast cancer: a new indication for sentinel node biopsy: a multi-institutional validation study. J Clin Oncol 2006;24:3374–80.
36. Tousimis E, Van Zee KJ, Fey JV, et al. The accuracy of sentinel lymph node biopsy in multicentric and multifocal invasive breast cancers. J Am Coll Surg 2003;197: 529–35.
37. Gentilini O, Veronesi P, Botteri E, et al. Sentinel lymph node biopsy in multicentric breast cancer: five-year results in a large series from a single institution. Ann Surg Oncol 2011;18:2879–84.
38. Goyal A, Newcombe RG, Mansel RE, et al. Sentinel lymph node biopsy in patients with multifocal breast cancer. Eur J Surg Oncol 2004;30:475–9.
39. Chung MH, Ye W, Giuliano AE. Role for sentinel lymph node dissection in the management of large (> or = 5 cm) invasive breast cancer. Ann Surg Oncol 2001;8:688–92.
40. Wong SL, Chao C, Edwards MJ, et al. Accuracy of sentinel lymph node biopsy for patients with T2 and T3 breast cancers. Am Surg 2001;67:522–6 [discussion: 7–8].
41. Bedrosian I, Reynolds C, Mick R, et al. Accuracy of sentinel lymph node biopsy in patients with large primary breast tumors. Cancer 2000;88:2540–5.
42. Albertini JJ, Lyman GH, Cox C, et al. Lymphatic mapping and sentinel node biopsy in the patient with breast cancer. JAMA 1996;276:1818–22.
43. Giuliano AE, Hunt KK, Ballman KV, et al. Axillary dissection vs no axillary dissection in women with invasive breast cancer and sentinel node metastasis: a randomized clinical trial. JAMA 2011;305:569–75.
44. Giuliano AE, McCall L, Beitsch P, et al. Locoregional recurrence after sentinel lymph node dissection with or without axillary dissection in patients with sentinel lymph node metastases: the American College of Surgeons Oncology Group Z0011 randomized trial. Ann Surg 2010;252:426–32 [discussion: 32–3].
45. de Boer M, van Deurzen CH, van Dijck JA, et al. Micrometastases or isolated tumor cells and the outcome of breast cancer. N Engl J Med 2009;361:653–63.
46. Weaver DL, Ashikaga T, Krag DN, et al. Effect of occult metastases on survival in node-negative breast cancer. N Engl J Med 2011;364:412–21.
47. American Society of Breast Surgeons position statement on management of the axilla in patients with invasive breast cancer. 2011. Available at: https://www.breastsurgeons.org/statements/PDF_Statements/Axillary_Management.pdf. Accessed July 6, 2012.
48. Land SR, Kopec JA, Julian TB, et al. Patient-reported outcomes in sentinel node-negative adjuvant breast cancer patients receiving sentinel-node biopsy or axillary dissection: National Surgical Adjuvant Breast and Bowel Project phase III protocol B-32. J Clin Oncol 2010;28:3929–36.
49. Montgomery LL, Thorne AC, Van Zee KJ, et al. Isosulfan blue dye reactions during sentinel lymph node mapping for breast cancer. Anesth Analg 2002;95: 385–8, table of contents.
50. Soran A, D'Angelo G, Begovic M, et al. Breast cancer-related lymphedema: what are the significant predictors and how they affect the severity of lymphedema? Breast J 2006;12:536–43.
51. Goyal A, Newcombe RG, Chhabra A, et al. Morbidity in breast cancer patients with sentinel node metastases undergoing delayed axillary lymph node

dissection (ALND) compared with immediate ALND. Ann Surg Oncol 2008;15: 262–7.

52. van Bemmel AJ, van de Velde CJ, Schmitz RF, et al. Prevention of seroma formation after axillary dissection in breast cancer: a systematic review. Eur J Surg Oncol 2011;37:829–35.

53. Roses DF, Brooks AD, Harris MN, et al. Complications of level I and II axillary dissection in the treatment of carcinoma of the breast. Ann Surg 1999;230: 194–201.

54. Purushotham AD, Upponi S, Klevesath MB, et al. Morbidity after sentinel lymph node biopsy in primary breast cancer: results from a randomized controlled trial. J Clin Oncol 2005;23:4312–21.

55. Fleissig A, Fallowfield LJ, Langridge CI, et al. Post-operative arm morbidity and quality of life. Results of the ALMANAC randomised trial comparing sentinel node biopsy with standard axillary treatment in the management of patients with early breast cancer. Breast Cancer Res Treat 2006;95:279–93.

56. Petrek JA, Senie RT, Peters M, et al. Lymphedema in a cohort of breast carcinoma survivors 20 years after diagnosis. Cancer 2001;92:1368–77.

57. McLaughlin SA, Wright MJ, Morris KT, et al. Prevalence of lymphedema in women with breast cancer 5 years after sentinel lymph node biopsy or axillary dissection: patient perceptions and precautionary behaviors. J Clin Oncol 2008;26:5220–6.

58. McLaughlin SA, Wright MJ, Morris KT, et al. Prevalence of lymphedema in women with breast cancer 5 years after sentinel lymph node biopsy or axillary dissection: objective measurements. J Clin Oncol 2008;26:5213–9.

59. Herd-Smith A, Russo A, Muraca MG, et al. Prognostic factors for lymphedema after primary treatment of breast carcinoma. Cancer 2001;92:1783–7.

60. Liljegren G, Holmberg L. Arm morbidity after sector resection and axillary dissection with or without postoperative radiotherapy in breast cancer stage I. Results from a randomised trial. Uppsala-Orebro Breast Cancer Study Group. Eur J Cancer 1997;33:193–9.

61. Erickson VS, Pearson ML, Ganz PA, et al. Arm edema in breast cancer patients. J Natl Cancer Inst 2001;93:96–111.

62. Paskett ED, Naughton MJ, McCoy TP, et al. The epidemiology of arm and hand swelling in premenopausal breast cancer survivors. Cancer Epidemiol Biomarkers Prev 2007;16:775–82.

63. Kiel KD, Rademacker AW. Early-stage breast cancer: arm edema after wide excision and breast irradiation. Radiology 1996;198:279–83.

64. Neuman H, Ollila D. Sentinel lymph node biopsy controversy: before or after chemotherapy. Curr Breast Cancer Rep 2009;1(2):71–7.

65. Gianni L, Eiermann W, Semiglazov V, et al. Neoadjuvant chemotherapy with trastuzumab followed by adjuvant trastuzumab versus neoadjuvant chemotherapy alone, in patients with HER2-positive locally advanced breast cancer (the NOAH trial): a randomised controlled superiority trial with a parallel HER2-negative cohort. Lancet 2010;375:377–84.

66. Fisher B, Bryant J, Wolmark N, et al. Effect of preoperative chemotherapy on the outcome of women with operable breast cancer. J Clin Oncol 1998;16: 2672–85.

67. Wolmark N, Wang J, Mamounas E, et al. Preoperative chemotherapy in patients with operable breast cancer: nine-year results from National Surgical Adjuvant Breast and Bowel Project B-18. J Natl Cancer Inst Monogr 2001;(30):96–102.

68. Mauri D, Pavlidis N, Ioannidis JP. Neoadjuvant versus adjuvant systemic treatment in breast cancer: a meta-analysis. J Natl Cancer Inst 2005;97:188–94.

69. van der Hage JA, van de Velde CJ, Julien JP, et al. Preoperative chemotherapy in primary operable breast cancer: results from the European Organization for Research and Treatment of Cancer trial 10902. J Clin Oncol 2001;19:4224–37.

70. Mamounas EP, Brown A, Anderson S, et al. Sentinel node biopsy after neoadjuvant chemotherapy in breast cancer: results from National Surgical Adjuvant Breast and Bowel Project Protocol B-27. J Clin Oncol 2005;23:2694–702.

71. Hunt KK, Le-Petross HT, Suman V, et al. A phase II study evaluating the role of sentinel lymph node surgery and axillary lymph node dissection following preoperative chemotherapy in women with node-positive breast cancer (T1-4, N1-2, M0) at initial diagnosis: ACOSOG Z1071. J Clin Oncol 2010;28:15s.

72. Fisher B, Jeong JH, Anderson S, et al. Twenty-five-year follow-up of a randomized trial comparing radical mastectomy, total mastectomy, and total mastectomy followed by irradiation. N Engl J Med 2002;347:567–75.

73. Spruit PH, Siesling S, Elferink MA, et al. Regional radiotherapy versus an axillary lymph node dissection after lumpectomy: a safe alternative for an axillary lymph node dissection in a clinically uninvolved axilla in breast cancer. A case control study with 10 years follow up. Radiat Oncol 2007;2:40.

74. Hwang RF, Gonzalez-Angulo AM, Yi M, et al. Low locoregional failure rates in selected breast cancer patients with tumor-positive sentinel lymph nodes who do not undergo completion axillary dissection. Cancer 2007;110:723–30.

75. Straver ME, Meijnen P, van Tienhoven G, et al. Sentinel node identification rate and nodal involvement in the EORTC 10981-22023 AMAROS trial. Ann Surg Oncol 2010;17:1854–61.

76. Kuehn T, Santjohanser C, Grab D, et al. Endoscopic axillary surgery in breast cancer. Br J Surg 2001;88:698–703.

77. Langer I, Kocher T, Guller U, et al. Long-term outcomes of breast cancer patients after endoscopic axillary lymph node dissection: a prospective analysis of 52 patients. Breast Cancer Res Treat 2005;90:85–91.

78. Hussein O, El-Nahhas W, El-Saed A, et al. Video-assisted axillary surgery for cancer: non-randomized comparison with conventional techniques. Breast 2007;16:513–9.

79. Ponzone R, Mininanni P, Cassina E, et al. Axillary reverse mapping in breast cancer: can we spare what we find? Ann Surg Oncol 2008;15:390–1 [author reply: 2–3].

80. Thompson M, Korourian S, Henry-Tillman R, et al. Axillary reverse mapping (ARM): a new concept to identify and enhance lymphatic preservation. Ann Surg Oncol 2007;14:1890–5.

81. Nos C, Lesieur B, Clough KB, et al. Blue dye injection in the arm in order to conserve the lymphatic drainage of the arm in breast cancer patients requiring an axillary dissection. Ann Surg Oncol 2007;14:2490–6.

82. Boneti C, Korourian S, Diaz Z, et al. Scientific Impact Award: axillary reverse mapping (ARM) to identify and protect lymphatics draining the arm during axillary lymphadenectomy. Am J Surg 2009;198:482–7.

83. Vassallo P, Wernecke K, Roos N, et al. Differentiation of benign from malignant superficial lymphadenopathy: the role of high-resolution US. Radiology 1992; 183:215–20.

84. Deurloo EE, Tanis PJ, Gilhuijs KG, et al. Reduction in the number of sentinel lymph node procedures by preoperative ultrasonography of the axilla in breast cancer. Eur J Cancer 2003;39:1068–73.

85. Abe H, Schmidt RA, Kulkarni K, et al. Axillary lymph nodes suspicious for breast cancer metastasis: sampling with US-guided 14-gauge core-needle biopsy–clinical experience in 100 patients. Radiology 2009;250:41–9.

86. Yang WT, Metreweli C, Lam PK, et al. Benign and malignant breast masses and axillary nodes: evaluation with echo-enhanced color power Doppler US. Radiology 2001;220:795–802.

87. Houssami N, Ciatto S, Turner RM, et al. Preoperative ultrasound-guided needle biopsy of axillary nodes in invasive breast cancer: meta-analysis of its accuracy and utility in staging the axilla. Ann Surg 2011;254(2):243–51.

88. Van Zee KJ, Manasseh DM, Bevilacqua JL, et al. A nomogram for predicting the likelihood of additional nodal metastases in breast cancer patients with a positive sentinel node biopsy. Ann Surg Oncol 2003;10:1140–51.

89. Kohrt HE, Olshen RA, Bermas HR, et al. New models and online calculator for predicting non-sentinel lymph node status in sentinel lymph node positive breast cancer patients. BMC Cancer 2008;8:66.

90. Unal B, Gur AS, Ahrendt G, et al. Can nomograms predict non-sentinel lymph node metastasis after neoadjuvant chemotherapy in sentinel lymph node-positive breast cancer patients? Clin Breast Cancer 2009;9:92–5.

91. Mittendorf EA, Hunt KK, Boughey JC, et al. Incorporation of sentinel lymph node metastasis size into a nomogram predicting nonsentinel lymph node involvement in breast cancer patients with a positive sentinel lymph node. Ann Surg 2012;255: 109–15.

# Breast Reconstruction

Frank J. DellaCroce, MD[a],*, Emily T. Wolfe, MD[b]

## KEYWORDS

- Breast reconstruction • Mastectomy • Breast implant
- Superior gluteal artery perforator flap • Lumpectomy
- Deep inferior epigastric perforator flap • Breast cancer

## KEY POINTS

- A collaborative approach within the diagnostic, oncologic, and surgical team with the reconstructive specialist is essential to develop a treatment plan that optimizes the patient's care from the very beginning.
- Only 33% of women who are otherwise candidates for immediate reconstruction at the time of mastectomy choose reconstruction.
- The type of mastectomy the patient undergoes directly influences the reconstructive outcome and aesthetics.
- Careful handling of the skin, gentle retraction, pristine dissection between the gland and the overlying subcutaneous fat layer, minimized cautery settings, and an understanding of the associated thermal plume are essential to reliably healthy skin flaps.

## INTRODUCTION

An estimated 300,000 women are affected by breast cancer every year in the United States, and another 2.6 million are living posttreatment. As diagnostic technology has progressed and the understanding of the disease process has evolved, the number of mastectomies performed in the United States has increased. Breast reconstructive techniques have commensurately become more sophisticated along the same timeline. The result is that those facing mastectomy have the potential to simultaneously retain physical beauty and wholeness. Despite these advances, only 33% of women who are otherwise candidates for immediate reconstruction at the time of mastectomy choose reconstruction. The 2 reasons most attributed to this remarkable statistic are failure of the treatment team to refer the patient to a plastic surgeon at the time of diagnosis/decision for mastectomy and the resultant lack of understanding on the patient's part regarding her reconstructive options.

Disclosures: None.
[a] Department of Plastic Surgery, Center for Restorative Breast Surgery, 1717 Saint Charles Avenue, New Orleans, LA 70130, USA; [b] Department of Surgery, Ochsner Health Care System, 1514 Jefferson Highway, Jefferson, LA 70121, USA
* Corresponding author.
E-mail address: drd@breastcenter.com

Surg Clin N Am 93 (2013) 445–454
http://dx.doi.org/10.1016/j.suc.2012.12.004
0039-6109/13/$ – see front matter © 2013 Elsevier Inc. All rights reserved.

A collaborative approach within the diagnostic, oncologic, and surgical team with the reconstructive specialist is essential to develop a treatment plan that optimizes the patient's care from the very beginning. One facet of this team-based mindset is the mastectomy itself. Where will the incision be placed? What portion of the breast skin will be preserved? Will we reconstruct at the time of mastectomy or not? Will we preserve the nipple-areolar complex?

The type of mastectomy the patient undergoes will directly influence her reconstructive outcome and aesthetics. Mastectomy planning has become a surgical art in this regard. This procedure begins with incision placement. The convention of large horizontal incisions has become archaic in centers that use team-based planning before mastectomy. Incision placement that allows adequate exposure for mastectomy and simultaneous maximized reconstructive outcome may vary from vertical incision from nipple to fold, lateral incision from nipple to flank, straight, serpentine, fold hidden, and anywhere in between. The rule is complete preservation of the skin envelope in all but those with advanced disease or tumor cells near the skin surface. Even in these cases, the design may be carried out in a way that preserves peripheral landmarks in the breast and avoids a large medial extension that would otherwise be visible in drop-neck clothing. Basic considerations, such as preservation of the inframammary fold are a given, but the surgical oncologist must approach the breast skin as though it were a facelift. Careful handling of the skin, gentle retraction, pristine dissection between the gland and the overlying subcutaneous fat layer, minimized cautery settings, and an understanding of the associated thermal plume are essential to reliably healthy skin flaps. Perhaps even more important within these considerations is the avoidance of dissection beyond the peripheral boundaries of the breast because the medial and lateral intercostal blood flow is critical to meaningful perfusion of preserved breast skin.

Nipple-sparing mastectomy is a concept in evolution and one more level of sophistication with respect to mastectomy planning. For those who are candidates, this approach further elevates the standard, allowing outcomes that reach toward an "untouched" look after mastectomy. These concepts push the reconstructive result and in many cases, can produce a superior aesthetic to "breast preservation" (lumpectomy) protocols.

Tissue expander/implant reconstruction remains the most common form of reconstruction because of quicker recovery potential, avoidance of donor site morbidity, ease of procedure for the operating surgeon, and resultant wide availability. The implant or expander is placed beneath the pectoralis muscle to camouflage its upper pole and help protect the overlying skin. Acellular dermal matrix may be used to complete this pocket and further support the implant position and add thickness to the lower pole coverage.

Concerns with tissue expander/implant reconstruction include capsular contracture, infection, deflation, and the need for resultant additional surgery.

Autologous reconstruction allows one to use the patient's own tissue to reconstruct her breast. The pedicled transverse rectus abdominis myocutaneous (TRAM) flap, developed over 30 years ago, was the most significant step forward in autologous reconstruction. At present, autologous tissue breast reconstruction has evolved allowing free tissue transplantation to recreate the breast. These techniques no longer require use or loss of the rectus or other musculature and may be taken from any place on the body where musculo/fascio cutaneous perforating vascular pedicles enter overlying fat.

Most commonly, the abdomen is the source of tissue for autologous reconstruction with several options including pedicled TRAM, free TRAM, or deep inferior epigastric perforator (DIEP) flaps. Other options include gluteal artery perforator (GAP) flaps, latissimus flaps, and transverse gracilis (TUG) flaps. Considerations with autologous tissue reconstruction include donor site morbidity, increased complexity of the procedure, longer operative times, an added 2 days hospitalization (on average), and less widespread availability.

## BACKGROUND

Breast cancer affects 1 in 8 women in the United States. Often, the treatment plan includes mastectomy, which may offer a chance for cure, but has a tradeoff of scars and disfigurement. Modern breast reconstruction allows women facing mastectomy not only to avoid disfigurement but also, in many cases, to achieve an outcome that may enhance the beauty of the breast and the overall body shape. Breast reconstruction helps these women retain their femininity, physical wholeness, and emotional sense of well-being.[1] Reconstruction is an important part of the healing process; it avoids leaving an injured look as a consequence of treatment and thereby occupies an integral place in the overall treatment strategy for breast cancer.

There has been an increase in the number of mastectomies in the United States for a variety of reasons. The advent of genetic testing for *BRCA1* and *BRCA2* allows women with a genetic predisposition to breast cancer to understand their risk and address it should they choose. Women with *BRCA1* mutation have a 65% chance of developing breast cancer by the age of 70 years, and women with *BRCA2* have a 45% risk.[2] In addition, many women are electing prophylactic mastectomies whether it is for genetic reasons or for their own personal cancer history and the associated desire to reduce the chance of experiencing breast cancer for a second time.[3] Prophylactic mastectomy has been demonstrated to be an effective strategy to minimize the risk of developing breast cancer in patients with high-risk genetic profiles.[4] Add to this, the improvements made in diagnostic imaging, a better understanding of multifocal disease patterns, and improvements in reconstructive techniques that restore a lost breast in the same operation and the reasons for an increased number of mastectomies recommended becomes more clear.

There has been much progress and evolution in the techniques used to provide the patient with an aesthetic result indistinguishable from the natural breast. The ultimate goal of reconstruction is symmetry between the native breast and the newly reconstructed breast or symmetry between 2 newly created breasts. The art of breast reconstruction has undergone significant evolution over the past 20 years.

Because the goal of breast reconstruction is creating a natural appearing and symmetric outcome, the surgeon must consider the size of the reconstructed breast. The plastic surgeon must make an estimate of the volume that will be required to reconstitute the breast shape and projection when mastectomy is complete. The surgeon may weigh the removed breast tissue and the tissue used for reconstruction to help achieve symmetry during the operation, but the reconstructive plan must be fully developed before entering the operative suite. To achieve symmetry in a unilateral reconstruction, the opposing breast may need to be altered with mastopexy, implant addition, or reduction. The Federal Women's Health and Cancer Right Act of 1998 states that surgery performed to produce a symmetric or balanced appearance must be covered by insurance if they offer coverage for the mastectomy.

Patients have multiple options for reconstruction including alloplastic techniques such as tissue expanders/implants or autologous reconstruction and the many variations that are found within each of these 2 major approaches. The choice of reconstruction is largely dependent on the dialogue between the patients and their plastic surgeon. Immediate reconstruction should be considered the standard. Delayed reconstruction may be more appropriate for patients with advanced disease or patients not committed to the process. Many patients will present to the plastic surgeon well informed on the various options, and it should be the goal of the surgeon to direct them in a way best suited for their particular situation. It is the job of the diagnostic and oncologic team to provide information and referral to a plastic surgeon for in-depth discussion of their options before mastectomy so that outcomes may be optimized.

## MASTECTOMY

Reconstruction begins with the mastectomy. The incision placement and portion of skin/nipple-areolar complex that are preserved determine, in large part, how natural the new breast will look. The traditional mastectomy and the modified radical mastectomy involve removal of an ellipse of skin including the nipple-areolar complex, with a horizontal pattern that extends the scar into the medial breast leaving a visible signature in all but the most carefully chosen apparel. This approach remains commonly used, even though it is rarely the best choice from an aesthetic standpoint. The skin-sparing mastectomy preserves the skin envelope of the breast with a more limited incision that typically involves removal of the nipple/areola. The nipple-sparing mastectomy allows for preservation of not only the breast skin but also the nipple/areola with an incision placed vertically, laterally, or in the inframammary fold. Careful handling of the skin, gentle retraction, pristine dissection between the gland and the overlying subcutaneous fat layer, minimized cautery settings, and an understanding of the associated thermal plume are essential to reliably healthy skin flaps. Avoidance of dissection beyond the peripheral boundaries of the breast is also critical because the medial and lateral intercostal blood flow is imperative if skin necrosis is to be avoided.

## ALLOPLASTIC RECONSTRUCTION
### History

The silicone breast implant was introduced in 1961 by Thomas Cronin and Frank Gerow. This implant was intended to be used only for breast augmentation, but eventually its use in breast reconstruction evolved. Modern implants are filled with either silicone or saline, and most reconstructive surgeons prefer silicone because they tend to have a more natural overall texture. Saline implants typically have more palpable wrinkling particularly in the lower pole of the breast. Implants are placed beneath the pectoralis major with or without completing the submuscular pocket with a sheet of collagen (Alloderm [Lifecell Corporation, Bridgewater, NJ, USA], Allomax [Davol, a BARD Company, Warwick, RI, USA], Stratus [Lifecell Corporation, Bridgewater, NJ, USA], etc).

Tissue expanders are used when skin has been excised during the mastectomy to an extent that closure of the skin over the desired implant is not possible. Expanders may also be used in an immediate reconstruction when the reconstructive surgeon is concerned about the vitality of the skin after mastectomy. The skin is subsequently expanded postoperatively, and once an adequate pocket is developed, it is exchanged to a definitive implant in a separate procedure. Implant reconstruction remains more common than autologous reconstruction based on 2008 statistics by the American Society of Plastic Surgeons.[5] This fact may be attributed to a shorter recovery potential compared with flap procedures, avoidance of donor site morbidity, technical simplicity for the operating surgeon, and resultant wide availability.

### Advantages/Disadvantages

Tissue expander/implant reconstruction is less complex than autologous reconstruction and does not carry donor site morbidity potential. This procedure offers surgical simplicity for the operative team with a reduced operative time and a more rapid recovery. Modern flap techniques allow for solutions in the thin patient, so implants are not the only choice in that scenario. Women with smaller breast size tend to heal more uneventfully after implant reconstruction than those with large breasts.

Complications after implant reconstruction can occur. Use of an artificial device under a compromised skin covering opens the potential for extrusion and infection. If a wound forms in the skin over an implant, it may need to be removed for a period to allow the soft tissue to recover before further attempts at reconstruction are undertaken. In addition, aesthetic results may be compromised by capsular contracture and implant failure, possibly prompting implant exchange.[6] Other-less appealing facets of implant reconstruction include frequent clinic visits for expansion followed by a second surgery to replace the expander with the implant. It may be more difficult to match the ptosis and pliability of a natural breast when a one-sided implant reconstruction has been performed as well. Implant reconstruction is generally not considered for patients who will or have previously undergone radiation therapy because the soft tissue fibrosis limits the outcome potential and increases the rate of capsular contracture dramatically. It has been found that there is a higher patient aesthetic satisfaction rate with autologous reconstruction compared with implant reconstruction.[7]

### Acellular Dermal Matrix

It is preferable to perform implant reconstruction at the time of the mastectomy. This timing offers the benefit of a preserved skin envelope without the need for expansion in those undergoing skin-sparing mastectomy. Expansion may be a painful process, and limiting the need for a subsequent exchange from an expander to an implant is an important benefit. The "straight to implant" or "dermal-matrix-assisted implant" reconstruction is used for women with healthy preserved skin envelopes with no need for skin expansion. The implant is placed at the time of the mastectomy in a subpectoral pocket that is completed from the lower border of the pectoralis to the inframammary fold with a sheet of acellular collagen matrix. This procedure avoids the need for expander placement and the associated painful fill sessions in the clinic and allows the patient to sidestep an exchange procedure. The dermal sheeting allows the implant to be supported with respect to positioning in the breast pocket and provides a layer of thickness that helps camouflage the implant's palpability.[8,9] When a tissue expander is placed, it is serially inflated over several weeks and then replaced by the definitive implant at a second surgery.

### Surgery

The mastectomy is performed with gentle technique, preserving the peripheral boundaries of the breast and the associated blood supply to the skin. The implant is then placed beneath muscle to add coverage for the implant and soften the appearance of the upper pole. Attempts at complete muscular coverage by elevating the serratus anterior as well as placing the expander beneath these muscles has largely been supplanted by adding a sheet of dermal matrix from the pectoralis down to the inframammary fold. The pocket should never be dissected too medially or cross the midline. Drains are typically left in the axilla and mastectomy space.

When tissue expansion is required, the process begins 2 to 3 weeks postoperatively with injection of approximately 50–100 mL of sterile saline every 1 to 2 weeks until the desired volume is reached. Tissue expanders have been shaped anatomically to expand the lower pole of the breast to create a natural ptosis. About 1 to 2 months after the final expansion, the expander should be exchanged for the implant, which may require capsulectomy for the desired cosmesis to be achieved.

### Acellular dermal matrix

Acellular dermal matrix is basically a sheet of collagen with intervening cellular content. In breast reconstruction, it is used as a soft tissue replacement to cover the tissue expander or implant. Acellular dermal matrix is used to maintain the implant position and inframammary fold height and offers better overall control of the implant.[9] This matrix compartmentalizes the implant and helps to improve aesthetic outcomes.

### Complications

Common complications of tissue expander/implant reconstruction are infection, capsular contraction, skin flap necrosis, and deflation. Infection can result in implant loss. It has been suggested that use of acellular dermal matrices may have a higher rate of infection, although this is disputed.[10] Infections need to be aggressively treated with antibiotics, but they typically require removal of the implant to eliminate the infective process. Capsular contraction rates may be decreased by using textured implants and may increase in patients who require radiotherapy. Skin flap necrosis may result in full-thickness excision of eschar prompting additional surgery to achieve good cosmesis. Patients should be counseled that implants are not to be considered lifetime devices and that they may need to be replaced for leakage or other problems at some point.[11] The cosmetic outcome of implants seems to deteriorate over time, resulting in less-satisfied patients at 5 years as opposed to 2 years postoperatively.[12]

## AUTOLOGOUS RECONSTRUCTION
### Background

Autologous reconstruction offers some distinct benefits over alloplastic reconstruction for women with breast cancer. Most importantly, it allows the patient to use her own tissue, which is as close a replacement for breast tissue as modern technology provides. Free tissue transfer was first used in 1976 by Fujino.[13] The pedicled TRAM flap used by Hartrampf[14] in 1982 was the most significant step toward producing an aesthetic result indistinguishable from the nature breast. This step was followed by free perforator flaps that were originally pioneered in Japan in 1989 by Koshima.[15] These flaps have reduced donor site morbidity compared with TRAM and latissimus flaps because they do not sacrifice the underlying muscle. Currently, there are many techniques available for use in autologous reconstruction, and the decision of which type to use should be based on the patients' anatomy and the surgeons' experience with the particular methods.

### Types of Flaps

Flaps may be musculocutaneous containing both the vascularized muscle with the overlying fat and skin. The flaps may be used as pedicled flaps, where they are transposed into position with the vascular supply intact, or as free flaps, where the vascular supply from the donor tissue is anastomosed to the internal mammary or the thoracodorsal vessels. The perforator-free flaps are based on the same vascular supply but spare the underlying muscle to decrease donor site morbidity.

Pedicled TRAM flaps have served as the basis of today's autologous reconstruction. The flap is composed of an ellipse of skin and subcutaneous tissue with the rectus muscle. The vascular supply comes from the superior epigastric vessels. The flap is rotated into the breast pocket with the rectus attached at the costal margin. One or both rectus muscles may be used depending on the volume of tissue required. Pedicled TRAM flaps have a higher partial flap loss rate than any other flap option. The design flaw results from the fact that there must be a reversal of flow through "choke vessels" in the rectus abdominus; in addition, there is potential for kinking or compression of the pedicle at the subcostal rotation point. Blood flow insufficiency in a pedicled TRAM flap may be addressed by "supercharging" the flap with an extra microvascular anastomosis from its distal pedicle to the thoracodorsal or internal mammary system. The blood supply may also be augmented by using a preliminary delay procedure, where the inferior epigastric vessels are ligated before the reconstruction, causing the superior epigastric vessels to dilate due to the hypoperfusion. The free version of this flap detaches the tissue from the lower abdomen and insets it into the mastectomy site with anastomosis of the vessels.

The latissimus dorsi flap, which is also a pedicled flap, is tunneled through the axilla leaving the thoracodorsal artery and vein intact as the vascular pedicle. The flap itself does not usually have adequate volume to serve as the reconstruction alone. Many times it is combined with an implant or tissue expander to provide the volume and projection needed to create an aesthetically pleasing reconstruction. These flaps may also be used in patients to repair defects created by lumpectomy and radiation therapy or in cases of partial tissue loss from previous autologous tissue reconstruction.

Multiple free flaps have been developed to reconstruct the breast after mastectomy. The abdomen is the first choice for autologous breast reconstruction. The DIEP is based on the deep inferior epigastric system that penetrates the rectus abdominus and its fascia. These vessels provide the vascular pedicle for the flap without sacrificing the rectus abdominus or requiring mesh placement in the abdomen as is required with the TRAM flap. The incision placement is aesthetically favorable, and usually the soft tissue volume is adequate. The superficial inferior epigastric artery (SIEA) flap uses the same fatty abdominal tissue with reliance on the superficial inferior epigastric pedicle for its vascular supply. Occasionally, the flow from the SIEA may be more robust than its deep counterpart. The SIEA is used as an alternative to the deep inferior epigastric artery when the perforators of the deep artery are judged to be of insufficient size or the deep artery cannot be used because of previous surgeries. The superficial artery is usually much smaller in caliber and more tortuous, making its anastomosis to recipient vessels and inset of the flap more difficult.

Patients who do not have enough abdominal tissue or have had prior abdominoplasty or other prohibitive surgery may be candidates for GAP flaps. These flaps evolved as a refinement of the gluteal myocutaneous flap first described by Fujino in 1975.[16] These flaps were originally used for the management of sacral pressure sore.[17] There is typically a substantial amount of fatty tissue even in very thin patients, and the avoidance of the gluteal muscle decreases morbidity and shortens recovery time. This flap may be based on the superior or the inferior gluteal artery. The inferior flap is not used as often because of the additional dissection required around the sciatic nerve and the potential morbidity associated with this. More importantly, taking fat from the lower buttock can defat weight-bearing surfaces and square of the gluteal shape leaving a masculine appearance. Historically, this flap has been regarded as more technically complex because of the delicate nature of the pedicle dissection. For experienced microsurgeons, this procedure serves as a powerful second option when the abdominal tissue is not available.[18]

Additional options for the thin patient include the stacked DIEP free flap. This procedure allows 2 independent flaps to be linked to one another and layered into the breast reconstruction site. The technique although technically demanding, is reproducible and safe for patients seeking autologous breast reconstruction with otherwise inadequate abdominal adipose tissue.[19]

When bilateral reconstruction is necessary in a thin patient, the stacked abdomen/hip flap allows for a DIEP flap to be layered with a GAP flap for patients with inadequate volume in the abdominal and gluteal donor regions.[20]

### Advantages/Disadvantages

Advantages include a natural texture and appearance to the new breast. Once healed, flap procedures are considered a lifetime solution compared with implants, which may require maintenance surgeries over time. The operative time may be longer, and longer hospital stays are required, but the payoff of long-term result durability often outweighs these issues. Musculocutaneous flaps have the additional disadvantage of donor site morbidity including weakness and potential for abdominal contour bulges and/or overt hernia. The need for mesh placement in the abdominal donor site also reduces the appeal of the TRAM flap compared with the DIEP flap.

### Contraindications

Patients who have had procedures that may have injured the vessels that perforate the rectus sheath such as abdominoplasty are not candidates for DIEP or SIEA flaps. Abdominal procedures such as hysterectomy, appendectomy, laparoscopic cholecystectomy, and cesarean deliveries are not contraindications. Smoking, although not an overt contraindication, is prone to cause wound healing delays, and patients should discontinue their habit at least 3 weeks before surgery.[21] In addition, patients who are morbidly obese or have diabetes need close postoperative follow-up because their healing particularly in the donor site may be slow.

### Surgery

#### TRAM

There are 2 dominant vascular pedicles in the TRAM flap: the superior and the inferior epigastric arteries. The pedicled TRAM flap relies on the superior vessel, whereas the free TRAM flap relies on the inferior epigastric arteries. The harvest of the flap is approached the same in both flaps with the dissection of a transverse skin flap down to the fascia. The anterior rectus fascia is entered, which exposes the rectus muscle, and the vascular pedicle of interest is dissected. For the pedicled TRAM flap, the lower rectus is transected and tunneled subcutaneously to the chest wall defect leaving the superior portion anchored to the costal margin. The free TRAM flap completely transects the lower rectus abdominus, and the inferior epigastric vessels are anastomoses to the internal mammary or thoracodorsal vessels using microsurgical technique.

#### DIEP flap

The harvest of the free flap is similar to that of the TRAM flap. The skin is marked with an elliptical incision, and harvest begins along the lower half of the arc to identify and inspect the SIEA and veins to determine if the superficial system is more dominant. Next, the upper arc of the incision is completed and the flap is elevated in a plane superficial to the fascia. The lateral row of perforators is encountered. If it is well developed, it is used as the supplying vasculature; otherwise the medial perforators are used. The dissection then continues to the deep inferior epigastric trunk through a fascial incision. The muscle is gently teased away from the pedicle, and then the flap is harvested via ligation and transection of the pedicle at its proximal origin point. The fascial incision is then closed followed by the abdominal wound. The internal mammary vessels or the thoracodorsal vessels are then exposed and prepared, and the microvascular anastomosis is completed. The flap is then contoured and inset to create the new breast mound. The nipple and areolar reconstruction is completed in the following weeks in those who have not undergone nipple-sparing mastectomy.

### Superior gluteal artery perforator flap (SGAP)
The patient is initially placed in the prone position, and the perimeter of the flap is defined with electrocautery. The superficial fascia of the gluteus maximus is incised, and perforators are identified in the subfasical plane. The dominant perforators are chosen and followed through the muscle and the deep gluteal fascia to reach the larger vessels in the subgluteal fat pad where they emerge from the sacral formina. The superior GAP flap chosen is then ligated and transected. The flaps are harvested and passed off the field, and donor sites are closed. The patient is then returned to the supine position, and the flaps are contoured and deepithelialized followed by completion of the microvascular anastomosis to the internal mammary vessels. The flaps are then inset, and nipple-areolar complex reconstruction takes place in the following weeks along with recontouring of the donor site to produce a smooth and aesthetically proper gluteal shape.

### Nipple-areolar complex
Typically, the nipple-areolar complex is created 3 to 4 months after the initial reconstruction. The complex may be recreated in a variety of manners with the most common being local skin flap rearrangement followed by tattooing.

### Complications
Wound-related complications are composed of simple infections, seromas, hematomas, skin flap necrosis, and delayed healing of the donor or recipient site. Ischemic complications may occur, resulting in partial flap necrosis or fat necrosis, particularly with the pedicled TRAM flap. Complete flap failure is usually due to venous or arterial thrombus. Experienced teams have flap failure rates of less than 3%. Seromas are typically treated by simple aspiration. Neoadjuvant therapy and obesity may contribute to wound healing complications.[22] Donor site morbidity is greater in flaps in which the muscle is harvested with the flap.

## SUMMARY

Breast reconstruction is a very important part of the healing process for patients with breast cancer. The options are vast and should be decided in combination with the patient's surgeon. Patients generally have a high level of satisfaction with the option they choose, contributing to a feeling of overall recovery and physical and emotional wholeness.

## REFERENCES

1. Stevens LA, McGrath MH, Druss RG, et al. The psychological impact of immediate breast reconstruction for women with early breast cancer. Plast Reconstr Surg 1984;73(4):619–28.
2. Metcalfe KA, Narod SA. Breast cancer prevention in women with a BRCA1 or BRCA2 mutation. Open Med 2007;1(3):e184–90.
3. Stucky CC, Gray RJ, Wasif N, et al. Increase in contralateral prophylactic mastectomy: echoes of a bygone era? Surgical trends for unilateral breast cancer. Ann Surg Oncol 2010;17(Suppl 3):330–7.

4. Rebbeck TR, Friebel T, Lynch HT, et al. Bilateral prophylactic mastectomy reduces breast cancer risk in *BRCA1* and *BRCA2* mutation carriers: the PROSE Study Group. J Clin Oncol 2004;22(6):1055–62.

5. American Society of Plastic Surgeons. Report of the 2008 National Clearinghouse of Plastic Surgery Statistics. Available at: http://www.plasticsurgery.org/Media/stats/2008-US-cosmetic-reconstructive-plastic-surgery-minimally-invasive-statistics.pdf.

6. Yeh KA, Lyle G, Wei JP, et al. Immediate breast reconstruction in breast cancer: morbidity and outcome. Am Surg 1998;64(12):1195–9.

7. Alderman AK, Kuhn LE, Lowery JC, et al. Does patient satisfaction with breast reconstruction change over time? Two-year results of the Michigan Breast Reconstruction Outcomes Study. J Am Coll Surg 2007;204(1):7–12.

8. Namnoum JD. Expander/implant reconstruction with AlloDerm: recent experience. Plast Reconstr Surg 2009;124(2):387–94.

9. Spear SL, Parikh PM, Reisin E, et al. Acellular dermis-assisted breast reconstruction. Aesthetic Plast Surg 2008;32(3):418–25.

10. Kim JY, Davila AA, Persing S, et al. A meta-analysis of human acellular dermis and submuscular tissue expander breast reconstruction. Plast Reconstr Surg 2012;129(1):28–41.

11. Stevens WG, Stoker DA, Fellows DR, et al. Acceleration of textured saline breast implant deflation rate: results and analysis of 645 implants. Aesthet Surg J 2005;25(1):37–9.

12. Clough KB, O'Donoghue JM, Fitoussi AD, et al. Prospective evaluation of late cosmetic results following breast reconstruction: I. Implant reconstruction. Plast Reconstr Surg 2001;107(7):1702–9.

13. Fujino T, Harashina T, Enomoto K. Primary breast reconstruction after a standard radical mastectomy by free flap transfer: case report. Plast Reconstr Surg 1976;58:371–4.

14. Hartrampf CR, Scheflan M, Black PW. Breast reconstruction with a transverse abdominal island flap. Plast Reconstr Surg 1982;69(2):216–25.

15. Koshima I, Soeda S. Inferior epigastric artery skin flaps without rectus abdominis muscle. Br J Plast Surg 1989;42(6):645–8.

16. Fugino T, Harasina T, Aoyagi F. Reconstruction for aplasia of the breast and pectoral region by microvascular transfer of a free flap from the buttock. Plast Reconstr Surg 1975;56:178.

17. Koshima I, Moriguchi T, Soeda S, et al. The gluteal perforator-based flap for repair of sacral pressure sores. Plast Reconstr Surg 1993;91(4):678–83.

18. DellaCroce F, Sullivan S. Application and refinement of the superior gluteal artery perforator free flap for bilateral simultaneous breast reconstruction. Plast Reconstr Surg 2005;116(1):97–103.

19. DellaCroce FJ, Sullivan SK, Trahan C. Stacked deep inferior epigastric perforator flap breast reconstruction: a review of 110 flaps in 55 cases over 3 years. Plast Reconstr Surg 2011;126(3):1093–9.

20. DellaCroce FJ, Sullivan SK, Trahan C, et al. Body lift perforator flap breast reconstruction: a review of 100 flaps in 25 cases. Plast Reconstr Surg 2012;129(3):551–61.

21. Gill PS, Hunt JP, Guerra AB, et al. A 10-year retrospective review of 758 DIEP flaps for breast reconstruction. Plast Reconstr Surg 2004;113(4):1153–60.

22. Mehrara BJ, Santoro TD, Arcilla E, et al. Complications after microvascular breast reconstruction: experience with 1195 flaps. Plast Reconstr Surg 2006;118(5):1100–9 [discussion: 1110–1].

# Radiation Therapy in the Management of Breast Cancer

T. Jonathan Yang, MD, Alice Y. Ho, MD*

## KEYWORDS

- Breast cancer • Radiation therapy • Ductal carcinoma in situ
- Breast-conserving therapy • Postmastectomy irradiation

## KEY POINTS

- Adjuvant radiation therapy (RT) after wide local excision (WLE) for ductal carcinoma in situ (DCIS) reduces the relative risk of ipsilateral breast tumor recurrence (IBTR) at 10 years by 54%. The addition of tamoxifen (TAM) to RT further decreases the cumulative incidence of IBTR as well as contralateral recurrence.
- Six randomized trials established the equivalence of breast-conserving therapy (BCT) (breast-conserving surgery [BCS] followed by RT) and mastectomy on overall survival in patients with early-stage breast cancer at 20-year follow-up. The addition of RT to BCS decreased the 10-year risk of local recurrence by 16%, which translated into a 15-year reduction in the risk of breast cancer death by 4%.
- Alternative methods of irradiation for early-stage breast cancer have been developed, to abbreviate treatment times, enhance convenience, and/or decrease exposure to the normal tissues. These methods include hypofractionated therapy, prone breast irradiation, and accelerated partial breast irradiation (APBI). A large phase III trial comparing the efficacy of APBI versus whole-breast irradiation (WBI) is underway.
- According to the Early Breast Cancer Trialists' Collaborative Group (EBCTCG) meta-analysis, postmastectomy irradiation (PMRT) proportionally decreased the risk of locoregional recurrence (LRR) by 73% in node-positive patients. This finding translated into an increase in breast cancer–specific survival at 15 years by 5.4%.

## INTRODUCTION

Radiation therapy plays an essential role in the management of breast cancer by eradicating subclinical disease after surgical removal of grossly evident tumor. Radiation reduces local recurrence rates and increases breast cancer–specific survival in patients with early-stage breast cancer after BCS and in node-positive patients who have undergone mastectomy.[1] This article reviews the following topics: (1) the rationale for

Department of Radiation Oncology, Memorial Sloan-Kettering Cancer Center, 1275 York Avenue, New York, NY 10065, USA
* Corresponding author.
E-mail address: HoA1234@mskcc.org

Surg Clin N Am 93 (2013) 455–471
http://dx.doi.org/10.1016/j.suc.2013.01.002
0039-6109/13/$ – see front matter © 2013 Elsevier Inc. All rights reserved.

adjuvant RT and the evidence for its use in noninvasive and invasive breast cancer, (2) RT delivery techniques for breast-conserving therapy such as hypofractionated RT, partial breast irradiation, and prone irradiation, and (3) indications for PMRT.

## DUCTAL CARCINOMA IN SITU

The efficacy of radiation in reducing local recurrence in DCIS has been demonstrated by 4 randomized trials comparing outcomes in patients who received lumpectomy plus RT versus lumpectomy alone (**Table 1**).[2–6] In 2010, the EBCTCG published a meta-analysis including more than 3000 women with DCIS treated in 4 of these trials. Radiation was found to reduce the relative risk of IBTR at 10 years by 54% (absolute reduction 15.2%, $P<.00001$) in all patients. A significant reduction in the risk of local recurrence was seen, regardless of the age at diagnosis, margin status, and differences in tumor characteristics such as size, grade, and multifocality. The use of RT did not significantly affect breast cancer–related mortality.[7]

To investigate the benefit of adding hormonal therapy to patients receiving radiation, the National Surgical Adjuvant Breast and Bowel Project (NSABP) B-24 trial randomized 1804 women with DCIS treated with lumpectomy and RT to TAM versus placebo between 1991 and 1994. At 15 years, the addition of TAM to RT decreased the cumulative incidence of IBTR from 10.0% (RT + placebo) to 8.5% ($P = .025$). The addition of TAM is equally effective in preventing contralateral breast cancer recurrence, with a 15-year cumulative incidence of 10.8% in patients who received RT and placebo versus 7.3% in patients who received RT and TAM ($P = .023$).[3]

Although adjuvant RT after lumpectomy for DCIS has been shown to improve local control in all subsets of patients, it remains controversial whether or not patients with low-risk characteristics require treatment, as the toxicities of treatment may potentially

**Table 1**
**Phase III trials of radiation therapy after wide local excision for ductal carcinoma in situ**

| Study | Accrual Dates | Patients Enrolled (n) | Median Follow-up (yr) | Radiation Therapy Dose | Relative Risk Reduction in IBTR in RT Arm |
|---|---|---|---|---|---|
| NSABP B-17 | 1985–1990 | 818 | 17.3 | 50 Gy in 2 Gy fractions[a] | DCIS = 47% Invasive disease = 52% |
| EORTC 10853 | 1986–1996 | 1010 | 10.4 | 50 Gy in 2 Gy fractions[b] | DCIS = 48% Invasive disease = 42% |
| SweDCIS | 1987–1999 | 1067 | 8.4 | 50 Gy in 2 Gy fractions or 48 Gy in 2.4 Gy fractions or 54 Gy in 2 Gy fractions | DCIS = 67% Invasive disease = 41% |
| UK/ANZ DCIS | 1990–1998 | 1030 | 12.7 | 50 Gy in 2 Gy fractions | DCIS = 38% Invasive disease = 32% |

*Abbreviations:* EORTC, European Organisation for Research and Treatment of Cancer; NSABP, National Surgical Adjuvant Breast and Bowel Project; SweDCIS, Swedish Breast Cancer Group DCIS trial; UK/ANZ DCIS, United Kingdom, Australia, and New Zealand DCIS trial.
[a] Nine percent of patients randomized to lumpectomy + radiation therapy received boost.
[b] Five percent of patients randomized to lumpectomy + radiation therapy received boost.

outweigh the benefits. In 2006, Wong and colleagues[8] investigated whether WLE alone was adequate in treating small ($\leq$2.5 cm mammographically) grade 1 to 2 DCIS with negative margins (defined as absence of DCIS $\geq$1 cm from the inked margin). The use of chemotherapy or TAM was not permitted in this trial. At 5 years, the cumulative IBTR rate was 12.5%. Given the high rate of local recurrence, the trial was terminated early. Investigators concluded that WLE alone was not sufficient for local control, even in patients with favorable histology. In 2009, the Eastern Cooperative Oncology Group published the results of a prospective trial of 701 women with DCIS treated with WLE alone. Surgical microscopic margins were required to be 3 mm or more. Patients were categorized into low-risk (low or intermediate histologic grade DCIS 2.5 cm or smaller) versus high-risk groups (high-grade DCIS 1 cm or smaller). Median follow-up was 6.2 years. Although the low-risk women had acceptably low IBRT rates (6.1%) at 5 years, patients in the high-risk group had a 15.3% rate of IBTR at 5 years, suggesting that excision alone was inadequate as sole therapy in this patient subset.[9]

## EARLY-STAGE BREAST CANCER
### Breast-Conserving Therapy

To date, 6 prospective randomized trials comparing BCT with mastectomy have been performed (**Table 2**).[10–16] Although patient selection criteria and length of follow-up between these trials differed, all 6 trials established the equivalence of BCT and mastectomy on survival outcomes. Two of the largest trials with 20 years follow-up include the NSABP B-06 and Milan trials.[13,16] NSABP B-06 included 1851 women with invasive tumors that were 4 cm or less and randomized to total mastectomy, lumpectomy alone, or lumpectomy with postoperative WBI. Negative margins were required and defined as no tumor at the inked margin. At 20 years, the LRR rate in the mastectomy group was 14.8%, versus 17.5% in the lumpectomy alone group and 8.1% in the lumpectomy followed by postoperative RT group. Local failure in this study was defined by recurrence in the chest wall or scar, but ipsilateral breast failure in patients who underwent lumpectomy was not considered as local failure. No significant differences in disease-free survival, distant-disease-free survival, or overall survival were observed among groups who underwent mastectomy and BCT.[13] Similar results were reported by the Milan Cancer Institute trial. At 20 years, the rate of death from all causes was 41.7% in the BCT cohort and 41.2% in the mastectomy cohort ($P$ = 1.0), demonstrating that the long-term survival rate with BCT is equivalent to mastectomy.[16]

Multiple randomized trials have demonstrated that the addition of RT to the whole breast after BCS significantly reduces local relapse.[17–20] With a median follow-up of 20 years, the NSABP B-06 trial demonstrated that the cumulative incidence of IBTR in women who underwent BCS alone was 39% versus 14% ($P$<.001) for women who received RT after BCS.[13] The long-term survival impact of this reduction in local control was recently published by the EBCTCG group, who conducted a meta-analysis that included 10,801 women in 17 randomized trials of RT versus no RT after BCS. The addition of RT was found to reduce the 10-year risk of any first recurrence from 35% to 19%. This benefit in local control translated into a 15-year reduction in the risk of breast cancer death from 25% to 21%. These benefits were observed across all patients, regardless of nodal status. For patients with node-negative disease, adjuvant RT reduced any recurrence by 15.4% (95% confidence interval [CI], 13.2–17.6; $P$<.00001) and improved survival by 3.3% (95% CI, 0.8–5.8; $P$ = .005). For patients with node-positive disease, adjuvant RT reduced any recurrence by reduction 21.2% (95% CI, 14.5–27.9; $P$<.00001) and improved survival by 8.5% (95% CI, 1.8–15.2; $P$ = .01). Overall, 1 breast cancer death was avoided for every 4 local recurrences prevented by the addition of RT.[21]

**Table 2**
Phase III trials comparing breast-conserving therapy and mastectomy

| | IGR | Milan | NSABP B-06 | NCI | EORTC 10801 | DBCG-82TM |
|---|---|---|---|---|---|---|
| Enrollment | 1972–1980 | 1973–1980 | 1976–1984 | 1979–1987 | 1980–1986 | 1983–1989 |
| Eligible patients (n) | 179 | 701 | 1211 | 237 | 868 | 793 |
| **Eligibility** | | | | | | |
| Tumor (cm) | ≤2 | ≤2 | ≤4 | ≤5 | ≤5 | Not specified |
| Axilla | cN0-1a, Nb | cN0 | cN0-1 | cN0-1 | Apex pN0 (optional) | Not specified |
| Age (y) | <70 | <70 | No age limit | No age limit | <70 | <70 |
| Surgery | Modified radical M vs Tumorectomy + Ax + RT | Halsted M vs Quad + Ax + RT | Total M + Ax vs Lump + Ax + RT | Modified radical M vs Lump + Ax + RT | Modified radical M vs Lump + Ax + RT | Modified radical M vs Lump + Ax + RT |
| Boost | 15 Gy | 10 Gy | No boost | 10–20 Gy | 25 Gy | 10–25 Gy |
| Median follow-up (y) | 15 | 20 | 20 | 18 | 10 | 20 |
| **Endpoint** | | | | | | |
| LR (BCT vs M) | 13% vs 18% P = .44 | 9% vs 2% P<.001 | 3% vs 10%[a] No analysis | 22% vs 0% No analysis | 20% vs 12%[b] P = .01 | 5% vs 7% P = .16 |
| OS (BCT vs M) | 73% vs 65% P = .19 | 59% vs 58% P = 1.0 | 46% vs 47% P = .23 | 54% vs 58% P = .67 | 65% vs 66% P = .11 | 58% vs 51% P = .20 |

*Abbreviations:* Ax, axillary dissection; c/pN, clinical/pathologic nodal stage; DBCG, The Danish Breast Cancer Cooperative Group; IGR, Institut Gustave-Roussy Breast Cancer Group; LR, local recurrence; Lump, lumpectomy; M, mastectomy; NCI, National Cancer Institute; OS, overall survival; Quad, quadrantectomy; other abbreviations same as **Table 1**.
[a] Local failure was defined by recurrence in the chest wall or scar.
[b] locoregional recurrence.

The aforementioned trials are important for understanding the context in which the rationale for irradiation after BCS was derived. Over time, local control rates with whole-breast RT after BCS have continued to improve, reflecting changes in pathologic analysis of surgical margins, increased use of systemic therapy, and improvements in imaging, surgical, and RT techniques.

## Selection Criteria for BCT

Contraindications to RT in the setting of BCT are categorized as absolute or relative. Absolute contraindications include pregnancy, inability to obtain negative margins, multicentric cancer, or diffuse malignant-appearing calcifications. Relative contraindications include a history of prior RT and collagen vascular disease (CVD). Mastectomy remains the standard of care in patients who experience an in-breast recurrence after BCT. However, the feasibility of re-irradiation with APBI for select patients with small, recurrent breast cancer is currently being investigated in a Radiation Therapy Oncology Group (RTOG) trial.[22] RT can also be offered on a case-by-case basis to patients with CVD, with the caveat that these patients may be at enhanced risk of soft tissue fibrosis and subcutaneous toxicities after treatment. Data identifying patients with breast cancer and CVD who are at the greatest risk of RT-induced toxicity is limited to single-institution series. In a retrospective analysis of 209 patients with CVDs treated with RT to various sites, rheumatoid arthritis (RA) was not found to be associated with an elevated risk of late toxicity, while systemic lupus erythematosus (SLE) and scleroderma were associated with increased late RT toxicity.[23] To date, there is only 1 matched case-control study investigating BCT in the setting of active CVDs.[24] Thirty-six patients with CVDs (RA 47%, SLE 14%, scleroderma 11%, Raynaud phenomenon 11%, polymyositis 11%, and Sjögren disease 6%) and their double matched controls with respect to age, RT technique, systemic therapy, histologic features, and treatment dates were identified. No significant difference was found between patients with CVDs and control group patients in acute toxicity (14% vs 8%, $P = .40$). At the median follow-up of 12.5 years, a significant increased risk of late complication was found in patients with CVDs (17% vs 3%, $P<.001$); however, in subset analysis based on specific CVD, the statistically significant difference was noted only in patients with scleroderma.

## Use of a Boost

The rationale for adding a boost to the tumor bed after WBI for invasive breast cancer was established by the European Organization for the Research and Treatment of Cancer (EORTC) 22881-10882 trial.[25] This trial included 5318 women age 70 years or less with T1-2N0-1M0 breast cancer who received WLE and whole-breast RT (50 Gy) and were randomized to a boost to the lumpectomy cavity (16 Gy) or observation. All patients were required to have a 1-cm margin of macroscopically normal breast tissue. At a median follow-up of 10.8 years, a local relapse rate of 10.2% (95% CI, 8.7%–11.8%) was observed in the no boost versus 6.2% (95% CI, 4.9%–7.5%) in the boost cohort ($P<.0001$).[26] Although a proportional risk reduction in local recurrence of 39% was seen across all age groups, the absolute reduction in local recurrence with boost was the largest in patients 40 years or younger (from 23.9% to 13.5%, $P = .0014$). Based on these results, a boost after whole-breast RT is most frequently used in women younger than 60 years with invasive breast cancer or in the setting of close or positive margins. Indications for boost in older women or in those with DCIS are less well defined, given the lack of data demonstrating a local control benefit in these subgroups.[3,4,25]

### Omission of RT in Elderly Women with T1N0 Estrogen Receptor–Positive Breast Cancer

Select patient groups have been identified as having a low risk of local recurrence after BCS without RT. Two randomized trials evaluated the incremental value of RT in older women with small, node-negative, estrogen receptor (ER)-positive tumors treated with BCS and hormonal therapy. The Cancer and Leukemia Group B (CALGB) conducted a trial of 636 women who were 70 years or older and underwent BCS and TAM for ER-positive, T1N0 disease. Patients were randomized to RT versus observation. The 5-year LRR rate was significantly lower in patients who received RT (1% vs 4% in no RT, P<.001).[27] Updated results with longer follow-up (median 10.2 years) were reported, demonstrating a 2% local recurrence rate in the RT + TAM versus 9% in the TAM alone arm.[28] There was no significant difference in the rates of mastectomy for local recurrence, distant metastases, or overall survival between the 2 groups.

A second trial from Canada published in parallel with the CALGB study had an identical design but broader inclusion criteria. This study randomized 769 women 50 years or older with T1-2N0 breast cancer treated with BCS and TAM ± RT. At 5 years, the addition of RT significantly reduced the rate of local recurrence (0.6% vs 7.7% in the TAM only cohort, P<.001).[29]

The local control rates demonstrated in the patients who did not receive RT in these trials are considered acceptable to warrant the omission of RT in women 70 years or older with small, node-negative, ER-positive breast cancer who plan on receiving hormonal therapy. Patient preference, ability to tolerate hormonal therapy, treatment goals, and competing comorbidities are all important factors to be considered when making this decision.

### Techniques of Breast Irradiation

A standard course of RT to the whole breast consists of 50 to 50.4 Gy delivered in 25 to 26 fractions, followed by a 10- to 16 Gy boost to the tumor bed. Several alternative methods of radiation delivery have been developed, all with the purpose of abbreviating treatment times, enhancing convenience, and/or decreasing exposure to the normal tissues. Each technique and fractionation schema should be individualized to the patient's anatomy, tumor characteristics, and availability of institutional resources.

#### Hypofractionation

Hypofractionation (HFx) is defined as the delivery of larger-than-standard doses of radiation over a shorter period of time. A concept originally conceived in the 1960s, HFx was initially associated with a high rate of late complications, therefore resulting in abandonment of its use.[30] As the understanding of the radiobiologic principles that govern normal tissue responses improved, HFx regimens regained popularity in the United States. To date, there have been 3 randomized trials that have established equivalent local control and cosmetic outcomes between HFx and standard fractionation (SFx) regimens.[31–33]

The most influential among these trials is the one conducted by the Ontario Clinical Oncology Group. This study included 1234 women with node-negative invasive breast cancer who received WLE and axillary node dissection, randomized to SFx (25 treatments over 5 weeks) or HFx RT to the whole breast. The HFx arm consisted of 16 treatments using a higher dose per day—a regimen now commonly used in the United States and referred to as the "Canadian fractionation." With a median follow-up of 12 years, there was no significant difference in local recurrence (6.7% for the standard fractionated group vs 6.2% for the HFx group) or cosmesis (71.3% of women in the standard fractionation group vs 69.8% of women in the HFx group had good or excellent cosmetic outcome).

These results were corroborated by the Standardization of Breast Radiotherapy (START) A and B trials from the United Kingdom, which tested various HFx regimens against SFx in women with both node-negative and node-positive breast cancer. The START A trial included 2 different HFx schedules: 41.6 Gy delivered in 13 fractions over 3 weeks and 39 Gy delivered in 13 fractions over 3 weeks. With a median follow-up of 5.1 years, the LRR rates were equivalent in the SFx cohort (3.6%) and the 41.6 Gy HFx cohort (3.5%), whereas the 39 Gy HFx group demonstrated a significantly higher local recurrence rate (5.2%).[31] The START B trial compared SFx to a HFx regimen of 40 Gy delivered in 15 fractions over 3 weeks. With a median follow-up of 6 years, the HFx group demonstrated a lower but not statistically significant recurrence rate (2.2%) compared with the SFx arm.[33]

Despite the uniformity of the results, several differences in patient selection, length of follow-up, and use of systemic therapy and boost RT among the 3 trials should be noted (**Table 3**). In the Canadian trial, most patients had tumors with low-risk features (T1-2, grade 1–2, and ER+), none of the patients received boost RT, only 10.9% of patients received adjuvant systemic therapy, and women with large breast separations (ie, very thick breasts) were excluded. In contrast, the START A and B trials included patients with larger tumors and node-positive disease, 36% of patients received adjuvant systemic therapy, and there was no exclusion criteria based on breast size. Moreover, the use of a boost was not standardized, information on hormonal receptors status was unavailable, and the median follow-up was short.

These differences have precluded the widespread acceptance of HFx regimens into practice in the United States. In an effort to formalize guidelines on selection criteria for HFx RT, the American Society of Therapeutic Radiology and Oncology (ASTRO) published a consensus statement issued by a panel of experts in 2010.[34] The group agreed that HFx RT was appropriate in patients who met all the following criteria:

**Table 3**
**Randomized trials of hypofractionation for whole-breast irradiation**

|  | Canadian Trial | START A | START B |
|---|---|---|---|
| Sample size (*n*) | 1234 | 2236 | 2215 |
| Stage | T1-2 pN0 | T1-3, pN0-1 | T1-3, pN0-1 |
| Median follow-up | 12 y | 5 y | 5 y |
| Surgery type | All BCS | 15% mastectomy | 8% mastectomy |
| Hypofractionation regimen | 42.5 Gy/16 fx over 3 wk | 41.6 Gy/13 fx over 3 wk or 39 Gy/13 fx over 3 wk | 40 Gy/15 fx over 3 wk |
| Systemic therapy | 11% chemotherapy (CMF) | 36% (anthracycline based) | 22% (anthracycline based) |
| Use of boost | None | 61% | 44% |
| Exclusion criteria based on breast size | Excluded >25 cm | None | None |
| Regional nodal irradiation | None | Yes | Yes |
| Receptor status | Majority were ER+/PR+ | Not reported | Not reported |

*Abbreviations:* CMF, cyclophosphamide, methotrexate, and 5-fluorouracil; PR, progesterone receptor; T, tumor stage; other abbreviations same as **Table 2**.

*Data from* Ho A, Morrow M. The evolution of the locoregional therapy of breast cancer. Oncologist 2011;16:1367–79.

age 50 years or older at diagnosis, pathologic stage T1-T2 N0 disease treated with BCS, no chemotherapy, and a radiation plan with 7% dose inhomogeneity. A consensus on the applicability of HFx to young patients and those who received chemotherapy and boost was unable to be reached, based on the lack of mature clinical data on these patient subsets.

### Prone breast irradiation

Standard tangential WBI in the supine position with standard fractionation was the predominant position used in the seminal trials of both conventional and HFx RT.[1,31–33] Prone positioning was developed in the early 1990s as an alternative treatment of women with large breasts, with the goal of decreasing toxicities resulting from increased breast thickness, dose inhomogeneity, and the presence of skin folds.

The prone position requires patients to lie with the treated breast suspended through an aperture in the breast board, which displaces the breast away from the chest wall (**Fig. 1**). In single-institution series, prone RT has been shown to deliver a lower radiation dose to the lung and heart without compromising tumor control.[35–37] One disadvantage of this technique is the lesser coverage of level I and II axillary lymph nodes.[35] Other suboptimal candidates for prone RT include patients with tumors near the chest wall or elderly or obese patients who are unable to tolerate the position.

### Accelerated partial breast irradiation

APBI has gained significant popularity as a radiation technique in women opting for BCT. APBI delivers larger-than-standard doses of daily radiation to the postsurgical cavity plus a 1- to 2-cm margin over 1 to 2 weeks, therefore lowering RT exposure to normal tissues and expediting overall treatment times. The rationale for APBI is that most local recurrences after BCT occur in the immediate vicinity of the original tumor. Prospective randomized trials comparing lumpectomy with or without postoperative RT have shown that 80% to 90% of local recurrences are located at the site of

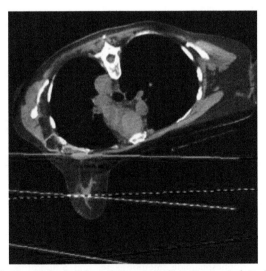

**Fig. 1.** Prone irradiation. (*Adapted from* Setton J, Cody H, Tan L, et al. Radiation field design and regional control in sentinel lymph node-positive breast cancer patients with omission of axillary dissection. Cancer 2012;118:1994–2003; with permission.)

lumpectomy,[20,38,39] whereas the rate of "elsewhere failures" at sites far removed from the tumor bed were 4%, which approaches the risk for developing contralateral breast cancer. Pathologic studies have also shown that tumor cells rarely extend 4 cm beyond the index lesion in patients who underwent mastectomy without an extensive intraductal component.[40] Taken together, these results suggest that RT offers the highest local control benefit when doses are directed to the tumor bed.

APBI can be administered with a variety of methods including multicatheter brachytherapy (MIB), intracavitary balloon brachytherapy such as MammoSite (Hologic Inc., Bedford, MA, USA), intraoperative RT (IORT), and external beam conformal therapy (EBRT) (**Fig. 2**). Each of these techniques has its own unique advantages and disadvantages, emphasizing the importance of individualizing the technique to patient anatomy, preferences, and resources. Data from modern randomized trials comparing WBI and APBI have just become available, or trials are actively accruing patients (**Table 4**).[41–47] The largest among these trials is the NSABP B-39/RTOG 0413,[42] which is aiming to accrue 4300 patients and permits APBI with MIB, EBRT, or MammoSite. By enrolling patients with all grades of DCIS, invasive cancers with 1 to 3 positive lymph nodes, and ER-negative breast cancers, this trial will provide data on the efficacy of APBI in a higher-risk population of patients than those included in prior studies.

MIB represents the ABPI technique with the longest follow-up. The ability to differentially load multiple catheters throughout the tumor bed allows for the greatest dosing flexibility.[48,49] However, it is an invasive procedure and requires considerable training and expertise, which limits use of this technique. In contrast, intracavitary brachytherapy is the most popular form of ABPI currently used in the United States. This technique involves placement of a balloon-based catheter applicator within the lumpectomy cavity, which is subsequently inflated to securely fit against the cavity. Postoperatively, the balloon is filled with saline, and a high dose rate brachytherapy (HDR) afterloading device inserts an iridium-192 source into the center of the balloon. The

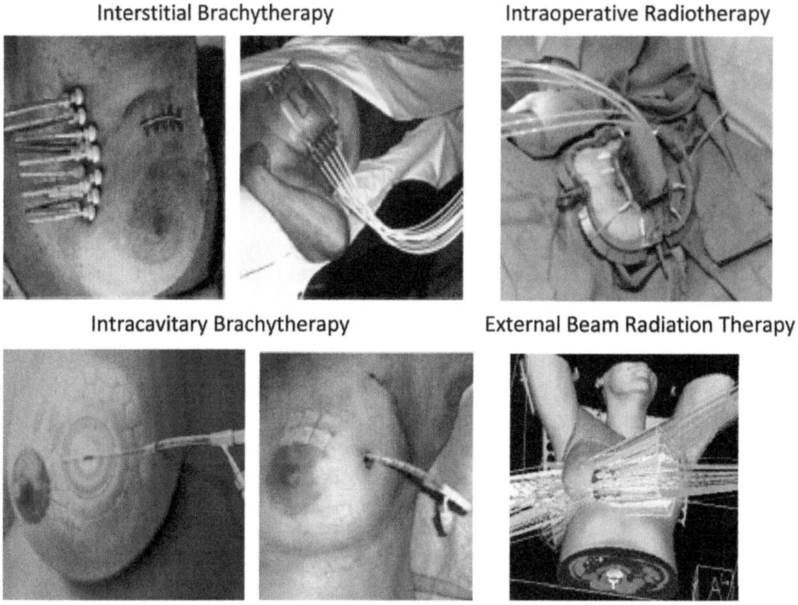

Interstitial Brachytherapy    Intraoperative Radiotherapy

Intracavitary Brachytherapy    External Beam Radiation Therapy

**Fig. 2.** Four methods of accelerated partial breast irradiation delivery.

**Table 4**
**Modern phase III trials of APBI versus WBI**

| Institution/Trial | Total n/Target Accrual (y) | Control Arm | Experimental Arm |
|---|---|---|---|
| National Institute of Oncology, Budapest, Hungary | 258 (1998–2004) | WBI 50 Gy in 25 fx | MIB (36.4 Gy in 7 fx) Electrons (50 Gy in 25 fx) |
| European Institute of Oncology EIO | 1200 (2000–2007) | WBI 50 Gy in 25 fx ± 10 Gy Boost | IORT (21 Gy in 1 fx) |
| European Brachytherapy Breast Cancer GEC-ESTRO Working Group | 1170 (2004–2009) | WBI 50–50.4 Gy in 25–28 fx + 10 Gy Boost | Brachytherapy only 32.0 Gy 8 fx HDR or 30.3 Gy 7 fx HDR or 50 Gy pulsed dose rate |
| TARGIT-A | 2232 (2000–2010) | WBI 40–56 Gy ± 10–16 Gy boost | IORT (20 Gy in 1 fx) |
| Medical Research Council—UK IMPORT LOW | 1935 (2007–2010) | WBI 2.67 Gy × 15 fx | WBI 2.4 Gy × 15 PBI 2.67 Gy × 15 PBI only 2.67 Gy × 15 |
| Ontario Clinical Oncology Group Canadian Trial RAPID | 2128 (2006–2011) | WBI ± 10 Gy boost: 42.5 Gy in 16 fx for small breasts or 50 Gy in 25 fx for large breasts | 3D-CRT only (38.5 Gy in 10 fx) |
| NSABP B-39/ RTOG 0413 | Accrual goal: 4300 (2005–present) | WBI 50–50.4 Gy ± 10–16 Gy Boost | MIB (34 Gy in 10 fx) or MammoSite (34 Gy in 10 fx) or 3D-CRT (38.5 Gy in 10 fx) |

*Abbreviations:* GEC-ESTRO, The Groupe Européen de Curiethérapie and the European Society for Therapeutic Radiology and Oncology; IMPORT LOW, Intensity Modulated and Partial Organ Radiotherapy trial; RAPID, Randomized Trial of Accelerated Partial Breast Irradiation; TARGIT, Targeted Intraoperative Radiotherapy for Breast Cancer trial; other abbreviations same as **Table 1**.

radiation dose is prescribed to a 1 cm distance from the balloon surface. Treatment is delivered over a total of 10 fractions, twice a day over 5 consecutive days. Compared with MIB, it is easier to perform and less invasive. The MammoSite Registry Trial, a prospective study by the American Society of Breast Surgeons, represents the largest body of evidence for patients treated with this technique. Among the 1449 patients enrolled, the actuarial IBTR rate was 3.8% at 5 years and 90.6% of patients demonstrated good/excellent cosmesis.[50]

IORT consists of a single dose of RT administered to the operative bed at the time of lumpectomy. It is the most convenient to deliver of all the APBI techniques but is limited by lack of availability of centers in the United States equipped to perform this treatment. Another disadvantage is the lack of knowledge of final margin pathology and lymph node status before treatment delivery. Interest in IORT was renewed by the publication of the Targeted Intraoperative Radiotherapy for Breast Cancer trial,[45] in which 2232 women 45 years or older were randomized to receive either WBI or IORT after WLE using a single dose of 20 Gy delivered to the tumor bed using a device called INTRABEAM (Carl Zeiss, Oberkochen, Germany), a miniature x-ray source that delivers a point source of orthovoltage x-rays. Most patients had node-negative, low- or intermediate-grade invasive tumors 2 cm or less. Fourteen percent of patients in the IORT group received additional WBI if final pathology revealed prespecified high-risk features. At 4 years, the local recurrence rates were equivalent between both groups (1.2% in IORT vs 0.95% in WBI, $P = .41$), as was the incidence of major toxicity (3.3% in IORT vs 3.9% in WBI, $P = .44$). Criticisms of this trial include the short follow-up (median 4 years) and the potential for low therapeutic efficacy of a single dose delivered to the distant margins of the target volume.

EBRT is the most common technique used for APBI in the NSABP/RTOG trial.[42] Compared with other APBI techniques, its advantages include its noninvasive nature, excellent dose homogeneity, availability, and ease of use. The first randomized trial comparing WBI and APBI using EBRT was conducted at Christie Hospital (Manchester, UK) between 1982 and 1987.[51] A total of 708 patients with invasive ductal or lobular carcinoma measuring 4 cm or less were included. All patients received lumpectomy without axillary dissection. Microscopic evaluation of the surgical margins was not performed, and chemotherapy was not administered. At 8 years, the in-breast recurrence rate was significantly higher in the APBI arm compared with the WBI arm (25% vs 13%, $P<.0001$). In retrospect, the high local recurrence rates were attributed to poor patient selection, outdated RT techniques, inadequate management of the axilla, lack of systemic therapy, and incomplete pathologic examination of margins. With radiation technique and technological advancements, the ability to visualize the target cavity and to deliver adequate dose consistently and precisely with external beam therapy have improved. One of the prospective studies with the longest follow-up using modern EBRT APBI technique was conducted at the William Beaumont Hospital.[52] In this study, 94 patients with stage 0–II breast cancer with lesions 3 cm or less, negative margins, and negative nodes were treated with 3-dimensional conformal RT to the tumor bed at 3.85 Gy per fraction to a total of 38.5 Gy. At a median follow-up of 4.2 years, the investigators reported 1.1% IBTR, demonstrating with appropriate RT technique and patient selection, EBRT APBI can achieve adequate local control.

At present, data on long-term outcomes with APBI and the best technique for its delivery are limited. Recognizing that mature results from randomized trials will not be available for some time, the ASTRO Task Force developed a consensus statement to help guide patient selection for the practice of APBI outside of a clinical trial. Patients who were "suitable," "cautionary," or "unsuitable" for APBI performed off-protocol were defined. The last 2 groups were defined based on lack of data to support treatment of these subsets, rather than known lack of efficacy or toxicities (**Table 5**).[34] It is important to acknowledge that these guidelines are subject to evolve as further data become available.

## POSTMASTECTOMY IRRADIATION

PMRT is used to treat regions that are at risk for local and regional recurrence but are not excised during modified radical mastectomy, such as the chest wall lymphatics and upper axillary, supraclavicular, and internal mammary lymph nodes. The most influential study to establish the efficacy of PMRT in node-positive patients comes from the Early Breast Cancer Trialists Collaborative Group Overview, a meta-analysis that included more than 9000 patients from randomized trials of RT after mastectomy plus varying extent of axillary surgery. In this meta-analysis, PMRT was found to proportionally decrease the risk of LRR by 73% (annual odds ratio 0.28), with the 5-year risk of local recurrence of 5.8% versus 22.8% in node-positive patients treated with and without PMRT. This reduction in LRR translated

**Table 5**
**ASTRO guidelines for use of ABPI off-protocol**

| Factors | Suitable Group: Suitable for APBI if all Criteria are Present | Cautionary Group: Any of These Criteria Should Involve Concern When Considering PBI | Unsuitable Group: Unsuitable for APBI Outside a Clinical Trial if Any of These Criteria Are Present |
|---|---|---|---|
| **Patient** | | | |
| Age (y) | ≥60 | 50–59 | <50 |
| BRCA 1/2 mutation | Not present | — | Present |
| **Pathologic** | | | |
| Tumor size (cm) | ≤2 | 2.1–3.0 | 3 |
| T stage | T1 | T0 or T2 | T3–4 |
| Margins | Negative by at least 2 mm | Close (<2 mm) | Positive |
| Grade | Any | — | — |
| LVSI | Not present | Limited/focal | Extensive |
| ER status | Positive | Negative | — |
| Multicentricity | Unicentric only | — | Present |
| Multifocality | Clinically unifocal with total size ≤2 cm | Clinically unifocal with total size 2.1–3.0 cm | In microscopically multifocal >3 cm in total size or if clinically multifocal |
| Histology | Favorable subtypes | Invasive lobular | — |
| Pure DCIS | Not allowed | ≤3 cm | If >3 cm in size |
| EIC | Not allowed | ≤3 cm | If >3 cm in size |
| Associated LCIS | Allowed | — | — |
| **Nodal** | | | |
| N stage | pN0 (i, i+) | — | pN1, pN2, pN3 |
| Nodal surgery | SN Bx or ALND | — | None performed |
| **Treatment** | | | |
| Neoadjuvant therapy | Not allowed | — | If used |

*Abbreviations:* ALND, axillary lymph node dissection; BRCA, breast cancer; LCIS, lobular carcinoma in situ; LVSI, lymphovascular space involvement; SN Bx, sentinel node biopsy; other abbreviations same as **Tables 1–5.**
*Data from* Smith BD, Arthur DW, Buchholz TA, et al. Accelerated partial breast irradiation consensus statement from the American Society for Radiation Oncology (ASTRO). J Am Coll Surg 2009;209:269–77.

into a 5.4% benefit in 15-year breast cancer–specific survival and a 4.4% benefit in overall survival.[1]

Three randomized trials of PMRT contributed most patients included in the EBCTCG meta-analysis and represent the first PMRT trials to have routinely used modern radiotherapy techniques and systemic therapy and report long-term follow-up. These include the Danish 82b and 82c and Vancouver British Columbia trials.[53–55] The 2 largest of these trials, the Danish trials, were performed simultaneously from

1982 to 1989. Danish 82b included 1705 premenopausal women who received cyclophosphamide, 5-fluorouracial, and methotrexate (CMF). Danish 82c recruited 1375 postmenopausal patients who received TAM. The 18-year rates of LRR (with or without simultaneous distant metastases) were 49% and 14% in the control and PMRT arms, respectively.[56] In a subsequent subgroup analysis of patients who had greater than 8 lymph nodes dissected, the 15-year overall survival was 29% and 39% in the control and PMRT groups, respectively.[57]

The British Columbia Cancer Agency trial, which was conducted between 1976 and 1985, randomized 318 premenopausal women with node-positive breast cancer to RT or observation after mastectomy. All patients received CMF chemotherapy. With a median of 20 years of follow-up, the addition of PMRT resulted in improved LRR-free survival (74% control vs 90% PMRT), breast cancer–specific survival (38% control vs 53% PMRT) and overall survival (37% control vs 47% PMRT).[55]

Despite their importance in establishing the efficacy of PMRT, several caveats to these trials must be considered when using these data to formulate current practice guidelines. In all 3 trials, rates of locoregional failure in the control arms were higher than would be expected with standard axillary dissection. The Danish trial had a low median number of axillary lymph nodes removed,[7] which may have contributed to high axillary failure rates and also limit detailed analysis of patient subgroups with 1 to 3+ lymph nodes.

### PMRT in 1 to 3+ Lymph Nodes

It is well accepted that PMRT is standard in patients with 4 or more involved axillary lymph nodes, primary tumors greater than 5 cm with any number of positive nodes, or any T4 tumors, based on consistent LRR rates of 15% or greater in these subgroups.[58–60] Indications for PMRT in patients with 1 to 3 positive lymph nodes are more controversial, as this patient subgroup carries a lower risk of LRR.

The British Columbia trial, the combined 2 Danish trials, and the EBCTCG meta-analysis that includes all 3 trials demonstrated a similar proportional survival benefit of PMRT for women with 1 to 3 or 4 or more positive lymph nodes.[1,55,57] In the EBCTCG meta-analysis, the "benefit ratio" of reduced breast cancer–specific mortality was 0.4 for patients with 1 to 3 and 0.21 for 4 or more positive nodes. However, the aforementioned limitations of these studies have prevented routine extrapolation of these recommendations to the 1 to 3 positive node patient group. Moreover, the EBCTCG meta-analysis included trials that used outdated radiotherapy techniques, had limited or no information on prognostic factors such as histologic grade and lymphovascular invasion, and did not distinguish between trials that did and did not use systemic therapy.

Several large retrospective studies have examined the combined effect of clinical and pathologic variables in subsets of 1 to 3 nodes positive who have not received PMRT.[61–63] Based on these results, factors such as patient age, tumor grade, tumor size, receptor status, extranodal extension, margin status, and lymphovascular invasion are used by clinicians to assess the risk of LRR in patients with 1 to 3+ nodes and thereby guide recommendations for PMRT. Gene expression profiling to predict the risk of locoregional failure (LRF) after mastectomy has been studied by a group in Taiwan, who found that a 34-gene model segregated groups of patients into 2 categories: those with a 3-year LRR of 32% and another with no LRRs.[64] Although promising, this approach requires significant validation before it can be used to tailor treatment recommendations.

Prospective data on the use of PMRT in this subgroup are forthcoming from the Selective Use of Postoperative Radiotherapy after Mastectomy trial, which randomizes high-risk node-negative or 1 to 3 node-positive patients who underwent mastectomy to PMRT or observation. In the meantime, all patients with 1 to 3 positive nodes should have an informed discussion with a radiation oncologist regarding the benefits and risks of treatment.

## REFERENCES

1. Clarke M, Collins R, Darby S, et al. Effects of radiotherapy and of differences in the extent of surgery for early breast cancer on local recurrence and 15-year survival: an overview of the randomised trials. Lancet 2005;366:2087–106.
2. Fisher B, Dignam J, Wolmark N, et al. Lumpectomy and radiation therapy for the treatment of intraductal breast cancer: findings from National Surgical Adjuvant Breast and Bowel Project B-17. J Clin Oncol 1998;16:441–52.
3. Wapnir IL, Dignam JJ, Fisher B, et al. Long-term outcomes of invasive ipsilateral breast tumor recurrences after lumpectomy in NSABP B-17 and B-24 randomized clinical trials for DCIS. J Natl Cancer Inst 2011;103:478–88.
4. Bijker N, Meijnen P, Peterse JL, et al. Breast-conserving treatment with or without radiotherapy in ductal carcinoma-in-situ: ten-year results of European Organisation for Research and Treatment of Cancer randomized phase III trial 10853–a study by the EORTC Breast Cancer Cooperative Group and EORTC Radiotherapy Group. J Clin Oncol 2006;24:3381–7.
5. Holmberg L, Garmo H, Granstrand B, et al. Absolute risk reductions for local recurrence after postoperative radiotherapy after sector resection for ductal carcinoma in situ of the breast. J Clin Oncol 2008;26:1247–52.
6. Cuzick J, Sestak I, Pinder SE, et al. Effect of tamoxifen and radiotherapy in women with locally excised ductal carcinoma in situ: long-term results from the UK/ANZ DCIS trial. Lancet Oncol 2011;12:21–9.
7. Correa C, McGale P, Taylor C, et al. Overview of the randomized trials of radiotherapy in ductal carcinoma in situ of the breast. J Natl Cancer Inst Monogr 2010;2010:162–77.
8. Wong JS, Kaelin CM, Troyan SL, et al. Prospective study of wide excision alone for ductal carcinoma in situ of the breast. J Clin Oncol 2006;24:1031–6.
9. Hughes LL, Wang M, Page DL, et al. Local excision alone without irradiation for ductal carcinoma in situ of the breast: a trial of the Eastern Cooperative Oncology Group. J Clin Oncol 2009;27:5319–24.
10. Arriagada R, Le MG, Rochard F, et al. Conservative treatment versus mastectomy in early breast cancer: patterns of failure with 15 years of follow-up data. Institut Gustave-Roussy Breast Cancer Group. J Clin Oncol 1996;14:1558–64.
11. Blichert-Toft M, Rose C, Andersen JA, et al. Danish randomized trial comparing breast conservation therapy with mastectomy: six years of life-table analysis. Danish Breast Cancer Cooperative Group. J Natl Cancer Inst Monogr 1992;(11):19–25.
12. Blichert-Toft M, Nielsen M, During M, et al. Long-term results of breast conserving surgery vs. mastectomy for early stage invasive breast cancer: 20-year follow-up of the Danish randomized DBCG-82TM protocol. Acta Oncol 2008;47:672–81.
13. Fisher B, Anderson S, Bryant J, et al. Twenty-year follow-up of a randomized trial comparing total mastectomy, lumpectomy, and lumpectomy plus irradiation for the treatment of invasive breast cancer. N Engl J Med 2002;347:1233–41.
14. Poggi MM, Danforth DN, Sciuto LC, et al. Eighteen-year results in the treatment of early breast carcinoma with mastectomy versus breast conservation therapy: the National Cancer Institute Randomized Trial. Cancer 2003;98:697–702.

15. van Dongen JA, Voogd AC, Fentiman IS, et al. Long-term results of a randomized trial comparing breast-conserving therapy with mastectomy: European Organization for Research and Treatment of Cancer 10801 trial. J Natl Cancer Inst 2000; 92:1143–50.

16. Veronesi U, Cascinelli N, Mariani L, et al. Twenty-year follow-up of a randomized study comparing breast-conserving surgery with radical mastectomy for early breast cancer. N Engl J Med 2002;347:1227–32.

17. Clark RM, Whelan T, Levine M, et al. Randomized clinical trial of breast irradiation following lumpectomy and axillary dissection for node-negative breast cancer: an update. Ontario Clinical Oncology Group. J Natl Cancer Inst 1996;88: 1659–64.

18. Fisher B, Bryant J, Dignam JJ, et al. Tamoxifen, radiation therapy, or both for prevention of ipsilateral breast tumor recurrence after lumpectomy in women with invasive breast cancers of one centimeter or less. J Clin Oncol 2002;20:4141–9.

19. Liljegren G, Holmberg L, Adami HO, et al. Sector resection with or without postoperative radiotherapy for stage I breast cancer: five-year results of a randomized trial. Uppsala-Orebro Breast Cancer Study Group. J Natl Cancer Inst 1994;86: 717–22.

20. Liljegren G, Holmberg L, Bergh J, et al. 10-Year results after sector resection with or without postoperative radiotherapy for stage I breast cancer: a randomized trial. J Clin Oncol 1999;17:2326–33.

21. Darby S, McGale P, Correa C, et al. Effect of radiotherapy after breast-conserving surgery on 10-year recurrence and 15-year breast cancer death: meta-analysis of individual patient data for 10,801 women in 17 randomised trials. Lancet 2011; 378:1707–16.

22. Radiation Therapy Oncology Group (RTOG) 1014 Protocol. A phase II study of repeat breast preserving surgery and 3D-conformal partial breast rirradiation (PBRI) for local recurrence of breast carcinoma. 2010. Available at: http://www. rtog.org/ClinicalTrials/ProtocolTable/StudyDetails.aspx?study=1014.

23. Morris MM, Powell SN. Irradiation in the setting of collagen vascular disease: acute and late complications. J Clin Oncol 1997;15:2728–35.

24. Chen AM, Obedian E, Haffty BG. Breast-conserving therapy in the setting of collagen vascular disease. Cancer J 2001;7:480–91.

25. Bartelink H, Horiot JC, Poortmans P, et al. Recurrence rates after treatment of breast cancer with standard radiotherapy with or without additional radiation. N Engl J Med 2001;345:1378–87.

26. Bartelink H, Horiot JC, Poortmans PM, et al. Impact of a higher radiation dose on local control and survival in breast-conserving therapy of early breast cancer: 10-year results of the randomized boost versus no boost EORTC 22881-10882 trial. J Clin Oncol 2007;25:3259–65.

27. Hughes KS, Schnaper LA, Berry D, et al. Lumpectomy plus tamoxifen with or without irradiation in women 70 years of age or older with early breast cancer. N Engl J Med 2004;351:971–7.

28. Hughes KS, Schnaper LA, Cirrincione C, et al. Lumpectomy plus tamoxifen with or without irradiation in women age 70 or older with early breast cancer. J Clin Oncol 2010;28:15s. [abstract 507].

29. Fyles AW, McCready DR, Manchul LA, et al. Tamoxifen with or without breast irradiation in women 50 years of age or older with early breast cancer. N Engl J Med 2004;351:963–70.

30. Fletcher GH. Hypofractionation: lessons from complications. Radiother Oncol 1991;20:10–5.

31. Bentzen SM, Agrawal RK, Aird EG, et al. The UK Standardisation of Breast Radiotherapy (START) Trial A of radiotherapy hypofractionation for treatment of early breast cancer: a randomised trial. Lancet Oncol 2008;9:331–41.
32. Whelan TJ, Pignol JP, Levine MN, et al. Long-term results of hypofractionated radiation therapy for breast cancer. N Engl J Med 2010;362:513–20.
33. Bentzen SM, Agrawal RK, Aird EG, et al. The UK Standardisation of Breast Radiotherapy (START) Trial B of radiotherapy hypofractionation for treatment of early breast cancer: a randomised trial. Lancet 2008;371:1098–107.
34. Smith BD, Bentzen SM, Correa CR, et al. Fractionation for whole breast irradiation: an American Society for Radiation Oncology (ASTRO) evidence-based guideline. Int J Radiat Oncol Biol Phys 2011;81:59–68.
35. Alonso-Basanta M, Ko J, Babcock M, et al. Coverage of axillary lymph nodes in supine vs. prone breast radiotherapy. Int J Radiat Oncol Biol Phys 2009;73:745–51.
36. Kirby AM, Evans PM, Donovan EM, et al. Prone versus supine positioning for whole and partial-breast radiotherapy: a comparison of non-target tissue dosimetry. Radiother Oncol 2010;96:178–84.
37. Stegman LD, Beal KP, Hunt MA, et al. Long-term clinical outcomes of whole-breast irradiation delivered in the prone position. Int J Radiat Oncol Biol Phys 2007;68:73–81.
38. Veronesi U, Marubini E, Mariani L, et al. Radiotherapy after breast-conserving surgery in small breast carcinoma: long-term results of a randomized trial. Ann Oncol 2001;12:997–1003.
39. Fisher B, Jeong JH, Anderson S, et al. Twenty-five-year follow-up of a randomized trial comparing radical mastectomy, total mastectomy, and total mastectomy followed by irradiation. N Engl J Med 2002;347:567–75.
40. Holland R, Veling SH, Mravunac M, et al. Histologic multifocality of Tis, T1-2 breast carcinomas. Implications for clinical trials of breast-conserving surgery. Cancer 1985;56:979–90.
41. European Institute of Oncology Intraoperative Radiotherapy with Electrons (EIO) Trial 2000. Available at: http://www.ieo.it/Italiano/Pages/Default.aspx.
42. NSABP B-39/RTOG 0413 phase III randomized study of adjuvant whole-breast versus partial-breast irradiation in women with ductal carcinoma in situ or stage I or II breast cancer. 2005. Available at: http://www.cancer.gov/clinicaltrials/search/view?cdrid=409590&version=HealthProfessional.
43. Ontario Clinical Oncology Group (OCOG) Trial NCT00282035. RAPID: randomized trial of accelerated partial breast irradiation. 2006. Available at: http://www.clinicaltrials.gov/ct2/show/NCT00282035?term=NCT00282035&rank=1.
44. Polgar C, Fodor J, Major T, et al. Breast-conserving treatment with partial or whole breast irradiation for low-risk invasive breast carcinoma–5-year results of a randomized trial. Int J Radiat Oncol Biol Phys 2007;69:694–702.
45. Vaidya JS, Joseph DJ, Tobias JS, et al. Targeted intraoperative radiotherapy versus whole breast radiotherapy for breast cancer (TARGIT-A trial): an international, prospective, randomised, non-inferiority phase 3 trial. Lancet 2010;376:91–102.
46. Medical Research Council- UK IMPORT LOW Trial. 2007. Available at: http://www.mrc.ac.uk/index.htm.
47. European Brachytherapy Breast Cancer GEC-ESTRO Working Group APBI Trial. 2007. Available at: http://www.apbi.uni-erlangen.de/.
48. Offersen BV, Overgaard M, Kroman N, et al. Accelerated partial breast irradiation as part of breast conserving therapy of early breast carcinoma: a systematic review. Radiother Oncol 2009;90:1–13.

49. Zwicker RD, Arthur DW, Kavanagh BD, et al. Optimization of planar high-dose-rate implants. Int J Radiat Oncol Biol Phys 1999;44:1171–7.

50. Vicini F, Beitsch P, Quiet C, et al. Five-year analysis of treatment efficacy and cosmesis by the American Society of Breast Surgeons MammoSite Breast Brachytherapy Registry Trial in patients treated with accelerated partial breast irradiation. Int J Radiat Oncol Biol Phys 2011;79:808–17.

51. Magee B, Swindell R, Harris M, et al. Prognostic factors for breast recurrence after conservative breast surgery and radiotherapy: results from a randomised trial. Radiother Oncol 1996;39:223–7.

52. Chen PY, Wallace M, Mitchell C, et al. Four-year efficacy, cosmesis, and toxicity using three-dimensional conformal external beam radiation therapy to deliver accelerated partial breast irradiation. Int J Radiat Oncol Biol Phys 2010;76:991–7.

53. Overgaard M, Hansen PS, Overgaard J, et al. Postoperative radiotherapy in high-risk premenopausal women with breast cancer who receive adjuvant chemotherapy. Danish Breast Cancer Cooperative Group 82b Trial. N Engl J Med 1997;337:949–55.

54. Overgaard M, Jensen MB, Overgaard J, et al. Postoperative radiotherapy in high-risk postmenopausal breast-cancer patients given adjuvant tamoxifen: Danish Breast Cancer Cooperative Group DBCG 82c randomised trial. Lancet 1999; 353:1641–8.

55. Ragaz J, Olivotto IA, Spinelli JJ, et al. Locoregional radiation therapy in patients with high-risk breast cancer receiving adjuvant chemotherapy: 20-year results of the British Columbia randomized trial. J Natl Cancer Inst 2005;97:116–26.

56. Nielsen HM, Overgaard M, Grau C, et al. Study of failure pattern among high-risk breast cancer patients with or without postmastectomy radiotherapy in addition to adjuvant systemic therapy: long-term results from the Danish Breast Cancer Cooperative Group DBCG 82 b and c randomized studies. J Clin Oncol 2006; 24:2268–75.

57. Overgaard M, Nielsen HM, Overgaard J. Is the benefit of postmastectomy irradiation limited to patients with four or more positive nodes, as recommended in international consensus reports? A subgroup analysis of the DBCG 82 b&c randomized trials. Radiother Oncol 2007;82:247–53.

58. Harris JR, Halpin-Murphy P, McNeese M, et al. Consensus Statement on post-mastectomy radiation therapy. Int J Radiat Oncol Biol Phys 1999;44:989–90.

59. Recht A, Edge SB, Solin LJ, et al. Postmastectomy radiotherapy: clinical practice guidelines of the American Society of Clinical Oncology. J Clin Oncol 2001;19: 1539–69.

60. National Comprehensive Cancer Network (NCCN) Guidelines. Available at: www.nccn.org.

61. Recht A, Gray R, Davidson NE, et al. Locoregional failure 10 years after mastectomy and adjuvant chemotherapy with or without tamoxifen without irradiation: experience of the Eastern Cooperative Oncology Group. J Clin Oncol 1999;17: 1689–700.

62. Katz A, Buchholz TA, Thames H, et al. Recursive partitioning analysis of locoregional recurrence patterns following mastectomy: implications for adjuvant irradiation. Int J Radiat Oncol Biol Phys 2001;50:397–403.

63. Wallgren A, Bonetti M, Gelber RD, et al. Risk factors for locoregional recurrence among breast cancer patients: results from International Breast Cancer Study Group Trials I through VII. J Clin Oncol 2003;21:1205–13.

64. Cheng SH, Horng CF, West M, et al. Genomic prediction of locoregional recurrence after mastectomy in breast cancer. J Clin Oncol 2006;24:4594–602.

# Adjuvant Systemic Therapies in Breast Cancer

Leonel F. Hernandez-Aya, MD[a],
Ana M. Gonzalez-Angulo, MD, MSc[b,c,d],*

## KEYWORDS

- Adjuvant • Breast cancer • Adjuvant endocrine • Adjuvant chemotherapy
- Adjuvant HER-2-targeted therapy

## KEY POINTS

- Adjuvant systemic therapy has improved survival of patients with breast cancer.
- Most guidelines have recommended systemic treatment for node-positive disease and/or tumors larger than 1 cm, irrespective of other tumor characteristics.
- Oncotype DX is a validated genomic predictor of outcome and response to adjuvant chemotherapy in node-negative, estrogen receptor–positive breast cancer.
- Taxane-containing and anthracycline-containing regimens are standard adjuvant therapies for lymph node–positive and possibly in high-risk lymph node–negative patients with BC.
- Current guidelines recommend incorporating aromatase inhibitors either as up-front therapy or as sequential treatment after tamoxifen for 5 years in all patients with endocrine-sensitive tumors.
- Anti-HER2 adjuvant therapy with trastuzumab combined with chemotherapy has shown significant improvement in clinical outcomes compared with chemotherapy alone.

## INTRODUCTION

The multidisciplinary approach for the treatment of breast cancer (BC) has been fundamental for the recent advances in the management of this disease. BC is the most common malignancy in women, accounting for nearly 1 in 3 cancers diagnosed among women in the United States, and it is one of the top causes of cancer-related deaths.[1] Over the past 5 decades, innovative and dedicated research has generated

[a] Division of Hematology/Oncology, Comprehensive Cancer Center, University of Michigan Health System, Ann Arbor, MI, USA; [b] Section Clinical Research and Drug Development, MD Anderson Cancer Center, The University of Texas, 1515 Holcombe Boulevard, Houston, TX 77030-4009, USA; [c] Department of Breast Medical Oncology, MD Anderson Cancer Center, The University of Texas, 1515 Holcombe Boulevard, Houston, TX 77030-4009, USA; [d] Department of Systems Biology, MD Anderson Cancer Center, The University of Texas, 1515 Holcombe Boulevard, Houston, TX 77030-4009, USA
* Corresponding author. Department of Breast Medical Oncology, The University of Texas, MD Anderson Cancer Center, Unit 1354, 1515 Holcombe Boulevard, Houston, TX 77030-4009.
*E-mail address:* agonzalez@mdanderson.org

Surg Clin N Am 93 (2013) 473–491
http://dx.doi.org/10.1016/j.suc.2012.12.002
0039-6109/13/$ – see front matter © 2013 Elsevier Inc. All rights reserved.
surgical.theclinics.com

major advances in the diagnosis and treatment of BC with significant survival impact. A substantial portion of the success in improving clinical outcomes of patients with BC is related to the standardized use of adjuvant therapies **Table 1**.[2,3] Cumulative evidence has demonstrated benefits in short-term and long-term outcomes by adjuvant treatments, especially when the 10-year risk of recurrence is at least 10%.[4] A recent meta-analysis, including randomized clinical trials conducted since adjuvant therapies became widely used in the 1990s, reported a decrease in annual relative risk of relapse and mortality of 23% and 17% respectively.[5]

The use of adjuvant therapy in BC has evolved as meaningful basic and clinical research contributes to the understanding of the complexity of breast tumors. For many years, the treatment recommendations for adjuvant therapies were based on classic anatomic and pathologic factors, such as tumor size, tumor grade, and lymph node (LN) status. With the development of immunohistochemistry (IHC), the identification of hormonal and human epidermal growth factor receptor 2 (HER2) in breast tumors allowed the classification of BC based on the expression of these markers and the development of specific receptor-targeted therapies with major clinical benefits. Furthermore, the past decade in BC research has been influenced by the development of genomic profiling techniques and the identification of tumor subtypes based on molecular expression patterns.[6,7] These recent advances have raised the idea of tailoring treatments even further, personalizing therapies for those most likely to respond and avoiding unnecessary side effects from treatment in the "nonresponders." The latter is preponderant in the adjuvant setting, given the constant challenge of distinguishing between those patients who need adjuvant treatment and those who do not.

## RATIONALE OF ADJUVANT CHEMOTHERAPY

Before the era of adjuvant therapies, the treatment of early BC relied only on loco-regional therapies. For almost a century, a purely anatomic and mechanistic perception governed the treatment of BC with the Halsted en bloc radical mastectomy.[8] Although some women with early BC may be cured with loco-regional treatment alone, up to 20% of patients with early-stage BC will ultimately experience treatment

**Table 1**
**Summary of classical and current chemotherapy regimens studied in adjuvant breast cancer therapy**

| | |
|---|---|
| CMF[a] | 6 cycles of C 100 × 14 + M 40 × 2 + 5-FU 600 × 2, given q 28 d. |
| AC[a] | 4 cycles of A 60 + C 600, given IV q 21 d. |
| EC[a] | 4 cycles of E 90 + C 600, given IV q 21 d. |
| FAC[a] | 6 cycles of 5-FU 500 × 2 + A 50 × 1 + C 500 IVx1, q-3 wk. |
| FEC[a] | 6 cycles of 5-FU 500 × 2 + E 60 × 2 + C 500 IVx1, q-4 wk. |
| AC → P | 4 cycles of A 60 C 600 q-3 wk → 12 cycles of P 80 q-wk |
| AC → D | 4 cycles of A 60 C 600 q-3 wk → 4 cycles of D 100 q 3-wk |
| FEC → D | 3 cycles of F 500 E 100 C 500 q-3 wk → 3 cycles of D 100 q 3-wk |
| FEC → P | 3 cycles of F 600 E 90 C 600 q-3 wk → 8 cycles of P 100 q-wk |
| Dose-dense AC → P | 4 cycles of A 60 C 600 q-2 wk → 4 cycles of P 175 q-2 wk + filgastrim days 3–10. |

Data are drug dose, mg/m$^2$ × frequency per cycle: ×14 = days, 1–14 oral; ×2 = days, 1 and 8 IV; ×1 = day 1 IV; q- = every.
*Abbreviations:* A, doxorubicin; C, cyclophosphamide; D, docetaxel; E, epirubicin; F, fluorouracil; IV, intravenous; M, methotrexate; P, paclitaxel.
[a] Classical and chemotherapy regimens.

failure and recurrence. The purpose of adjuvant systemic therapy is to improve the disease-free survival (DFS) and overall survival (OS) rates associated with treatment of BC by local therapies (surgery and/or radiation) alone. The elevated rates of recurrence are likely related to the presence of micrometastatic disease in 10% to 30% of LN-negative and in 35% to 90% of LN-positive patients at the time of diagnosis.[9–12] Adjuvant chemotherapy emerged as an instrument to eradicate the local or distant residual microscopic metastatic disease with potentially curative effects. In the 1970s, the understanding of BC as a systemic and biologically diverse disease grounded the development of clinical trials, the results of which changed dramatically the paradigm of BC treatment.[13] Early trials conducted by Fisher and colleagues,[14] at the National Surgical Adjuvant Breast and Bowel Project (NSABP), and by Bonadonna and colleagues,[15] at the Istituto Tumori Nationale in Milan, proved benefits in recurrence-free survival (RFS) and OS of adjuvant polychemotherapy in premenopausal women with node-positive BC. Following these initial studies, there were multiple prospective clinical trials conducted around the world investigating different adjuvant regimens.[16] The benefits of the early chemotherapy trials led to the recommendation of adjuvant chemotherapy to a wide range of population. The subgroups of patients in these early trials were classified based on anatomic/pathologic findings, mainly tumor size and LN status. The differences in treatment recommendations were dictated mainly by age and estrogen receptor (ER) status for the use of hormonal therapy, but in essence all patients with node-positive disease were considered potential candidates for cytotoxic chemotherapy.

By 2000, The National Institutes of Health's Consensus Development Conference on adjuvant therapy for BC recommended consideration of adjuvant chemotherapy for essentially all patients with tumors of 1 cm or larger.[17] The NSABP pooled analysis of more than 1250 cases with node-negative tumors up to 1 cm in size reported improved survival of adjuvant chemotherapy and hormone therapy in patients with node-negative tumors of 1 cm or smaller.[18] The most recent Early Breast Cancer Clinical Trialists' Collaborative Group (EBCTCG) overview of chemotherapy studies reported that proportional risk reduction from chemotherapy was little affected by age, nodal status, tumor diameter or differentiation, ER status, or tamoxifen use, and that information was lacking about tumor gene expression markers or quantitative IHC that might help to predict risk, chemosensitivity, or both.[19] Most guidelines have recommended systemic treatment for node-positive disease and/or tumors larger than 1 to 2 cm, irrespective of other tumor characteristics; however, the patients in these initial trials were unselected for their tumor biologic characteristics and the meta-analyses combine heterogeneous studies providing treatment benefits in a diverse population studied. Side effects of adjuvant chemotherapy can be life-threatening in up to 1% of patients. As the threshold for giving adjuvant chemotherapy is lowered, more patients will suffer the side effects of the therapy without a meaningful clinical benefit. Over the past 2 decades, extensive research has been dedicated to investigate prognostic and predictive markers to classify patients in risk-based groups with more homogeneous features and potentially find the population with higher response rates to adjuvant treatments. The decision on whether to use adjuvant systemic therapy is based on an analysis of prognostic factors that predict the likelihood of recurrence and efficacy of the treatment, counterbalanced by the toxicities of the drugs.

## PROGNOSTIC AND PREDICTIVE FACTORS

Adjuvant chemotherapy has been used in oncology practice for almost all patients except those with small, node-negative, and well-differentiated invasive primary cancers.[20] Tumor size and nodal status have been the classic factors influencing the decision on adjuvant chemotherapy; however, the clear-cut classic indication of chemotherapy for all node-positive patients with tumors larger than 1 cm is now controversial and a treatment recommendation should not be provided based strictly on size.[21] In addition to axillary sentinel node biopsy to identify micrometastatic disease,[22] histologic grading systems have been used to categorize cancers further. The Nottingham Prognostic Index (NPI) includes the evaluation of histologic grades in addition to tumor size and node involvement.[23,24] Three grades of differentiation are used (low, intermediate, and high grade), based on 3 morphologic features: the percentage of tubule formation, the degree of nuclear pleomorphism, and the mitotic count. The variables noted in these indices have been generally adopted as prognostic markers and have influenced recommendations for adjuvant therapy as markers of "high" risk. In addition to the variables that constitute the NPI, lymphovascular invasion (LVI) is reported as a separate finding. Quantitative measurements of ER and progesterone receptor (PR) and identification of HER2 overexpression are recommended assays in all invasive tumors. Although there is still controversy in the minimum percentage of cells stained for the receptor that should be considered positive, most groups are considering any positivity as a "positive" value.[21] Appropriate HER2 testing is pivotal in the management of patients with BC. Overexpression can be indirectly assessed by quantifying HER2 receptors by IHC, or by directly measuring the number of HER2 gene copies using fluorescence in situ hybridization or bright field in situ hybridization.[25] These factors have been used as prognostic markers to classify patients in high-risk groups and influence recommendations for adjuvant treatments. Tumors with a high grade of differentiation (grade 3), HER2 overexpression, and lack of ER/PR expression are considered more aggressive. Patients with these tumors are classified as "high risk" and more likely to benefit from adjuvant chemotherapy. Other factors, such as proliferation (Ki-67), weak expression of hormone receptors, and lymphovascular invasion, may be considered, but the evidence is limited. In patients with more than 3 axillary lymph nodes positive for metastasis, the use of adjuvant chemotherapy is well accepted.[26] ER-positive BCs are considered to have better prognosis than those with ER-negative tumors; however, some patients with ER-positive, LN-negative tumors may benefit from chemotherapy. In recent adjuvant studies, a category of "high-risk" node-negative patients has been included. This group is defined by a tumor larger than 2 cm in diameter and positive for ER or PR or as a tumor larger than 1 cm in diameter and negative for both ER and PR.

During the past several years, the development of genomic profiling techniques has identified gene expression patterns in breast tumors with distinct molecular profiles, pathologic features, and clinical outcomes.[6,7,27] Expression patterns have defined 4 different subtypes: luminal A and B (estrogen- sensitive BC), HER2-enriched, and basal-like tumors (negative ER/PR and negative HER2). Because the genetic profiling is not widely available in a standardized method, defining surrogate subtypes using immunohistochemical determination of ER/PR, and in situ hybridization technology for detecting HER2 amplification has been used as an approximation to the intrinsic subtypes. The St Gallen Consensus Conference in 2011 considered the clinicopathologic determination of ER, PR, HER2, and Ki-67 as useful for defining subtypes and to guide therapeutic choices in the absence of an available standardized test system able to molecularly characterize these subtypes.[26] Luminal A tumors are classified by positive ER/PR, negative HER2, and low Ki-67, whereas luminal B tumors characteristically have positive ER/PR, negative HER2, and high Ki-67.[28,29] The additive prognostic value of Ki-67, a cell proliferation marker, to steroid and HER2 receptors is accepted, as many significant genes in gene expression profiles are proliferation related. Ki-67 marks the difference between luminal A and B tumors; however, Ki-67 is not yet routinely available and standard cutoffs are not well defined.

The molecular classification has stimulated a targeted approach for the current BC therapies, including the use of hormonal therapy for luminal A tumors, HER2-targeting therapy for HER2-enriched tumors, and chemotherapy for luminal B and basal tumors. The priority of the current studies in adjuvant therapy is to identify the responders to a particular therapy and the population that does not require treatment. At the recent St Gallen Consensus Conference, the idea of using intrinsic tumor subtype for identifying responders and nonresponders to a specific therapy was considered. The goal is to move beyond the traditional prognostic factors, such as tumor size and lymph node status, to a personalized era using predictive factors of response to therapy.[26] The subgroup of patients with BC with luminal A tumors has a good prognosis and shows response to hormonal therapies. Conversely, these patients have a low likelihood to respond to adjuvant chemotherapy, especially in node-negative disease.[30] In these patients, the commercially available Oncotype DX (Genomic Health Inc, Redwood City, CA) and MammaPrint (Agendia BV, Irvine, CA) have a role in the prediction of chemotherapy response. In retrospective analysis of the NSABP B-20 trial in patients with node-negative disease, there was no advantage of adding chemotherapy to tamoxifen except among those with the highest levels of recurrence score (RS) as measured by Oncotype DX.[31]

Recent data suggest that even LN-positive luminal A tumors may derive little or no benefit from cytotoxic therapy when compared with the use of hormonal therapy alone. Analysis from the IBCSG (International Breast Cancer Study Group) IX trial[32] and IBCSG VIII trial[33] showed no benefit of adjuvant cytotoxic therapy in premenopausal and postmenopausal patients with high endocrine receptor expression, negative HER2, and low proliferation (low Ki-67 labeling index). These features correspond to the surrogate definition of luminal A tumors. Similarly, the Southwest Oncology Group (SWOG) 8814[34] showed no advantage of cyclophosphamide, doxorubicin, and fluorouracil chemotherapy over tamoxifen among postmenopausal women with node-positive disease with high ER levels, negative HER2, and low RS. Penault-Llorca and colleagues[35] analyzed the PACS (French Adjuvant Study Group) 01 trial, suggesting an additional benefit of taxane in patients with ER-positive disease with higher Ki-67 expression. As suggested by Hayes,[36] emerging evidence suggests that this group of women with early BC with features similar to the luminal A type, may not benefit by adding chemotherapy to highly effective endocrine therapy; however, level I evidence is needed to support this thesis. Patients with luminal B breast tumors (both ER positive and HER2 positive) appear to benefit more from adjuvant chemotherapy and less from hormonal therapy. Because genetic profiling is not yet routinely performed in a standardized system, IHC is still considered standard for evaluating risk of relapse and response to therapy.

Several validated tools to define prognosis are undergoing evaluation.[37] Adjuvant! Online (www.adjuvantonline.com) for BC is a prognostic tool that uses OS data from women diagnosed with BC between 1988 and 1992 recorded in the Surveillance, Epidemiology, and End Results (SEER) registry (www.seer.cancer.gov) and applies risk reductions from the EBCTCG,[16] to determine prognosis and treatment benefits for hormone therapy and chemotherapy.[38] This tool has been validated in several case cohort studies,[39,40] and has been assisting oncologists and patients in the decision making of chemotherapy. Specific clinicopathologic data from a patient is entered to estimate the probability of 10-year survival with no therapy, and to calculate the patient's risk of recurrence given hormonal therapy, chemotherapy, or combined therapy. Other prognostic tools using known clinical and pathologic factors are under investigation. Predict+ uses mortality data from the United Kingdom and includes HER2 status and mode of detection in the clinical prognostication tool. A recent study showed that Predict+ was inferior to Adjuvant! In estimating all-cause mortality, but provided better BC-specific mortality estimates that Adjuvant![41]

Genomic data to predict recurrence risk in women with early BC is an active area of research. Multiple assays are currently available in the United States. The Oncotype DX RS[42] and the MammaPrint[43] are the most widely used and perform gene-expression profiling of node-negative cancers. Oncotype DX is a validated genomic predictor of outcome and response to adjuvant chemotherapy in ER-positive BC.[42] The 21-gene assay quantifies risk of distant recurrence in node-negative, ER-positive, tamoxifen-treated patients. It reports a continuous risk score between 1 and 100 and stratifies recurrence risk into low (0–18), intermediate (19–30), and high (>30). Women with a low 21-gene RS have a favorable prognosis that chemotherapy will not provide a meaningful benefit over the risks of toxicity, whereas chemotherapy will benefit the high-risk group. The MammaPrint is a 70-gene signature that uses microarray technology applied to fresh-frozen tissues to classify patients into good and poor prognosis categories. The high-risk group will be candidates for adjuvant chemotherapy and the low-risk group will avoid chemotherapy.[43] Oncotype DX and MammaPrint are both available to be performed on fixed tissue. Current guidelines support the use of these studies in cases in which the need for adjuvant chemotherapy is not clear, based on clinicopathologic variables or conflicting patient preference. These tests have no value (Oncotype DX) or very limited value (MammaPrint) in stratifying ER-negative disease.[21] Higher level of evidence is available supporting the prognostic value of Adjuvant! Online and Oncotype DX. Prospective studies using archived tissues conducted by the NSABP B-14 and B-20[31,42] and by the SWOG 8814[34] have shown the ability of the 21-gene RS to independently predict response to adjuvant chemotherapy. Using data from the randomized trials NSABP B-14 and NSABP B-20, Tang and colleagues[37] reported that both Adjuvant! Online and the 21-gene RS independently predicted distant recurrence and chemotherapy benefit. The 21-gene RS was found to be more predictive of both distant recurrence and response to adjuvant chemotherapy. This test is widely used in the evaluation of patients with node-negative, ER-positive BC, allowing less administration of chemotherapy in these women.[37,44] Multiple randomized controlled trials to add level I evidence to the use of the 21-gene signature are undergoing. During the 2011 St Gallen consensus meeting, only the multiparameter gene assay Oncotype DX was considered by most as potentially useful for decision making on adjuvant chemotherapy in cases in which other factors (eg, grade, HER2) do not help.

## ADJUVANT CHEMOTHERAPY REGIMENS IN BC

For almost 2 decades, multiple randomized clinical studies were conducted worldwide to find the most effective adjuvant regimen. In 1976, Bonadonna and colleagues[45] reported the efficacy of cyclophosphamide, methotrexate, and 5-fluorouracil (CMF) as adjuvant treatment for patients with node-positive BC. CMF was the leader in adjuvant chemotherapy, considered the standard for premenopausal women with node-positive disease. In women with node-negative and ER-positive tumors, tamoxifen was recommended, whereas in the ER-negative tumors, classical CMF for 6 cycles offered a significant advantage both on relapse-free survival (RFS) and OS.[46] The role of tamoxifen in premenopausal ER-positive patients was not yet clearly elucidated and the benefit in younger patients was attributed to the ovarian suppression of CMF.

In the mid-1980s, anthracyclines were included in the clinical trials. The initial trials comparing CMF and anthracyclines studied 6 to 12 months of CMF compared with

6 months of anthracycline-based treatment with combinations such as FAC (fluorouracil, adriamycin, cyclophosphamide) or FEC (fluorouracil, epirubicin, cyclophosphamide). These regimens achieved reductions in annual odds of recurrence of 24% and 35%, respectively, and in odds of death of 14% and 30%, respectively.[5,16,47] Greater benefits were seen in patients younger than 50 years old, with hormone receptor–negative and node-positive disease. Based on this evidence, during the 1990s, 6 cycles of a 3-drug anthracycline-containing combination became the standard of care in adjuvant chemotherapy.[5,47,48] In women older than 50, the initial trials (NSABP B-16) enrolling almost 1200 patients indicated greater benefit from tamoxifen plus anthracycline-containing regimen than from tamoxifen alone in hormone-responsive patients.

The most recently published meta-analysis of the EBCTCG of outcomes in 100,000 women with early BC, including more than 100 trials of old and modern adjuvant chemotherapy, confirmed the benefit of CMF and anthracycline-based therapies with proportional reduction in BC mortality rate of 20% to 25% with absolute reductions of BC mortality of 6.2% and 6.5% respectively at 10 years.[19] Importantly, for women with ER-positive disease, if adjuvant tamoxifen therapy is given after the anthracycline-based regimen, the average annual death rate from BC would be approximately cut in half.[5]

### The Taxane Era in Adjuvant Therapy

In the early 1990s, the taxanes (paclitaxel and docetaxel) showed a potent antitumor efficacy in advanced BC and rapidly were approved to be included in adjuvant chemotherapy trials. The Cancer and Leukemia Group B 9344 (CALGB) and the NSABP B-B28 trials compared the sequential or concurrent administration of taxanes and anthracycline-based therapies, with the standard doxorubicin and cyclophosphamide regimen. These studies reported a significant reduction of 17% in the risk of recurrence when paclitaxel was added to the standard regimens. Overall survival favored the paclitaxel combination, although without reaching statistical significance.[49,50] Similar results were observed comparing docetaxel, doxorubicin, and cyclophosphamide (DAC) regimen with fluorouracil, doxorubicin, and cyclophosphamide (FAC). The Breast Cancer International Research Group (BCIRG)-001 trial reported a 7% absolute improvement in RFS and a 6% improvement in OS with DAC.[51] The Grupo Español Para la Investigación del Cáncer de Mama (GEICAM) 9805 trial also showed higher DFS rates of DAC over FAC.

Given elevated rates of side effects observed in the concurrent studies, multiple randomized trials have been conducted evaluating sequential therapy with taxanes. The CALGB 9344[49] and the NSABP B-28[50] evaluated the use of paclitaxel after 4 cycles of AC (Doxorubicin and Cyclophasphamide) and showed significant benefit in DFS (CALGB 9344 and NSABP B-28) and OS (CALGB 9344) when paclitaxel was added to the standard AC. Subsequent trials confirmed the incremental benefit of sequential docetaxel with anthracycline-containing regimens in the adjuvant setting.[52–54] The Protocole Adjuvant dans le Cancer du Sein (PACS) 01 trial randomized 1999 patients with LN-positive disease to adjuvant therapy with six 21-day cycles of FEC or three 21-day cycles of FEC followed by three 21-day cycles of docetaxel. The addition of docetaxel to FEC resulted in a 27% reduction in the risk of death (hazard ratio [HR] 0.73, 95% confidence interval [CI] 0.56–0.94, $P = .017$). An update at 8 years' median follow-up demonstrated a continued benefit of docetaxel therapy for DFS (HR 0.85, 95% CI 0.73–0.99, $P = .035$) and OS (HR 0.79, 95% CI 0.65–0.97, $P = .024$).[52] The GEICAM 9906 trial randomized 1246 LN-positive BC patients to receive six 21-day cycles of FEC or four 21-day cycles of FEC followed by 8 weekly administrations of paclitaxel

(FEC-T). After 66 months of follow-up, 5-year DFS was superior for the FEC-T arm (HR 0.74, 95% CI 0.60–0.92, $P = .006$). FEC-T reduced the risk of relapse by 23%. There was no significant improvement in 5-year OS.[53] The addition of a taxane to AC improves DFS and reduces the risk of recurrence; however, there is a lesser impact on overall survival.

The ECOG 1199 trial was intended to solve the questions about the best taxane administration regimens. The trial included 5000 patients with node-positive or high-risk node-negative (tumor size >2 cm) BC randomized to a standard AC regimen to be followed by 1 of 4 taxane regimens: paclitaxel 175 mg/m$^2$ every 3 weeks for 4 cycles (control), 12 weekly doses of paclitaxel 80 mg/m$^2$, docetaxel 100 mg/m$^2$ every 3 weeks for 4 cycles, or 12 weekly doses of docetaxel 35 mg/m$^2$. After a median of 64 months of follow-up, 5-year DFS was significantly better in the group receiving weekly paclitaxel (HR 1.27, 95% CI 1.03–1.57) and in the group receiving docetaxel every 3 weeks (HR 1.23, 95% CI 1.00–1.52) when compared with the standard every-3-week pacli-taxel group. There was no significant benefit of receiving weekly docetaxel over paclitaxel every 3 weeks. Patients with HER2-negative disease treated with weekly paclitaxel had a significant improvement in DFS and OS over standard every-3-week administration of paclitaxel; this result was not seen with docetaxel administration.[54] Other studies have evaluated the use of taxanes without anthracycline in the adjuvant setting. The US Oncology (USO) trial 9735 compared 3-week cycles of AC versus docetaxel-cyclophosphamide (DC) in the adjuvant setting. After 7 years of median follow up, a higher DFS and OS was reported in the patients treated with DC compared with those treated with AC. A regimen of 4 cycles of AC is an inferior comparator and no longer an appropriate standard for treating node-positive patients. Therefore, DC may be considered in treating some node-negative patients (when chemotherapy is consid-ered) but is not appropriate adjuvant therapy for node-positive patients.[55]

New studies are undergoing to optimize taxane delivery. The CALGB 9741 trial showed that dose-dense regimens (every 2 weeks) were significantly better than the conventionally (every 3 weeks) timed regimens, improving DFS (HR = 0.74, $P = .0072$), as well as OS (RR = 0.69, $P = .014$). The 4-year DFS was 82% for the dose-dense regimens and 75% for the 3-weekly regimens. There was no difference in either DFS or OS between the concurrent and sequential schedules of treatment.[56] Updated results after a median 6.5 years of follow-up continue to show an improvement in DFS and OS in favor of dose-dense chemotherapy administration with greater benefit in ER-negative tumors. Growth factor support is needed for dose-dense paclitaxel to main-tain strict every-14-day scheduling.

A meta-analysis demonstrated that taxane-based regimens provide both DFS and OS benefit with an absolute 5-year risk reduction of 5% for DFS and 3% for OS when compared with standard anthracycline regimens irrespective of ER status, LN status, and age. Additionally, the improvements in DFS and OS were similar for both paclitaxel and docetaxel. This evidence supported the adoption of taxane-containing and anthracycline-containing regimens as the new standard adjuvant treatment for patients with BC with LN-positive and possibly in high-risk LN negative tumors.[55] Scheduling of these agents include weekly and every 2-week or 3-week regimens for periods of 2 to 6 months depending on tumor stage. Women with early-stage BC have traditionally been treated with 4 cycles of an anthracycline-based regimen, whereas patients with more advanced disease (eg, stage II or III) have been treated with anthracycline-based and taxane-based therapies for 4 to 6 months. The recently published CALGB trial 40101, including 3171 patients with node-negative and 1 to 3 positive LNs, compared 4 cycles versus 6 cycles of chemotherapy. The 4 arms of therapy included 6 cycles of AC versus 4 cycles of AC, and 4 cycles of single-agent paclitaxel versus 6 cycles of paclitaxel.[57] The results showed no superiority of 6 cycles over 4 cycles of therapy for either OS (HR 1.12, 95% CI 0.89–1.42) and DFS (HR 1.03, 95% CI 0.84–1.28) in this population. Hematological and cardiac toxicities from AC and neuropathy from paclitaxel were more common in the patients who received 6 cycles of therapy.[57] The results of the comparison of single-agent paclitaxel versus AC are not yet available.

More conclusive data are needed regarding the comparison between the 2 taxanes available, docetaxel and paclitaxel, the method of administration, and identification of subgroups of patients who may greatly benefit from taxane therapy based on their hormonal status or tumor biology. Studies of concurrent versus sequential taxane administration have favored the sequential use with benefits in DFS and better safety profile; however, more studies are needed in this regard. The latest meta-analysis by the EBCTCG including the taxane trials showed a small but significant BC mortality reduction of adjuvant taxane-anthracycline–based regimen (2.8% absolute gain at 8 years). Interestingly, this difference was not significant when higher doses of nontaxane regimens were given to the control group.[19] With the limitations of molecular heterogeneity in the groups compared, limited information about HER2, and trastuzumab effect, the results suggested that these more modern regimens compared with no chemotherapy, may reduce 10-year BC mortality by about a third independent of ER receptor status and patient age.[19,58] Ongoing clinical trials are evaluating other agents in combination with anthracyclines and taxanes. The Finnish Breast Cancer Group (FinXX) investigated the benefit of the addition of capecitabine to docetaxel. After a median follow-up of 59 months, the capecitabine-containing regimen did not improve DFS compared with regimens without capecitabine.[59] Ixabepilone, a microtubule inhibitor, is being compared with weekly paclitaxel after adjuvant AC in the TITAN III trial (available at: http://clinicaltrials.gov/NCT00789581, accessed September 2012).

## ADJUVANT ENDOCRINE THERAPY IN BC

Adjuvant hormone therapy is considered standard in all patients with endocrine-sensitive tumors defined by the expression of ER and PR by IHC. Approximately 70% of BCs have positive expression of the ER and are considered hormone sensitive. Adjuvant hormone therapy in BC evolved after the discovery of the ER in the 1960s. Initial studies showed that breast tumors with expression of ER and PR correlated with hormonal sensitivity in metastatic breast tumors.[60] Tamoxifen demonstrated activity in advanced BC and entered adjuvant trials, most prominently in Europe with the Nolvadex Adjuvant Trial Organization (NATO) trial.[61] Adjuvant studies with tamoxifen have demonstrated a significant benefit in hormone-sensitive patients. In premenopausal women, tamoxifen remains the only endocrine agent approved by the Food and Drug Administration in the adjuvant setting. Treatment with tamoxifen for 5 years reduces the risk of recurrence by 41% and BC mortality by 34%. Nevertheless, more than 30% of patients will develop a recurrent tumor in the first 15 years following diagnosis. Although an early peak of recurrence is seen in the first 2 to 3 years after surgery, late recurrence remains an important concern in adjuvant therapy. There is a persistent 2% to 3% annual recurrence risk in years 5 through 9, which has been lowered by tamoxifen (relative risk reduction, 32%). After 10 years, the annual risk of recurrence is approximately 2%, and there is no lasting risk reduction on a year-to-year basis for having received tamoxifen for the initial 5 years.[5]

The aromatase inhibitors (AI) prevent estrogen synthesis through inhibition of the aromatase enzyme. This enzyme results in the synthesis of estrogen in peripheral tissues, but not in the ovary. Therefore, AI therapy is used only in postmenopausal patients. Over the past decade extensive research has been conducted with AIs in postmenopausal women. Anastrozole was approved in 1996 for the treatment of metastatic endocrine-sensitive BC. Subsequently, multiple randomized phase III clinical trials using third-generation AIs (anastrozole, letrozole, exemestane) have demonstrated benefits in DFS of postmenopausal women with ER-positive BC with the use of AIs as upfront therapy or in sequence with tamoxifen.[62–66]

### Adjuvant Trials Using Aromatase Inhibitors

The Arimidex, Tamoxifen, Alone or in Combination (ATAC) trial, is a pivotal trial in adjuvant hormone therapy.[62] The ATAC trial compared the adjuvant use of anastrozole (n = 3125) with tamoxifen (n = 3116) or anastrozole plus tamoxifen (n = 3125) in postmenopausal women with early-stage BC. A recent updated report of the ATAC trial showed a continuous benefit of anastrozole over tamoxifen at 120 months of follow-up in all patients studied and more pronounced in the HR+ patients. At 10 years, anastrozole as initial therapy showed increased DFS (HR 0.86, $P = .003$), time to local and distant recurrence (HR 0.79, $P = .0002$; HR 0.85, $P = .02$, respectively), and reduced indices of contralateral BC (HR 0.62 $P = .003$) compared with tamoxifen. As in the initial results, there was no significant difference in overall mortality between the 2 groups.[67] The results of the ATAC trial influenced the changes in the adjuvant endocrine therapy and outcomes in women with early-stage BC. In December 2001, the NCCN Clinical Practice Guidelines in Oncology included anastrozole as an alternative to tamoxifen in the initial adjuvant treatment of postmenopausal women.

Since the ATAC trial, other important studies have been conducted using AIs in adjuvant endocrine therapy. The 3 different AIs (anastrozole, exemestane, and letrozole) have been studied up front or sequential after 2 to 3 years of tamoxifen and as extended therapy after 5 years of tamoxifen. The Breast International Group 01–98 (BIG 1–98) included 8010 postmenopausal patients to compare letrozole to tamoxifen in the adjuvant setting in 2 monotherapy arms and 2 sequential arms.[64] Letrozole as a monotherapy for 5 years significantly improved DFS (HR 0.81, $P = .003$), and time to distant recurrence (HR 0.73, $P = .001$), compared with tamoxifen. No significant differences were observed in OS (HR 0.86, $P = .16$). An analysis of predictors of early relapse in the BIG 1–98 trial (n = 7707) found that adjuvant letrozole therapy had a pronounced benefit in reducing the risk of distant metastases early on, at 2 years (87 vs 125 events). In the report of the sequential analysis at 71 months of follow-up, there were no significant differences in DFS or OS between sequential treatments in either order compared with letrozole monotherapy. Subgroup analyses revealed that letrozole was particularly effective in patients with more than 4 axillary lymph node metastases and in patients with highly proliferative BC.[68] Based on these results, the investigators suggested that adjuvant endocrine therapy should begin with letrozole, particularly in patients at high risk for local or distant recurrence.[64] Both the ATAC and the BIG trial showed reductions in DFS but no improvement in OS. The trials showed differences in the toxicity profile with tamoxifen being related to more thromboembolic events and AIs associated with more fractures and arthralgias.

In the Intergroup Exemestane Study (IES) trial, postmenopausal women with early BC who had already completed 2 to 3 years of adjuvant tamoxifen therapy were randomized to switch to exemestane or to continue on tamoxifen for a total of 5 years.[65] At a median follow-up of 91 months, a significant improvement in DFS was observed in patients who had switched to exemestane (HR 0.84; $P = .002$). A modest but statistically significant improvement in OS was observed with an absolute difference in survival outcome at 8 years of 2.4% (HR 0.86, 95% CI 0.74–0.99; $P = .04$) in favor of switching to exemestane compared with those continuing treatment with tamoxifen.[69] MA.17

examined the idea of extending endocrine therapy beyond 5 years of tamoxifen.[63] This trial randomized postmenopausal women who had completed 4.5 to 6.0 years of tamoxifen to letrozole versus placebo for a planned 5-year period. In the intent-to-treat analysis at 30 months of median follow-up, the DFS was 94.4% in the letrozole arm versus 89.8% in the placebo group ($P<.001$). When the analyses were restricted to those with ER-positive tumors, the HR for recurrence or contralateral BC substantially favored letrozole (HR 0.58, 95% CI 0.45–0.76). No OS advantage was noted; however, a survival advantage was reported in node-positive patients ($P = .04$).[70]

From the data reported and summarized in **Table 2**, AIs provide benefit in DFS compared with tamoxifen in postmenopausal women with early-stage BC. The benefits of anastrozole in DFS are maintained or extended with long-term follow-up. Although there has been lack of significant OS advantage in all studies reported (see **Table 2**), subgroup analyses of both MA.17 and BIG 1–98 demonstrated a survival benefit with AI therapy in node-positive patients. The lack of survival advantage has been attributed to the limited follow-up for a long-term disease, non-BC deaths, and the contribution of loco-regional or contralateral BC events to study end points, and late crossover from tamoxifen to AI treatments. With adjustment for that high rate of crossover, the MA.17 study and the BIG 1–98, reported a survival advantage for use of an AI instead of tamoxifen alone. These findings suggest that up-front adjuvant therapy with an AI may benefit a subgroup of patients with poor prognostic factors at the time of surgery (large and highly proliferative tumors, high number of axillary lymph node metastases).[71]

The best treatment regimen, up front or sequential after tamoxifen, and choice of AIs, remains to be defined. Also, multiple questions regarding the optimal duration of AI, long-term adverse effects of AIs, and the predictive value of molecular markers, such as PR, are being addressed by ongoing clinical trials.[72] At present, there are no clinical or biologic markers sufficiently reliable to determine whether duration should vary from patient to patient. The available evidence has led to major changes in oncologic practice, placing the AIs as the most commonly prescribed adjuvant endocrine therapy for postmenopausal women with early ER-positive BC.[63] Current guidelines from the American Society of Clinical Oncology recommend incorporating AI either as up-front

**Table 2**
**Summary of results from adjuvant aromatase inhibitor therapy trials in postmenopausal women with hormone receptor-positive**

| Trials | AI | Timing of AI | Results |
|---|---|---|---|
| ATAC[62] | Anastrozole | Up-front AI vs TAM | Benefit in DFS (HR 0.87, $P = .01$) No OS benefit |
| BIG 1–98[64] | Letrozole | Up-front AI vs TAM Sequential AI after TAM | Up-front AI: DFS ($P = .03$) T → AI vs AI: DFS (HR 1.05, 99% CI 0.84–1.32) No OS benefit |
| IES[65] | Exemestane | Sequential AI after TAM vs up-front AI | + Benefit in DFS ($P = .0001$) OS ($P = .05$) when restricted to ER+ |
| MA.17[70] | Letrozole | Extended after 5 y of TAM | + Benefit DFS ($P<.001$) OS ($P = .04$) in LN+. |
| TEAM[85] | Exemestane | Up-front Exemestane vs TAM → Exemestane | No difference in DFS ($P = .60$) |

*Abbreviations:* AI, aromatase inhibitor; DFS, disease-free survival; ER+, estrogen receptor–positive patients; HR, hazard ratio; LN+, lymph node–positive patients; OS, overall survival; TAM, tamoxifen.

therapy or as sequential treatment after tamoxifen for 5 years and acknowledge that the "optimal timing and duration of endocrine treatment remain unresolved." The St Gallen Consensus Conference panel in 2011 also considered appropriate to include AIs at some point in the adjuvant treatment of postmenopausal women, especially in LN-positive patients.[73]

## ADJUVANT THERAPY IN HER2 POSITIVE BCS

Approximately 15% to 20% of all BCs present with amplification of the HER2 gene. HER2 overexpression is reported to be an independent predictor of poor prognosis.[74,75] This poorer prognosis can be addressed by the incorporation of anti-HER2 therapy with trastuzumab, a monoclonal antibody targeting the extracellular domain of the HER2 protein, which in the adjuvant setting has shown significant improvement in clinical outcomes from adjuvant chemotherapy plus trastuzumab compared with chemotherapy alone. The initial trials led by the NSABP and the North Central Cancer Center Group showed benefits in DFS and OS with addition of trastuzumab, sequentially or concurrently with paclitaxel, after a regimen of doxorubicin and cyclophosphamide.[76] Based on results from 5 randomized clinical trials, a trastuzumab-containing regimen for up to 1 year is now considered standard for all patients with HER2-positive tumors larger than 1 cm.[77–79] Patients received either chemotherapy alone or chemotherapy with sequential treatment with trastuzumab for 12 months. One of these trials, the Herceptin Adjuvant (HERA) trial, included 5102 patients evaluating trastuzumab as adjuvant treatment for patients with HER2-positive BC. After a median follow-up of 4 years, the DFS was significantly higher in the trastuzumab group (HR 0.76, 95% CI 0.66–0.87) with no significant benefit in OS likely secondary to crossover of 52% of patients.

On the other hand, trials evaluating trastuzumab given concomitantly with chemotherapy have shown benefits in OS. The North Central Cancer Treatment Group (N9831) trial directly compared concomitant trastuzumab and paclitaxel versus sequential trastuzumab in the adjuvant setting. At a median follow-up of 6 years, the results favored the concomitant administration of trastuzumab with paclitaxel relative to sequential administration.[80] The Breast Cancer International Research Group 006 (BCIRG 006) trial evaluated trastuzumab combined with either docetaxel after AC (AC–TH) or docetaxel plus carboplatin (TCarboH), with a control arm of doxorubicin/ cyclophosphamide/docetaxel (ACT). The trial did not permit or facilitate crossover, and only 1.6% of patients in the control group crossed over to trastuzumab. At a median follow-up of 5.5 years, AC–TH and TCarboH were each associated with statistically significant improvements in DFS and OS compared with ACT.[79] In the combined analysis of the North Central Cancer Treatment Group trial N9831 and the NSABBP trial B-31, 20.9% of patients in the control group crossed over to trastuzumab.[77] An updated efficacy analysis (median follow-up of 2.9 years) showed that combining trastuzumab with paclitaxel after doxorubicin/cyclophosphamide (AC) significantly improved DFS (HR 0.49, 95% CI 0.41–0.58, $P<.0001$) and OS (HR 0.63, 95% CI 0.49–0.81, $P = .0004$) compared with chemotherapy alone.[80] These trials have led to the preferred use of trastuzumab concurrent with chemotherapy in the treatment patients with HER2-positive BC larger than 1 cm and medically fit to tolerate chemotherapy (**Table 3**).

The appropriate duration of anti-HER2 therapy is under investigation. Ongoing trials are evaluating 6 versus 12 months of adjuvant trastuzumab (http://www.clinicaltrials. gov/NCT00381901) and 9 weeks versus 1 year of trastuzumab in combination with chemotherapy (http://www.clinicaltrials.gov/NCT00593697). In the oncology practice, if there is easy access to the medication, 1 year of therapy is recommended. On the

| **Table 3** | |
| **Adjuvant regimens containing trastuzumab for HER2 overexpressed/amplified breast cancer** | |
| **Phase III Clinical Trials** | **Regimens with Improved Outcomes** |
| HERA[78] | Any Adjuvant therapy × 4 cycles → T (52 wk) |
| NSABP B-31[76] | A 60 C 600 × 4 →P 80 weekly × 12 + T (52 wk) |
| NCCTG N9831[77] | A 60 C 600 × 4 → P 80 weekly × 12 → T (52 wk) |
| | A 60 C 600 × 4 → P 80 weekly × 12 + T (52 wk) |
| BCIRG-006[79] | A 60 C 600 × 4 → D 100 q-3w × 4 + T (52 wk) |
| | A 60 C 600 × 4 → D 75 + C q-3wk × 6 + T (52 wk) |

Data are drug dose in mg/m$^2$ × (per number of cycles); q- = every; → (followed by); + (in addition to).
   *Abbreviations:* A, adriamycin; C, cyclophosphamide; D, docetaxel; P, paclitaxel; T, trastuzumab.

other hand, in the case of limited resources, shorter duration may be an option. Given the absence of conclusive data, adjuvant trastuzumab therapy over more than 1 year is not accepted as standard treatment.

Since the eligibility criteria for the phase III adjuvant trials of trastuzumab included tumor diameter of greater than 1 cm or positive LN, the effect of trastuzumab in very small tumors (pT1a/b, N0) is still under investigation. Several studies have reported worse DFS in HER2-positive small (<1 cm) tumors.[81] A subgroup analysis of the BCIRG 006 phase III trial evaluated patients with small (<1 cm), node-negative, and HER2-positive tumors. To be eligible, patients with small tumors needed to be younger than 35 years, with ER/PR negative or histologic and/or nuclear grade 2 to 3.[79] The estimated 5-year rates of DFS were 86% in the trastuzumab-containing arms (AC followed by docetaxel every 3 weeks plus 52 weeks of trastuzumab [AC-TH]; docetaxel and carboplatin plus 52 weeks of trastuzumab [TCH]) and 72% in the chemotherapy-only arm (doxorubicin and cyclophosphamide followed by docetaxel every 3 weeks [AC-T]). The HR for DFS for trastuzumab with anthracycline based chemotherapy was 0.36 ($P$ = .03), whereas for the trastuzumab and nonanthracycline-based chemotherapy, the HR was 0.45 ($P$ = .10).[79] The scarce data available, suggest benefit of trastuzumab in small HER2-positive tumors in patients with other risk factors, such as young age, high nuclear grades, or absence of HR expression. It has been proposed to consider a course of chemotherapy plus trastuzumab especially in patients with T1b or with unfavorable risk factors.[82] The main concerns in this population are the side effects from trastuzumab therapy. The rates of grade III/IV congestive heart failure (CHF) reported in the adjuvant trials have been up to 3.3%. The trastuzumab-related cardiotoxicity seems to be reversible and not related to cumulative doses.[83] Nonanthracycline regimens plus trastuzumab are being evaluated in early-stage BC to minimize the risk of CHF (http://www.clinicaltrials.gov/NCT00542451; accessed September 2012). In patients with HER2-enriched and ER-positive BC, MammaPrint's "low-risk" tumors have been associated with a good prognosis; therefore, it is attractive to omit adjuvant chemotherapy and trastuzumab in these patients in favor of hormone therapy alone; however, MammaPrint has no shown predictive value.

Ongoing trials are evaluating other novel HER2-targeting agents. Pertuzumab is a recombinant humanized monoclonal antibody directed against the dimerization domain II of HER2. This agent has shown beneficial effects in the metastatic setting combined with trastuzumab and chemotherapy.[84] In the adjuvant setting, phase III clinical trials are undergoing to evaluate pertuzumab combined with trastuzumab and chemotherapy in patients with operable HER2-positive BC (http://www.clinicaltrials.gov/NCT01358877; accessed September 2012).

## SUMMARY

The benefit of the adjuvant therapies in BC has been extensively proven over several decades. Polychemotherapy regimens, including taxanes and hormone-targeted and HER2-targeted medications, are part of the armamentarium of the multidisciplinary teams that care for women with operable BC. The emerging genomic data reflecting the heterogeneity of the disease with potential predictive value is currently the focus of extensive research with the purpose of evolving from a universal use of adjuvant therapy to a more personalized approach.

## REFERENCES

1. DeSantis C, Siegel R, Bandi P, et al. Breast cancer statistics, 2011. CA Cancer J Clin 2011;61(6):408–18.
2. Berry DA, Cronin KA, Plevritis SK, et al. Effect of screening and adjuvant therapy on mortality from breast cancer. N Engl J Med 2005;353(17):1784–92.
3. Berry DA, Inoue L, Shen Y, et al. Modeling the impact of treatment and screening on U.S. breast cancer mortality: a Bayesian approach. J Natl Cancer Inst Monogr 2006;(36):30–6.
4. Mincey BA, Palmieri FM, Perez EA. Adjuvant therapy for breast cancer: recommendations for management based on consensus review and recent clinical trials. Oncologist 2002;7(3):246–50.
5. Early Breast Cancer Trialists' Collaborative Group (EBCTCG). Effects of chemotherapy and hormonal therapy for early breast cancer on recurrence and 15-year survival: an overview of the randomised trials. Lancet 2005;365(9472):1687–717.
6. Perou CM. Molecular stratification of triple-negative breast cancers. Oncologist 2010;15(Suppl 5):39–48.
7. Sorlie T, Perou CM, Tibshirani R, et al. Gene expression patterns of breast carcinomas distinguish tumor subclasses with clinical implications. Proc Natl Acad Sci U S A 2001;98(19):10869–74.
8. Bland CS. The Halsted mastectomy: present illness and past history. West J Med 1981;134(6):549–55.
9. Valagussa P, Bonadonna G, Veronesi U. Patterns of relapse and survival in operable breast carcinoma with positive and negative axillary nodes. Tumori 1978; 64(3):241–58.
10. Hortobagyi GN, Buzdar AU. Current status of adjuvant systemic therapy for primary breast cancer: progress and controversy. CA Cancer J Clin 1995; 45(4):199–226.
11. Schabel FM Jr. Concepts for systemic treatment of micrometastases. Cancer 1975;35(1):15–24.
12. Fisher B, Fisher ER. The interrelationship of hematogenous and lymphatic tumor cell dissemination. Surg Gynecol Obstet 1966;122(4):791–8.
13. Fisher B. A biological perspective of breast cancer: contributions of the National Surgical Adjuvant Breast and Bowel Project clinical trials. CA Cancer J Clin 1991; 41(2):97–111.
14. Fisher B, Redmond C, Elias EG, et al. Adjuvant chemotherapy for breast cancer: an overview of NSABP findings. Int Adv Surg Oncol 1982;5:65–90.
15. Bonadonna G, Valagussa P, Moliterni A, et al. Adjuvant cyclophosphamide, methotrexate, and fluorouracil in node-positive breast cancer: the results of 20 years of follow-up. N Engl J Med 1995;332(14):901–6.
16. Polychemotherapy for early breast cancer: an overview of the randomised trials. Early Breast Cancer Trialists' Collaborative Group. Lancet 1998;352(9132):930–42.

17. Eifel P, Axelson JA, Costa J, et al. National Institutes of Health Consensus Development Conference Statement: adjuvant therapy for breast cancer, November 1-3, 2000. J Natl Cancer Inst 2001;93(13):979–89.
18. Fisher B, Dignam J, Tan-Chiu E, et al. Prognosis and treatment of patients with breast tumors of one centimeter or less and negative axillary lymph nodes. J Natl Cancer Inst 2001;93(2):112–20.
19. Early Breast Cancer Trialists' Collaborative Group (EBCTCG), Peto R, Davies C, et al. Comparisons between different polychemotherapy regimens for early breast cancer: meta-analyses of long-term outcome among 100,000 women in 123 randomised trials. Lancet 2012;379(9814):432–44.
20. Carlson RW, Allred DC, Anderson BO, et al. Invasive breast cancer. J Natl Compr Canc Netw 2011;9(2):136–222.
21. Schwartz GF, Bartelink H, Burstein HJ, et al. Adjuvant therapy in stage I carcinoma of the breast: the influence of multigene analyses and molecular phenotyping. Breast J 2012;18(4):303–11.
22. Schwartz GF, Giuliano AE, Veronesi U, et al. Proceedings of the consensus conference on the role of sentinel lymph node biopsy in carcinoma of the breast, April 19-22, 2001, Philadelphia, Pennsylvania. Cancer 2002;94(10): 2542–51.
23. Todd JH, Dowle C, Williams MR, et al. Confirmation of a prognostic index in primary breast cancer. Br J Cancer 1987;56(4):489–92.
24. Blamey RW, Ellis IO, Pinder SE, et al. Survival of invasive breast cancer according to the Nottingham Prognostic Index in cases diagnosed in 1990-1999. Eur J Cancer 2007;43(10):1548–55.
25. Wolff AC, Hammond ME, Schwartz JN, et al. American Society of Clinical Oncology/College of American Pathologists guideline recommendations for human epidermal growth factor receptor 2 testing in breast cancer. J Clin Oncol 2007;25(1):118–45.
26. Goldhirsch A, Wood WC, Coates AS, et al. Strategies for subtypes—dealing with the diversity of breast cancer: highlights of the St. Gallen International Expert Consensus on the Primary Therapy of Early Breast Cancer 2011. Ann Oncol 2011;22(8):1736–47.
27. Perou CM, Sorlie T, Eisen MB, et al. Molecular portraits of human breast tumours. Nature 2000;406(6797):747–52.
28. Cheang MC, Voduc D, Bajdik C, et al. Basal-like breast cancer defined by five biomarkers has superior prognostic value than triple-negative phenotype. Clin Cancer Res 2008;14(5):1368–76.
29. Cheang MC, Chia SK, Voduc D, et al. Ki67 index, HER2 status, and prognosis of patients with luminal B breast cancer. J Natl Cancer Inst 2009;101(10):736–50.
30. Colleoni M, Cole BF, Viale G, et al. Classical cyclophosphamide, methotrexate, and fluorouracil chemotherapy is more effective in triple-negative, node-negative breast cancer: results from two randomized trials of adjuvant chemoendocrine therapy for node-negative breast cancer. J Clin Oncol 2010;28(18):2966–73.
31. Paik S, Tang G, Shak S, et al. Gene expression and benefit of chemotherapy in women with node-negative, estrogen receptor-positive breast cancer. J Clin Oncol 2006;24(23):3726–34.
32. Aebi S, Sun Z, Braun D, et al. Differential efficacy of three cycles of CMF followed by tamoxifen in patients with ER-positive and ER-negative tumors: long-term follow up on IBCSG Trial IX. Ann Oncol 2011;22(9):1981–7.
33. Viale G, Regan MM, Maiorano E, et al. Chemoendocrine compared with endocrine adjuvant therapies for node-negative breast cancer: predictive value of

centrally reviewed expression of estrogen and progesterone receptors—International Breast Cancer Study Group. J Clin Oncol 2008;26(9):1404–10.

34. Albain KS, Barlow WE, Shak S, et al. Prognostic and predictive value of the 21-gene recurrence score assay in postmenopausal women with node-positive, oestrogen-receptor-positive breast cancer on chemotherapy: a retrospective analysis of a randomised trial. Lancet Oncol 2010;11(1):55–65.

35. Penault-Llorca F, Andre F, Sagan C, et al. Ki67 expression and docetaxel efficacy in patients with estrogen receptor-positive breast cancer. J Clin Oncol 2009; 27(17):2809–15.

36. Hayes DF. Targeting adjuvant chemotherapy: a good idea that needs to be proven! J Clin Oncol 2012;30(12):1264–7.

37. Tang G, Shak S, Paik S, et al. Comparison of the prognostic and predictive utilities of the 21-gene Recurrence Score assay and Adjuvant! for women with node-negative, ER-positive breast cancer: results from NSABP B-14 and NSABP B-20. Breast Cancer Res Treat 2011;127(1):133–42.

38. Ravdin PM, Siminoff LA, Davis GJ, et al. Computer program to assist in making decisions about adjuvant therapy for women with early breast cancer. J Clin Oncol 2001;19(4):980–91.

39. Olivotto IA, Bajdik CD, Ravdin PM, et al. Population-based validation of the prognostic model ADJUVANT! for early breast cancer. J Clin Oncol 2005;23(12): 2716–25.

40. Mook S, Schmidt MK, Rutgers EJ, et al. Calibration and discriminatory accuracy of prognosis calculation for breast cancer with the online Adjuvant! program: a hospital-based retrospective cohort study. Lancet Oncol 2009;10(11):1070–6.

41. Wishart GC, Bajdik CD, Dicks E, et al. PREDICT Plus: development and validation of a prognostic model for early breast cancer that includes HER2. Br J Cancer 2012;107(5):800–7.

42. Paik S, Shak S, Tang G, et al. A multigene assay to predict recurrence of tamoxifen-treated, node-negative breast cancer. N Engl J Med 2004;351(27): 2817–26.

43. van't Veer LJ, Paik S, Hayes DF. Gene expression profiling of breast cancer: a new tumor marker. J Clin Oncol 2005;23(8):1631–5.

44. Hornberger J, Alvarado MD, Rebecca C, et al. Clinical validity/utility, change in practice patterns, and economic implications of risk stratifiers to predict outcomes for early-stage breast cancer: a systematic review. J Natl Cancer Inst 2012;104(14):1068–79.

45. Bonadonna G, Brusamolino E, Valagussa P, et al. Combination chemotherapy as an adjuvant treatment in operable breast cancer. N Engl J Med 1976;294(8):405–10.

46. Fisher B, Redmond C, Dimitrov NV, et al. A randomized clinical trial evaluating sequential methotrexate and fluorouracil in the treatment of patients with node-negative breast cancer who have estrogen-receptor-negative tumors. N Engl J Med 1989;320(8):473–8.

47. Martin M, Villar A, Sole-Calvo A, et al. Doxorubicin in combination with fluorouracil and cyclophosphamide (i.v. FAC regimen, day 1, 21) versus methotrexate in combination with fluorouracil and cyclophosphamide (i.v. CMF regimen, day 1, 21) as adjuvant chemotherapy for operable breast cancer: a study by the GEI-CAM group. Ann Oncol 2003;14(6):833–42.

48. Fumoleau P, Kerbrat P, Romestaing P, et al. Randomized trial comparing six versus three cycles of epirubicin-based adjuvant chemotherapy in premenopausal, node-positive breast cancer patients: 10-year follow-up results of the French Adjuvant Study Group 01 trial. J Clin Oncol 2003;21(2):298–305.

49. Henderson IC, Berry DA, Demetri GD, et al. Improved outcomes from adding sequential Paclitaxel but not from escalating Doxorubicin dose in an adjuvant chemotherapy regimen for patients with node-positive primary breast cancer. J Clin Oncol 2003;21(6):976–83.
50. Mamounas EP, Bryant J, Lembersky B, et al. Paclitaxel after doxorubicin plus cyclophosphamide as adjuvant chemotherapy for node-positive breast cancer: results from NSABP B-28. J Clin Oncol 2005;23(16):3686–96.
51. Martin M, Pienkowski T, Mackey J, et al. Adjuvant docetaxel for node-positive breast cancer. N Engl J Med 2005;352(22):2302–13.
52. Coudert B, Asselain B, Campone M, et al. Extended benefit from sequential administration of docetaxel after standard fluorouracil, epirubicin, and cyclophosphamide regimen for node-positive breast cancer: the 8-year follow-up results of the UNICANCER-PACS01 trial. Oncologist 2012;17(7):900–9.
53. Martin M, Rodriguez-Lescure A, Ruiz A, et al. Randomized phase 3 trial of fluorouracil, epirubicin, and cyclophosphamide alone or followed by Paclitaxel for early breast cancer. J Natl Cancer Inst 2008;100(11):805–14.
54. Sparano JA, Wang M, Martino S, et al. Weekly paclitaxel in the adjuvant treatment of breast cancer. N Engl J Med 2008;358(16):1663–71.
55. Gajria D, Seidman A, Dang C. Adjuvant taxanes: more to the story. Clin Breast Cancer 2010;10(Suppl 2):S41–9.
56. Citron ML, Berry DA, Cirrincione C, et al. Randomized trial of dose-dense versus conventionally scheduled and sequential versus concurrent combination chemotherapy as postoperative adjuvant treatment of node-positive primary breast cancer: first report of Intergroup Trial C9741/Cancer and Leukemia Group B Trial 9741. J Clin Oncol 2003;21(8):1431–9.
57. Shulman LN, Cirrincione CT, Berry DA, et al. Six cycles of doxorubicin and cyclophosphamide or paclitaxel are not superior to four cycles as adjuvant chemotherapy for breast cancer in women with zero to three positive axillary nodes: cancer and leukemia group B 40101. J Clin Oncol 2012;30(33):4071–6.
58. Palmieri C, Jones A. The 2011 EBCTCG polychemotherapy overview. Lancet 2012;379(9814):390–2.
59. Joensuu H, Kellokumpu-Lehtinen PL, Huovinen R, et al. Adjuvant capecitabine, docetaxel, cyclophosphamide, and epirubicin for early breast cancer: final analysis of the randomized FinXX trial. J Clin Oncol 2012;30(1):11–8.
60. Jensen EV, Jacobson HI, Walf AA, et al. Estrogen action: a historic perspective on the implications of considering alternative approaches. Physiol Behav 2010; 99(2):151–62.
61. Singh L, Wilson AJ, Baum M, et al. The relationship between histological grade, oestrogen receptor status, events and survival at 8 years in the NATO ('Nolvadex') trial. Br J Cancer 1988;57(6):612–4.
62. Baum M, Buzdar A, Cuzick J, et al. Anastrozole alone or in combination with tamoxifen versus tamoxifen alone for adjuvant treatment of postmenopausal women with early-stage breast cancer: results of the ATAC (Arimidex, Tamoxifen Alone or in Combination) trial efficacy and safety update analyses. Cancer 2003; 98(9):1802–10.
63. Svahn TH, Niland JC, Carlson RW, et al. Predictors and temporal trends of adjuvant aromatase inhibitor use in breast cancer. J Natl Compr Canc Netw 2009; 7(2):115–21.
64. Breast International Group (BIG) 1-98 Collaborative Group, Thurlimann B, Keshaviah A, et al. A comparison of letrozole and tamoxifen in postmenopausal women with early breast cancer. N Engl J Med 2005;353(26):2747–57.

65. Coombes RC, Kilburn LS, Snowdon CF, et al. Survival and safety of exemestane versus tamoxifen after 2-3 years' tamoxifen treatment (Intergroup Exemestane Study): a randomised controlled trial. Lancet 2007;369(9561):559–70.

66. Kaufmann M, Jonat W, Hilfrich J, et al. Improved overall survival in postmeno-pausal women with early breast cancer after anastrozole initiated after treatment with tamoxifen compared with continued tamoxifen: the ARNO 95 Study. J Clin Oncol 2007;25(19):2664–70.

67. Cuzick J, Sestak I, Baum M, et al. Effect of anastrozole and tamoxifen as adjuvant treatment for early-stage breast cancer: 10-year analysis of the ATAC trial. Lancet Oncol 2010;11(12):1135–41.

68. BIG 1-98 Collaborative Group, Mouridsen H, Giobbie-Hurder A, et al. Letrozole therapy alone or in sequence with tamoxifen in women with breast cancer. N Engl J Med 2009;361(8):766–76.

69. Bliss JM, Kilburn LS, Coleman RE, et al. Disease-related outcomes with long-term follow-up: an updated analysis of the intergroup exemestane study. J Clin Oncol 2012;30(7):709–17.

70. Goss PE, Ingle JN, Pater JL, et al. Late extended adjuvant treatment with letrozole improves outcome in women with early-stage breast cancer who complete 5 years of tamoxifen. J Clin Oncol 2008;26(12):1948–55.

71. Sanchez-Munoz A, Ribelles N, Alba E. Optimal adjuvant hormonal therapy in postmenopausal women with hormone-receptor-positive early breast cancer: have we answered the question? Clin Transl Oncol 2010;12(9):614–20.

72. Mackey JR. Can quantifying hormone receptor levels guide the choice of adjuvant endocrine therapy for breast cancer? J Clin Oncol 2011;29(12):1504–6.

73. Gnant M, Harbeck N, Thomssen C. St. Gallen 2011: summary of the consensus discussion. Breast Care (Basel) 2011;6(2):136–41.

74. Slamon DJ, Clark GM, Wong SG, et al. Human breast cancer: correlation of relapse and survival with amplification of the HER-2/neu oncogene. Science 1987;235(4785):177–82.

75. Ravdin PM, Chamness GC. The c-erbB-2 proto-oncogene as a prognostic and predictive marker in breast cancer: a paradigm for the development of other macromolecular markers—a review. Gene 1995;159(1):19–27.

76. Romond EH, Perez EA, Bryant J, et al. Trastuzumab plus adjuvant chemotherapy for operable HER2-positive breast cancer. N Engl J Med 2005;353(16):1673–84.

77. Perez EA, Romond EH, Suman VJ, et al. Four-year follow-up of trastuzumab plus adjuvant chemotherapy for operable human epidermal growth factor receptor 2-positive breast cancer: joint analysis of data from NCCTG N9831 and NSABP B-31. J Clin Oncol 2011;29(25):3366–73.

78. Gianni L, Dafni U, Gelber RD, et al. Treatment with trastuzumab for 1 year after adjuvant chemotherapy in patients with HER2-positive early breast cancer: a 4-year follow-up of a randomised controlled trial. Lancet Oncol 2011;12(3):236–44.

79. Slamon D, Eiermann W, Robert N, et al. Adjuvant trastuzumab in HER2-positive breast cancer. N Engl J Med 2011;365(14):1273–83.

80. Perez EA, Suman VJ, Davidson NE, et al. Sequential versus concurrent trastuzumab in adjuvant chemotherapy for breast cancer. J Clin Oncol 2011;29(34):4491–7.

81. Gonzalez-Angulo AM, Litton JK, Broglio KR, et al. High risk of recurrence for patients with breast cancer who have human epidermal growth factor receptor 2-positive, node-negative tumors 1 cm or smaller. J Clin Oncol 2009;27(34):5700–6.

82. Burstein HJ, Winer EP. Refining therapy for human epidermal growth factor receptor 2-positive breast cancer: T stands for trastuzumab, tumor size, and treatment strategy. J Clin Oncol 2009;27(34):5671–3.

83. Russell SD, Blackwell KL, Lawrence J, et al. Independent adjudication of symptomatic heart failure with the use of doxorubicin and cyclophosphamide followed by trastuzumab adjuvant therapy: a combined review of cardiac data from the National Surgical Adjuvant breast and Bowel Project B-31 and the North Central Cancer Treatment Group N9831 clinical trials. J Clin Oncol 2010;28(21):3416–21.
84. Baselga J, Cortes J, Kim SB, et al. Pertuzumab plus trastuzumab plus docetaxel for metastatic breast cancer. N Engl J Med 2012;366(2):109–19.
85. van de Velde CJ, Rea D, Seynaeve C, et al. Adjuvant tamoxifen and exemestane in early breast cancer (TEAM): a randomised phase 3 trial. Lancet 2011; 377(9762):321–31.

# Neoadjuvant Chemotherapy in the Treatment of Breast Cancer

Meredith H. Redden, MD[a], George M. Fuhrman, MD[b],*

## KEYWORDS

- Neoadjuvant chemotherapy • Trastuzumab • Nodal disease • Breast cancer

## KEY POINTS

- Neoadjuvant chemotherapy is still the preferred approach for patients with locally advanced disease.
- Randomized prospective trials have demonstrated that early-stage patients with breast cancer who prefer breast conservation can benefit from neoadjuvant chemotherapy by achieving about a 25% complete and a greater than 80% partial pathologic response.
- Patients who opt for neoadjuvant chemotherapy should have a clinical and radiographic assessment of the axilla.
- If nodal disease is demonstrated at the time of diagnosis, then axillary staging requires a node dissection.
- Neoadjuvant trastuzumab seems to be an excellent option for patients with Her 2-neu–positive cancers.

Historically, neoadjuvant chemotherapy was used in an effort to improve the disease-free survival in patients with locally advanced breast cancer that was considered inoperable at presentation. These patients' primary tumors were large, fixed to the chest wall or skin, or had overwhelming axillary nodal disease that resulted in nodes becoming matted together and difficult or impossible to separate from axillary neurovascular structures. Neoadjuvant chemotherapy offered the hope that cancer cells in large and/or fixed primary tumors and bulky axillary lymph nodes could be downsized, if not eradicated, and facilitates a routine surgical procedure (eg, modified radical mastectomy) that in combination with radiotherapy would achieve local regional control of malignancy and enhanced survival.

The initial evidence to support neoadjuvant chemotherapy in the multimodality approach to locally advanced breast cancer is based on studies from MD Anderson, where patients with stages IIB, IIIA, IIIB, and regional IV disease were treated with

Funding Source: NIL.

Conflict of Interest: NIL.

[a] Atlanta Medical Center, 303 Parkway North East, Atlanta, GA 30312, USA; [b] Department of Surgery, Ochsner Clinic Foundation, Clinic Tower 8, 1514 Jefferson Highway, New Orleans, LA 70121, USA

* Corresponding author.

E-mail address: gfuhrman@ochsner.org

http://dx.doi.org/10.1016/j.suc.2013.01.006
0039-6109/13/$ – see front matter © 2013 Elsevier Inc. All rights reserved.

surgical.theclinics.com

initial chemotherapy followed by mastectomy, radiotherapy, and postoperative adjuvant chemotherapy.[1–4] This group was compared with a historical control group treated with surgery and radiotherapy only. At least a 50% reduction in the size of the tumor (partial response) was achieved in 67% of patients and complete responses were noted in 17% of patients. The 5-year and 10-year disease-free survival was 71% and 40% for the IIB and IIIA group and 33% and 30% for the stage IIIB and IV patients, respectively. These dramatic results for patients with historically poor prognosis for disease-free survival led to the enthusiastic development of National Surgical Adjuvant Breast and Bowel Project (NSABP) protocols to evaluate the potential benefits of neoadjuvant chemotherapy for patients with earlier stage breast cancer in comparison to postoperative adjuvant systemic treatment.

The first such protocol was the NSABP B-18 trial, which randomized patients to receive Adriamycin and cytoxan before or after definitive breast surgery (either mastectomy or breast-conservation surgery).[5,6] Disappointingly, there was no impact on disease-free or overall survival between the 2 treatment arms. Despite the apparent efficacy of neoadjuvant chemotherapy in the locally advanced setting, no survival benefit was apparent in the B-18 trial. However, the patients who received preoperative chemotherapy demonstrated a statistically significant ($P = .002$) increase in the use of breast conservation over mastectomy. The 36% rate of clinical complete response and 13% rate of pathologic complete response in the patients receiving neoadjuvant chemotherapy in the B-18 trial allowed for sufficient tumor shrinkage to permit an increased use of breast conservation surgery.

In the follow-up NSABP B-27 trial, the potential beneficial role of the addition of a taxane to anthracycline-based chemotherapy was investigated.[7] The trial was a 3-arm study comparing preoperative adriamycin and cytoxan followed by surgery to 2 groups that received a taxane in addition to the adriamycin and cytoxan (1 before and 1 after surgery). Once again no difference in disease-free or overall survival was demonstrated. Interestingly, in this trial the addition of a taxane increased the pathologic rate of complete response to 26%, thereby increasing the potential use of breast conservation. Although both the NSABP B-18 and the NSABP B-27 studies are used to justify the use of neoadjuvant chemotherapy to maximize the opportunity to use breast conservation, it is important to acknowledge that the preoperative determination of which patients will ultimately succeed in achieving breast conservation is inexact. Nevertheless, these trials provide the best available evidence to argue in favor of using neoadjuvant chemotherapy to downsize breast tumors that have an unfavorable tumor-to-breast size ratio to increase the use of breast conservation. Patients who achieve complete or significant partial responses can avoid mastectomy that would be recommended if surgery were to precede chemotherapy. It is important to restate that the use of neoadjuvant chemotherapy for earlier stage breast cancer (T1–2, N0–1) provides no survival advantage compared with the use of traditional postoperative adjuvant chemotherapy.

The evaluation of a response to neoadjuvant chemotherapy has 3 different components. A clinical complete response is the disappearance of all palpable malignancy from the breast and axilla based on physical examination. As expected, this is an inaccurate assessment and requires a more definitive assessment that includes imaging.[8–11] A complete radiographic response would be the disappearance of all radiographic evidence of malignancy. Although mammography and ultrasound have historically provided this assessment, more recently, breast magnetic resonance imaging (MRI) has been used and demonstrated to be the most accurate radiographic predictor of complete response. Unfortunately, a complete radiographic response might still be accompanied by persistence of cancer and excision of the focal point of breast malignancy is essential to determine definitively the extent of response. The discrepancy between a radiographic and pathologic response can be due to the persistence of intraductal cancer that is in association with the primary invasive cancer. Intraductal cancer is typically not affected by cytotoxic chemotherapy and will persist during treatment.[12] Also, invasive cancer that is no longer apparent on radiographic assessment after chemotherapy might still persist as microscopic islands of viable cancer in a background of eradicated cancer cells affected by the chemotherapy. These microscopic islands of tumor reflect a fragmented response to neoadjuvant chemotherapy that can challenge a surgeon's ability to achieve breast conservation.[13] Complete excision of these persistent areas of cancer after chemotherapy are essential to maximize treatment-related outcomes. Therefore, regardless of the extent of response to neoadjuvant chemotherapy, surgical excision of a portion of the breast should be performed after the patient recovers from the last planned neoadjuvant chemotherapy dose. Surgery is typically performed about 4 weeks after treatment to allow for recovery from the myelosuppresive toxicity of neoadjuvant chemotherapy. The extent of excision does not necessarily have to include the entire area of malignancy identified before chemotherapy. Instead, the central area of malignancy that should be marked with a clip before initiating chemotherapy becomes the target for excision after a complete or near complete response. The same principles that apply to breast conservation without neoadjuvant chemotherapy still apply, in that margins of excision should be assessed and considered negative.[14] One particularly difficult dilemma arises when scattered islands of viable tumor persist without radiographic identifiers and the entire area of preoperatively demonstrated cancer is not excised. In these situations a more extensive lumpectomy should be considered. Clearly, when a complete radiographically responded cancer is excised in part and no viable tumor is identified, then additional breast surgery is not required and radiotherapy can be added to achieve acceptable rates of local tumor control.

The importance of radiotherapy cannot be overstated for patients receiving neoadjuvant chemotherapy and opting for breast conservation. In the NSABP B-18 trial, the group of patients that was predicted to need mastectomy but was converted to breast conservation after achieving a response to neoadjuvant treatment suffered a 15.7% rate of breast recurrence, which was significantly higher than the group that was considered good breast conservation candidates before neoadjuvant treatment (9.9%).[6] This concern regarding a higher rate of local recurrence was also demonstrated in a meta-analysis that was flawed by the inclusion of patients who did not have surgery if they were considered to have achieved a complete radiographic response. Patients with persistent tumor that was not excised after neoadjuvant chemotherapy contributed to a higher than acceptable rate of local recurrence. Perhaps the most important evaluation of local recurrence after breast conservation achieved with the aid of neoadjuvant chemotherapy comes from the MD Anderson retrospective evaluation of breast conservation after neoadjuvant chemotherapy, demonstrating a low (9%) rate of local recurrence compared with breast conservation patients treated without neoadjuvant chemotherapy.[6] The 1 subgroup that was at particular risk of local failure was the group previously mentioned, whereby chemotherapy results in a fragmented pattern of persistent tumor. This group suffered a 20% rate of local recurrence. This fragmented pattern of tumor persistence should be considered a strong relative contraindication for breast conservation after neoadjuvant chemotherapy. The final decision as to whether to pursue breast conservation after breast conservation should be based on the ability to achieve negative margins and an esthetically satisfactory-appearing breast that can be treated with whole breast radiotherapy.[14]

Another important consideration for patients hoping to achieve breast conservation after neoadjuvant chemotherapy is placement of a radiographic marker near the center of the tumor before initiating chemotherapy.[15] This marker allows for detection of the appropriate breast excision site in the event of a complete radiographic response to treatment. The evaluation for complete clinical response requires both pretreatment and posttreatment imaging studies. In addition to standard mammography and ultrasound, the value of breast MRI has been reported. Although MRI is superior to clinical examination, mammography, and ultrasound, it still lacks the accuracy to select women for breast conservation reliably. There is no substitute for excellent clinical judgment that mandates that the surgeon clinically and radiographically evaluate patients before, during, and after neoadjuvant therapy to provide women the best opportunity for breast conservation. Ultimately, unless clinical and radiographic assessments clearly demonstrate an unfavorable tumor-to-breast ratio after chemotherapy, the decision to use breast conservation will be based on the pathologic assessment of a lumpectomy specimen to determine response to treatment and the adequacy of margins.

Women who receive neoadjuvant chemotherapy that does not respond present a management challenge. One of the theoretical advantages of neoadjuvant chemotherapy is the opportunity to assess a tumor's responsiveness to treatment and develop alternative strategies for nonresponders. In reality, resistance to the effects of a chemotherapy regimen predicts resistance to alternative drugs. In a trial of more than 600 patients who received 4 cycles of neoadjuvant anthracycline-based treatment that failed to respond, patients were randomized to 4 additional cycles versus a theoretically non-cross-resistant regimen of vinorelbine and capecitabine before surgery.[16] Neither group of patients had any significant benefit from additional chemotherapy, suggesting a broad resistance to cytotoxic systemic therapy. This cytotoxic systemic therapy should not be confused with the benefits of adding a taxane to anthracycline-based chemotherapy in the neoadjuvant setting as demonstrated in the B-27 trial. There is a difference between achieving an improved response by the addition of chemotherapy to patients likely to respond compared with adding alternative additional systemic treatment of nonresponders. In other words, tumors that are resistant to chemotherapy are broadly resistant.

Once a decision has been made to treat a woman with neoadjuvant chemotherapy, the next priority is an evaluation of the regional nodes in the axilla. When axillary nodal disease is detected on clinical examination or suggested on radiographic study, a confirmatory percutaneous biopsy (usually by fine-needle aspiration) is recommended.[16,17] For patients with involved nodes at the time of diagnosis, a node dissection (levels I and II) should be performed at the time of breast surgery, regardless of the response achieved by neoadjuvant chemotherapy. For patients without evidence of axillary disease that are planning neoadjuvant chemotherapy, a decision to stage the axilla before or after systemic treatment must be made.

The advantage of mapping before chemotherapy is that axillary status can be determined at the time of diagnosis and not confounded by the response to chemotherapy. The response to chemotherapy in the axilla could be uneven with a complete response to chemotherapy being achieved in the sentinel node and an incomplete response in nonsentinel nodes. A negative sentinel node after neoadjuvant chemotherapy could potentially be a false negative finding and axillary disease in nonsentinel nodes might be left untreated, especially if radiotherapy was not to be included (eg, mastectomy patients). Proponents of performing sentinel node biopsy before neoadjuvant chemotherapy argue that the accuracy of the technique and the important prognostic information obtained provide for superior treatment planning. This opinion was more prevalent in the 1990s and early 2000s, when reports of sentinel node accuracy after neoadjuvant chemotherapy were lower than the rates achieved for patients with breast cancer treated with initial surgery that included sentinel node mapping. An example of the inferior sentinel node mapping rates of accuracy after neoadjuvant chemotherapy can be found in the NSABP B-27.[18] A total of 428 patients had sentinel node mapping attempted after neoadjuvant chemotherapy and the sentinel node was identified in only 84% of cases. Furthermore, a total of 218 patients with negative sentinel nodes underwent a complete axillary node dissection; a false negative sentinel node was demonstrated in 10.7% of patients. These results were published at a time when surgeons treating early-stage breast cancer were identifying sentinel nodes in greater than 90% of cases and false negative sentinel nodes were found in less than 5% of cases. Subsequently, reports were published of better rates of node identification and fewer rates of false negative sentinel node after neoadjuvant chemotherapy. The accuracy of sentinel node mapping after neoadjuvant chemotherapy and the opportunity to avoid an unnecessary surgical procedure before starting breast cancer chemotherapy made axillary staging after neoadjuvant chemotherapy more attractive. Recently, the results from the American College of Surgeons Oncology Group Z-11 trial have provided even more enthusiasm to defer axillary staging until after neoadjuvant chemotherapy.[19] The Z-11 trial failed to demonstrate an impact on survival or axillary recurrence when patients with a positive sentinel node were treated with breast conservation and whole breast radiotherapy. It is important to point out that the Z-11 trial excluded patients treated by mastectomy and required a clinically negative axilla at the time of breast cancer diagnosis. Although the Z-11 trial is controversial, patients with a clinically negative axilla that undergo neoadjuvant chemotherapy to enhance opportunities for breast conservation, with a positive sentinel node, no longer require a complete axillary node dissection. An argument might be made that the Z-11 trial did not include patients treated with neoadjuvant chemotherapy and therefore all such patients should have an axillary dissection for staging. In practice, when neoadjuvant chemotherapy is used to optimize breast conservation and if the axilla is negative at the time of initial diagnosis, the results of Z-11 should still be valid.

Women with tumors that express hormone receptors can have treatment with neoadjuvant endocrine therapy. Both tamoxifen and aromatase inhibitors have been evaluated as neoadjuvant agents and have rates of response that approximate neoadjuvant chemotherapy for patients who have estrogen-positive and/or progesterone-positive tumors.[20,21] These rates of response reflect the fact that neoadjuvant chemotherapy is less effective in estrogen receptor–positive tumors compared with estrogen receptor–negative cancer. Rates of partial response of about 60% can be expected for neoadjuvant endocrine therapy in receptor-positive cases. Complete response to neoadjuvant endocrine therapy is uncommon with reported rates of 3% to 10%. Patients with estrogen-positive or progesterone-positive tumors and unfavorable tumor-to-breast size ratios for breast conservation who achieve a partial response to neoadjuvant endocrine therapy can be converted from requiring mastectomy to potential breast conservation candidate, which is similar to neoadjuvant chemotherapy.

An interesting group of patients for consideration of neoadjuvant endocrine therapy includes women with invasive lobular cancer. Invasive lobular cancer is nearly always estrogen receptor–positive and often these tumors are poorly visualized on mammography and therefore present at a larger size compared with invasive ductal cancer. These larger invasive lobular estrogen receptor–positive tumors do not respond as favorably to neoadjuvant chemotherapy and their larger size makes breast conservation challenging to accomplish.[22,23] For women who hope to achieve breast conservation, neoadjuvant endocrine therapy can provide an opportunity for tumor shrinkage and a more favorable tumor-to-breast size ratio that will allow for a cosmetically satisfactory posttreatment breast appearance.

An area of ongoing investigation that holds promise for enhanced rates of response to neoadjuvant chemotherapy is the treatment of the patient with overexpression of Her 2-neu receptors. Targeted therapy to the Her 2-neu receptor with trastuzumab has the potential to improve rates of complete response. Her 2-neu has consistently proven to be a marker of an inferior prognosis; however, like many markers that reflect an increased level of biologic aggressiveness, Her 2–rich tumors when treated with systemic therapies have an increased rate of chemosensitivity and rate of response. In 1 small trial (42 patients) that used trastuzumab in the neoadjuvant setting for Her 2–positive tumors, rates of complete response were 67% compared with 25% for the chemotherapy-only arm.[24]

In summary, neoadjuvant chemotherapy is still the preferred approach for patients with locally advanced disease. Randomized prospective trials have demonstrated that patients with early-stage breast cancer who prefer breast conservation can benefit from neoadjuvant chemotherapy by achieving about a 25% complete and a greater than 80% partial pathologic response. These responses do not translate into a survival advantage. For earlier stage patients, neoadjuvant chemotherapy's primary advantage is the ability to increase the use of breast conservation. Patients who opt for neoadjuvant chemotherapy should have a clinical and radiographic assessment of the axilla. If nodal disease is demonstrated at the time of diagnosis, then axillary staging requires a node dissection. When the axilla is considered negative at the time of diagnosis, sentinel node mapping should be performed after neoadjuvant chemotherapy. Negative sentinel nodes do not require node dissection. Patients with positive nodes can avoid node dissection if breast conservation with whole breast radiotherapy is planned. Neoadjuvant endocrine therapy is an option for estrogen receptor–positive patients. Neoadjuvant trastuzumab seems to be an excellent option for patients with Her 2-neu–positive cancers. The inability to predict the extent and pattern of response to chemotherapy requires that surgeons monitor patient's response during neoadjuvant chemotherapy to provide optimal surgical planning.

## REFERENCES

1. Hortobagyi GN, Blumenschein GR, Spanos W, et al. Multimodal treatment of locoregionally advanced breast cancer. Cancer 1983;51:763–8.
2. Hortobagyi GN, Ames FC, Buzdar AU, et al. Management of stage III primary breast cancer with primary chemotherapy, surgery, and radiation therapy. Cancer 1988;62:2507–16.
3. Hortobagyi GN, Buzdar AU. Locally advanced breast cancer: a review including the M.D. Anderson experience. In: Ragaz J, Ariel IM, editors. High-risk breast cancer-therapy. Berlin: Springer-Verlag; 1991. p. 382–415.
4. Hortobagyi GN. Multidisciplinary management of advanced primary and metastatic breast cancer. Cancer 1994;74:416–23.
5. Fisher B, Brown A, Mamounas E, et al. Effect of preoperative chemotherapy on local-regional disease in women with operable breast cancer: findings from National Surgical Adjuvant Breast and Bowel Project B-18. J Clin Oncol 1997;15:2483–93.
6. Wolmark N, Wang J, Mamounas E, et al. Preoperative chemotherapy in patients with operable breast cancer: nine-year results from National Surgical Adjuvant Breast and Bowel Project B-18. J Natl Cancer Inst Monographs 2001;30:96–102.
7. Bear HD, Anderson S, Smith RE, et al. Sequential preoperative or postoperative docetaxel added to preoperative doxorubicin plus cyclophosphamide for operable breast cancer: National Surgical Adjuvant Breast and Bowel Project B-27. J Clin Oncol 2006;24:2019–27.

8. Weatherall PT, Evans GF, Metzger GJ, et al. MRI vs. histologic measurement of breast cancer following chemotherapy: comparison with x-ray mammography and palpation. J Magn Reson Imaging 2001;13:868–75.

9. Esserman L, Hylton N, Yassa I, et al. Utility of magnetic resonance imaging in the management of breast cancer: evidence for improved preoperative staging. J Clin Oncol 1999;17:110–9.

10. Yeh E, Slanetz P, Kopans DB, et al. Prospective comparison of mammography, sonography, and MRI in patients who have undergone neoadjuvant chemotherapy for palpable breast cancer. AJR Am J Roentgenol 2005;184:868–77.

11. Berg WA, Gutierrez L, NessAiver ME, et al. Diagnostic accuracy of mammography, clinical examinations, US, and MR imaging in preoperative assessment of breast cancer. Radiology 2004;233:830–49.

12. Mazouni F, Peintinger S, Wan-Kau F, et al. Effect on patient outcome of residual DCIS in patients with complete eradication of invasive breast cancer after neoadjuvant chemotherapy. J Clin Oncol 2007;25(Suppl 18):530.

13. Chen AM, Meric-Bernstam F, Hunt KK. Breast conservation after neoadjuvant chemotherapy. Cancer 2005;103(4):689–95.

14. Verponesi U, Bonnadonna G, Zurrida S, et al. Conservation surgery after primary chemotherapy in large carcinomas of the breast. Ann Surg 1995;222:612–8.

15. Oh JL, Nguyen G, Whitman GJ, et al. Placement of radiopaque clips for tumor localization in patients undergoing neoadjuvant chemotherapy and breast conservation therapy. Cancer 2007;110:2420–7.

16. Leenders MW, Broeders M, Croese C, et al. Ultrasound and fine-needle aspiration cytology of axillary lymph nodes in breast cancer. To do or not to do? Breast 2012;21:578–83.

17. Orumari JU, Chung MA, Koelliker S, et al. Axillary staging using ultrasound-guided fine needle aspiration biopsy in locally advanced breast cancer. Am J Surg 2002;184:307–9.

18. Mamounas EP, Brown A, Anderson S, et al. Sentinel node biopsy after neoadjuvant chemotherapy for breast cancer: results from National Surgical Adjuvant Breast and Bowel Project B-27. J Clin Oncol 2005;23:2694–702.

19. Giuliano AE, McCall L, Beitsch P, et al. Locoregional recurrence after sentinel lymph node dissection with or without axillary dissection in patients with sentinel lymph node metastases: the American College of Surgeons Oncology Group Z0011 randomized trial. Ann Surg 2010;252:426–33.

20. Cataliotti L, Buzdar AU, Noguchi S, et al. Comparison of anastrozole versus tamoxifen as preoperative therapy in postmenopausal women with hormone receptor-positive breast cancer: the pre-operative "Arimidex" compared to Tamoxifen (PROACT)trial. Cancer 2006;106:2095–103.

21. Semiglazov VF, Amiglozoz V, Ivanov V, et al. The relative efficacy of neoadjuvant endocrine therapy versus chemotherapy in postmenopausal women with ER-positive breast cancer. J Clin Oncol 2004;23:7s.

22. Mathieu MC, Rouzier R, Llombart-Cussac A, et al. The poor responsiveness of infiltrating lobular breast carcinomas to neoadjuvant chemotherapy can be explained by their biological profile. Eur J Cancer 2004;40:342–51.

23. Cocquyt VF, Blondeel PN, Depypere HT, et al. Different responses to preoperative chemotherapy for invasive lobular and invasive ductal breast carcinoma. Eur J Surg Oncol 2003;29:361–7.

24. Buzdar AU, Ibrahim NK, Francis D, et al. Significantly higher pathologic complete remission rate after neoadjuvant therapy with trastuzumab, paclitaxel, and epirubicin chemotherapy: results of a randomized trial in human epidermal growth factor receptor 2-positive operable breast cancer. J Clin Oncol 2005;23:3676–85.

# Landmark Trials Affecting the Surgical Management of Invasive Breast Cancer

Dalliah M. Black, MD, Elizabeth A. Mittendorf, MD, PhD*

## KEYWORDS

- Breast cancer • Clinical trials • Breast-conserving therapy
- Sentinel lymph node biopsy

## KEY POINTS

- Large randomized trials have demonstrated no OS difference between mastectomy and breast-conserving therapy.
- SLND has replaced ALND as the recommended procedure for axillary staging of patients with clinically node-negative breast cancer.
- Select patients with one to two positive SLNs undergoing BCT can be spared ALND with no impact on local-regional recurrence or OS.
- Current cooperative group trials evaluating new radiation approaches, tumor ablative techniques, and systemic treatments along with the development of assays assessing tumor biology will continue to advance personalized local-regional treatment plans for individual patients.

## INTRODUCTION

Large cooperative group trials have defined surgical management of breast cancer. Until the late 1890s, breast cancer was a fatal disease. William Stewart Halsted challenged that theory by performing aggressive surgery to achieve local control.[1] Termed the Halsted radical mastectomy, the procedure involved removal of the breast, the underlying pectoralis major and minor muscles, and the regional lymph nodes. This extensive resection addressed Halsted's premise that cancer spread from the breast to the pectoralis muscles and regional lymph nodes first and then to distant sites. By the late 1960s, however, investigators had begun to question this "contiguous

Funding Support: This research is supported in part by the National Institutes of Health through MD Anderson's Cancer Center Support Grant CA016672.
Financial Disclosures: The authors have nothing to disclose.
Department of Surgical Oncology, The University of Texas MD Anderson Cancer Center, Unit 1484, 1400 Pressler Street, Houston, TX 77030, USA
* Corresponding author.
E-mail address: eamitten@mdanderson.org

spread" model and suggested instead that breast cancer was a systemic disease.[2–5] Around the same time, interest in using chemotherapy for a variety of malignancies increased. Thus, investigators also started to question the need to routinely perform a procedure as morbid as the radical mastectomy. Subsequently, large randomized clinical trials in the United States and Europe demonstrated that breast cancer could be successfully treated with less radical surgery combined with other modalities including systemic chemotherapy, endocrine therapy, and radiation. Advances from these trials resulted in personalized surgical management of breast cancer. This article reviews the most recently published data from landmark randomized trials that have guided current practices in surgical management of invasive breast cancer.

## FROM RADICAL MASTECTOMY TO BREAST-CONSERVING THERAPY
### National Surgical Adjuvant Breast and Bowel Project B-04: Radical Mastectomy to Total Mastectomy

Dissatisfaction with the significant morbidity of radical mastectomy along with new information regarding tumor biology and metastasis led to anecdotal reports of surgeons using less aggressive surgery to treat breast cancer.[2,6–8] This led investigators from the National Surgical Adjuvant Breast and Bowel Project (NSABP) to conduct the NSABP B-04 trial, which compared radical mastectomy with less extensive surgery.[9] The trial was set up as two parallel trials: one for patients with clinically node-negative disease and one for patients with node-positive disease (**Fig. 1**). Between 1971 and 1974, 1079 patients with clinically node-negative disease were randomized to radical mastectomy (N = 362); total mastectomy plus local-regional/axillary radiation (N = 352); or total mastectomy alone without axillary treatment (N = 365). During the same period, 586 patients with clinically node-positive disease were randomized to radical mastectomy (N = 292) or total mastectomy and radiation (N = 294).[9] Patients did not receive systemic therapy. The goal was to determine whether patients who received local-regional treatment other than radical mastectomy had similar outcomes to those undergoing radical mastectomy.

Initial reports from the NSABP B-04 trial at 3, 5, and 10 years showed no significant differences with respect to disease-free survival (DFS), distant-disease-free survival (DDFS), and overall survival (OS) among the three groups of patients with clinically node-negative disease or the two groups of patients with clinically node-positive disease.[2,9,10] The 25-year outcomes from the NSABP B-04 trial reported in 2002 also revealed no significant differences between groups with respect to any end point.[11] In the node-negative arm, patients who underwent total mastectomy plus radiation had a lower rate of local-regional recurrence (LRR; 5%) than did those

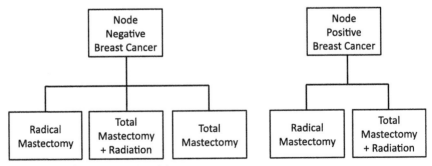

**Fig. 1.** Schema for NSABP B-04 trial.

who underwent radical mastectomy (9%) or total mastectomy alone (13%) ($P$ = .002). In the node-positive arm, the LRR rates were not significantly different: 16% in patients who underwent radical mastectomy versus 14% in patients who underwent total mastectomy plus radiation ($P$ = .67). When broken down by local versus regional recurrence, the rate of local recurrence was significantly different between those who underwent radical mastectomy (8%) and those who underwent total mastectomy plus radiation (3%); however, no significant differences in regional recurrence rates were found.

Of note, 40% of the patients with clinically node-negative disease who underwent radical mastectomy had lymph node involvement in their surgical specimens.[9] Thus, one can assume that 40% of patients with clinically node-negative disease who underwent total mastectomy also had nodal involvement. However, of the 365 patients with node-negative disease who underwent total mastectomy without radiation, only 68 (19%) subsequently developed nodal disease and underwent axillary lymph node dissection (ALND).[11] The median time from mastectomy to identification of axillary metastases was 15 months (range, 3–135 months), and most cases were identified within 2 years of the initial operation. These patients remained in the total mastectomy cohort for survival analyses. Therefore, because there was no significant difference with respect to OS between the arms of the trial, these data suggest that routine ALND for patients with a clinically node-negative axilla is unnecessary and omission of this procedure until there is clinically evident disease in the axilla does not have a significant negative impact on OS. This study also did not demonstrate an advantage of adding local-regional radiation to total mastectomy. Most importantly, the trial supported the paradigm shift to less radical surgery for breast cancer.

### NSABP B-06: Total Mastectomy Versus Breast-conserving Therapy

To further minimize the extent of surgery, several investigators evaluated breast-conserving surgery and reported encouraging results in small studies that included patients with small tumors.[12–14] To further evaluate this strategy, NSABP investigators conducted the NSABP B-06 study, a randomized prospective trial comparing lumpectomy and ALND with or without breast irradiation with total mastectomy and ALND (modified radical mastectomy) in patients with tumors 4 cm or less (**Fig. 2**).[15] Patients could enroll regardless of clinical nodal status, and all patients underwent level I and II

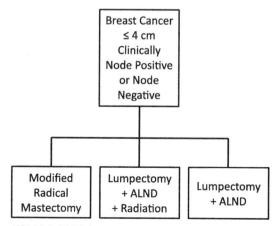

**Fig. 2.** Schema for NSABP B-06 trial.

ALND. Radiation was administered to 50 Gy without a boost to the lumpectomy bed or radiation to the axilla. Patients with positive axillary lymph nodes received adjuvant systemic therapy with fluorouracil and melphalan. The aim of this trial, which enrolled and randomized 2163 patients from 1976 to 1984, was to determine rates of ipsilateral breast cancer recurrence, DFS, DDFS, and OS. Initial reports of the trial at 5, 8, and 12 years included 1843 evaluable patients and showed no significant differences for any end point among the groups.[15–17]

The most recent publication from this trial reported 20-year follow-up data, which also showed no significant differences in DFS, DDFS, or OS among groups.[18] They did, however, identify differences among the three arms with respect to local control.[18] Chest wall recurrences were reported in 10% of patients who underwent mastectomy. The cumulative incidence of ipsilateral breast tumor recurrence (IBTR) in patients with tumor-free margins was 39% in patients who underwent lumpectomy alone and 14% in patients who underwent lumpectomy and radiation (P<.001). Patients who received radiation had fewer late recurrences; 73% of recurrences in the lumpectomy plus radiation group were within 5 years, whereas 9% occurred after 10 years compared with the lumpectomy-only group, in which 40% of the recurrences were within 5 years and 30% occurred after 10 years. Importantly, patients with positive margins in either lumpectomy group (~10% of patients) who subsequently underwent total mastectomy were followed in their respective lumpectomy group for survival outcome analyses.[18] Similarly, per protocol definition, an IBTR after lumpectomy was not considered an event in the DFS analysis because women who underwent total mastectomy were not at risk. Instead, an IBTR after lumpectomy was considered a cosmetic failure, and such patients who subsequently underwent mastectomy continued in their assigned lumpectomy group for data analyses.[18] The NSABP B-06 trial was critical for establishing the concept of breast-conserving therapy (BCT) and confirmed the importance of radiation as a component of such treatment. These results were confirmed by randomized clinical trials conducted by others, including the group from the Milan Cancer Institute.[19,20]

More modern series have reported even lower rates of local-regional failure after BCT. We recently reported our experience at The University of Texas MD Anderson Cancer Center with a cohort of 2331 patients who underwent BCT including lumpectomy and whole-breast irradiation (WBI) between 1987 and 2005. After a median follow-up of 8 years, the 5-year LRR-free rate was 97% (95% confidence interval [CI], 96%–98%) and the 10-year rate was 94% (95% CI, 93%–95%).[21] These results reflect improvements in imaging and pathologic evaluation; expanding indications for adjuvant therapy including systemic chemotherapy and endocrine therapy, which have been shown to decrease LRR rates in the breast; and improvements in systemic agents. An appreciation for the need to obtain a clearly negative margin at the time of surgery has also increased.[22] Although there is no consensus on the optimal margin width, "no ink on tumor" was considered to be a negative margin in the NSABP B-06 trial.

### Cancer and Leukemia Group B 9343: Radiation in Women 70 Years and Older

After studies demonstrated the feasibility of BCT, investigators began questioning whether radiation could be safely omitted in selected patients in whom the absolute risk of recurrence would be predicted to be low. One trial that investigated this was the Cancer and Leukemia Group B 9343, conducted between 1994 and 1999.[23,24] The trial enrolled 636 women 70 years and older who had undergone lumpectomy for stage I, ER-positive breast cancer. A negative surgical margin, defined as no tumor on the inked margin, was required. Patients were randomized to receive tamoxifen

(N = 319) or tamoxifen and radiation (N = 317). ALND was discouraged but was performed in approximately 36% of patients in both groups.[23] The primary end points were time to local or regional recurrence, frequency of mastectomy for recurrence, DFS, time to distant metastasis, and OS.

Initial results from the study were published in 2004 after a median follow-up of 5 years.[23] The investigators found no significant differences between the groups in the rates of subsequent mastectomy, distant metastases, or OS. The rate of local or regional recurrence was 1% in the tamoxifen plus radiation group and 4% in the tamoxifen-alone group, a difference that was statistically significant (P<.001). In 2005, after the initial report of the Cancer and Leukemia Group B 9343 results, the National Comprehensive Cancer Network (NCCN) amended their guidelines with a footnote that stated "Breast irradiation may be omitted in those 70 years of age or older with ER-positive, clinically node-negative T1 tumors who receive adjuvant hormonal therapy."[25] Updated data from this trial were presented in 2010.[24] After a median follow-up of 10.5 years, the LRR rate remained significantly different between the two groups: 9% in the tamoxifen-alone group and 2% in the tamoxifen plus radiation group. The difference was driven largely by a difference in IBTR: 8% in the tamoxifen-alone group and 2% in the tamoxifen plus radiation group. DDFS, breast cancer–specific survival, OS, and the ability to undergo BCT remained comparable between the two groups. Based on these findings, the authors concluded that lumpectomy with endocrine therapy and without radiation is an appropriate treatment option for women 70 years or older with node-negative, ER-positive breast cancer.

### Summary and Future Directions: Management of the Primary Breast Tumor

Taken together, the randomized clinical trials discussed previously have changed the paradigm of the surgical management of primary tumors of women with invasive breast cancer. As a result of these studies, most patients with early stage breast cancer undergo BCT that includes segmental resection followed by radiation. Because BCT is now well established, ongoing cooperative group trials are evaluating other modalities to treat the primary tumor and to minimize radiation. There is interest in managing the primary tumor without surgery using one of several described modalities, including percutaneous ablation, radiofrequency ablation, or cryoablation.[26] For example, the American College of Surgeons Oncology Group (ACOSOG) is conducting the Z1072 trial, a phase II study exploring cryoablation for the treatment of invasive breast cancer less than 2 cm.[27] The trial is currently accruing patients, and the estimated completion date is March 2013.

The previously discussed trials describing BCT all evaluated WBI. Because most IBTRs occur near the lumpectomy cavity, investigators have begun exploring other methods of delivering radiation including accelerated partial-breast irradiation (APBI). APBI is associated with several purported benefits, including a shorter interval for treatment completion, the potential for repeat breast-conserving surgery when an in-breast event occurs outside the irradiated cavity, and an alternative for women who are reluctant to undergo WBI. APBI is being evaluated in a large trial by the NSABP and Radiation Therapy Oncology Group (RTOG) (NSABP B-39/RTOG 0413).[28] The trial will enroll 4300 women with operable breast cancer treated with lumpectomy. Initial eligibility criteria included stage 0 ductal carcinoma in situ or stage I or II invasive cancer that was 3 cm or smaller with fewer than three positive axillary lymph nodes. The trial opened in 2005 and after brisk accrual of low-risk patients (women older than 50 years with ductal carcinoma in situ or node-negative and ER-positive invasive tumors), was closed to accrual of patients with these favorable characteristics. The trial continues to accrue higher-risk patients.

## FROM ALND TO SENTINEL LYMPH NODE DISSECTION

Axillary lymph node involvement has long been considered an important prognostic factor in breast cancer. To determine axillary status for staging purposes, to assist with adjuvant treatment recommendations, and to provide regional control, complete ALND was routinely performed. However, ALND is associated with potential morbidity, including lymphedema, shoulder dysfunction, pain, and paresthesias.[29,30] In addition, in women presenting with clinically node-negative disease, the rate of nodal metastases is only 20% to 35%.[31–33] Removing healthy lymph nodes renders no benefit; therefore, sentinel lymph node dissection (SLND), a more selective approach to managing the axilla, was developed. The concept of the SLN as the first draining lymph node was popularized in melanoma in the late 1980s and early 1990s.[34,35] In 1994, Giuliano and colleagues[36] published findings on the feasibility and accuracy of SLND for early stage breast cancer in 114 patients and reported a 65% identification rate and 96% accuracy. This report led to the design and conduct of larger trials evaluating SLND as a staging procedure for clinically node-negative breast cancer.

### SLND for Axillary Staging

#### NSABP B-32
To determine whether SLND renders the same survival benefit and regional control that ALND does but with fewer side effects in patients with clinically node-negative disease, NSABP investigators conducted the NSABP B-32 trial. Between 1999 and 2004, the trial enrolled 5611 patients and randomized them to undergo SLND plus ALND (group one) or SLND with ALND only if the SLN was positive (group two; **Fig. 3**). The primary end points were OS, regional control, and morbidity. The secondary end points were accuracy and technical success.[37]

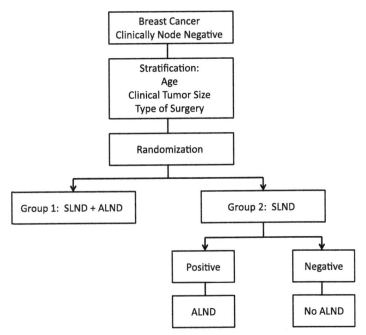

**Fig. 3.** Schema for NSABP B-32 trial.

SLNs were defined as nodes that were radioactive, blue, or hard and highly suspicious for metastatic disease. Radioactive nodes were removed until the count in the axilla was less than 10% of the hottest ex vivo SLN.[31] Pathologic evaluation included sectioning at 2-mm intervals and staining with hematoxylin and eosin (H&E). Routine immunohistochemistry (IHC) was not allowed. The initial publication reported on technical success and accuracy in 5536 patients in whom data were available.[31] An SLN was identified in 5379 (97%). The SLN was positive in 26% of patients in both groups. In group one, the accuracy of SLND was 97%, and the false-negative rate was 9.8%. Factors associated with a higher false-negative rate included tumor location, the type of biopsy performed, and the number of SLNs removed.[31] Patient-reported outcomes and morbidity related to lymphedema, range of motion, sensory deficits, and pain have also been published and for all outcomes, morbidity was greater in patients who underwent ALND.[38,39]

Data for the primary survival end points of the trial were published in 2010.[37] Per protocol, analysis included patients with a pathologically negative SLN in whom follow-up information was available (N = 3986). The two groups were well balanced with respect to age, clinical tumor size, and surgical treatment. The use of systemic therapy and radiation was similar between groups. The 5-year Kaplan-Meier estimates for OS were 97% and 95% for groups one and two, respectively, and the 8-year estimates were 92% and 90%, respectively (P = .12). Differences in DFS were also not statistically significant; the 8-year estimates of DFS were 82% in both groups. Rates of regional control were also similar. Eight regional nodal recurrences as first events, including two in the axilla, were reported in group one. Fourteen regional nodal recurrences as first events, including eight in the axilla, were reported in group two. Because the OS, DFS, and regional control rates between the treatment groups were statistically equivalent, the NSABP investigators concluded that when the SLN is negative, SLND alone without further ALND is appropriate for patients with clinically negative lymph nodes.

The findings of the NSABP B-32 trial were confirmed by a single center randomized trial conducted at the European Institute of Oncology. This trial enrolled patients with primary tumors that were 2 cm or smaller who underwent BCT. Patients were randomized to SLND plus ALND (ALND arm; N = 257) or SLND and ALND only if the SLN was positive for metastatic disease (SLND arm; N = 259).[33,40,41] In 2010, the 10-year follow-up data from this trial were published.[41] The ALND and SLND groups were well matched with respect to clinicopathologic characteristics and use of adjuvant systemic therapy. After a median follow-up of 102 months, no significant differences in OS were found. Taken together, the NSABP B-32 and EIO trials confirmed that SLND is effective for staging the axilla in patients with clinically node-negative breast cancer and that SLND alone is safe when the SLN is negative.

### Role of Completion ALND in the Setting of a Positive SLN

After SLND was shown to be safe in patients with clinically node-negative disease, omission of ALND in patients with a negative SLN became standard practice. For patients with a positive SLN, most consensus statements, including one from the American Society of Clinical Oncology, and NCCN guidelines recommended completion ALND for patients with a positive SLN.[42,43] However, recalling the results of the NSABP B-04 trial, a study that showed no survival advantage for patients who underwent ALND at the time of their initial surgery, and recognizing improvements in systemic therapy options and radiation delivery, the use of completion ALND in all patients with a positive SLN was questioned.

To determine whether all patients with a positive SLN need an ALND, ACOSOG conducted the Z0011 trial that enrolled patients with clinical T1 or T2, N0, M0 breast cancer who underwent BCT and were found to have one or two positive SLNs by H&E evaluation.[44,45] The patients were randomized to ALND or no further surgery. All patients received WBI (third-field axillary irradiation was not allowed), and recommendations for systemic adjuvant therapy were made at the discretion of the treating oncologist (**Fig. 4**). The primary end point was OS and secondary end point was DFS. Local-regional control was not a prespecified end point; however, because of concerns that the regional recurrence rates may be high without completion ALND, regional recurrences were monitored.

The trial, which was designed to enroll 1900 patients, began accrual in 1999. Because of slow accrual and a lower than anticipated event rate, the study was closed early in 2004 after 891 patients were randomized (446 in the SLND-alone arm and 445 in the SLND plus ALND arm). Clinicopathologic characteristics were similar between the two groups and overall reflected a population of patients with favorable characteristics (**Table 1**).[45] Micrometastases were identified in the SLN of 38% of patients in the SLND-alone arm and in the SLN of 45% of patients in the ALND arm ($P = .05$). Additional positive lymph nodes were identified in 27% of patients in the ALND arm.[44] Adjuvant systemic therapy was administered in 97% of patients in the SLND-only arm, including chemotherapy in 58% and hormonal therapy in 47%. In the ALND arm, 96% of patients received adjuvant systemic therapy, including chemotherapy in 58% and hormonal therapy in 46%.[44]

After a median follow-up of 6.3 years, only 29 LRRs were reported in the entire population. The local recurrence rate was 2% in the SLND arm and 4% in the ALND arm. Ipsilateral axillary recurrences were uncommon, occurring in four (0.9%) patients in the SLND arm and two (0.5%) patients in the ALND arm.[44] The authors found no differences in DFS or OS between the two groups.[45] Based on these results, the ACOSOG investigators concluded that routine use of ALND is not justified and may be safely omitted in selected patients with clinically node-negative disease who have one or two positive SLNs. Importantly, the Z0011 trial did not include patients with T3 tumors or patients who had undergone mastectomy, those receiving neoadjuvant chemotherapy, APBI, or WBI administered in the prone position where the low axilla is not treated. Therefore, the ACOSOG investigators have cautioned against broad extrapolation of the data indicating that, in such patients, ALND remains the standard practice when a positive SLN is identified.[45]

When the Z0011 data were published, several questions were raised regarding the trial and whether the results of the study would change practice.[46] The most significant

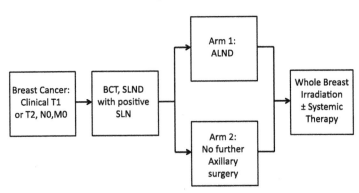

**Fig. 4.** Schema for ACOSOG Z0011 trial.

**Table 1**
**Baseline patient and tumor characteristics of patients enrolled in the American College of Surgeons Oncology Group Z0011 trial**

| Characteristic | ALND (N = 420) | SLND Alone (N = 436) |
|---|---|---|
| Age in years, median (range) | 56 (24–92) | 54 (25–90) |
| Clinical T stage | | |
| T1 | 284 (68%) | 303 (71%) |
| T2 | 134 (32%) | 126 (29%) |
| Missing | 2 | 7 |
| Tumor size, median (range), cm | 1.7 (0.4–7) | 1.6 (0–5) |
| ER positive | 317 (83%) | 324 (83%) |
| LVI | | |
| Present | 129 (41%) | 113 (35%) |
| Absent | 189 (59%) | 208 (65%) |
| Missing | 102 | 115 |
| Grade[a] | | |
| 1 | 71 (22%) | 81 (26%) |
| 2 | 158 (49%) | 148 (47%) |
| 3 | 94 (29%) | 87 (27%) |
| Missing | 97 | 120 |
| Histology | | |
| Infiltrating ductal | 344 (83%) | 356 (84%) |
| Infiltrating lobular | 27 (6%) | 36 (8.5%) |
| Other | 45 (11%) | 32 (7.5%) |
| Missing | 4 | 12 |
| Lymph node metastases | | |
| 0 | 4 (1%) | 29 (7%) |
| 1 | 199 (58%) | 295 (71%) |
| 2 | 68 (20%) | 76 (18%) |
| 3 | 25 (7%) | 11 (3%) |
| ≥4 | 47 (14%) | 4 (1%) |
| Missing | 77 | 21 |

*Abbreviations:* ALND, axillary lymph node dissection; ER, estrogen receptor; LVI, lymphovascular invasion; SLND, sentinel lymph node dissection.
[a] Grade was determined using the modified Bloom-Richardson score.
*Data from* Giuliano AE, Hunt KK, Ballman KV, et al. Axillary dissection vs no axillary dissection in women with invasive breast cancer and sentinel node metastasis. JAMA 2011;305:569–75.

concern was that the planned sample size was not reached. One reason for early closure was that the increased acceptance of screening mammography and improvements in systemic therapy led to an event rate that was lower than anticipated at the time of study design. In addition, the study was designed to demonstrate the noninferiority of SLND alone for OS with a P value of 0.008. Because the 95% CIs for the hazard ratios did not cross the predefined point at which the treatments would not be considered equal, the results would not be expected to change with a larger sample size. Finally, the end points of total LRRs, DFS, and OS all numerically favored the SLN group.[44–46]

The American Society of Breast Surgeons has issued a consensus statement on axillary management that incorporates the findings from the Z0011 trial.[47] Additionally, in the most recent version of its guidelines, the NCCN has changed their algorithm for the management of clinically node-negative disease in patients with a positive SLN to include the category 1 recommendation to consider no further surgery for patients who meet all of the following criteria: T1 or T2 tumor, one or two positive SLNs, undergoing BCT, planned to receive WBI, and did not receive neoadjuvant chemotherapy.[48] Emerging data confirm that the Z0011 data have been practice changing.[46,49–51]

The International Breast Cancer Study Group (IBCSG 23-01) trial will provide additional data regarding the necessity of ALND in patients with a positive SLN. This trial enrolled patients with clinically node-negative breast cancer and a primary tumor that was 5 cm or smaller who were found to have an SLN micrometastasis that was 2 mm or smaller. Patients were randomized to ALND or no further axillary surgery. Unlike the Z0011 trial, which required patients to undergo BCT, patients in the IBCSG 23-01 trial could undergo mastectomy. The primary end point was DFS, and the secondary end points were OS and systemic DFS. The trial was designed to accrue 1960 patients. It opened in 2001 and closed early in 2010 after enrolling 934 patients. Similar to the Z0011 trial, reasons for early closure included slow accrual and a lower than anticipated event rate.

Initial results from this trial were presented in 2011.[52] The mean age of enrolled patients was 54 years (range, 26–81 years), and 56% were postmenopausal. Most (67%) had tumors that were smaller than 2 cm; 89% had tumors that were ER positive, and 74% had grade 1 or 2 disease. Breast-conserving surgery was performed in 75%. In 85% of patients, one or two SLNs were identified. The SLN metastasis was 1 mm or smaller in approximately 70% of patients and 1.1 to 2 mm in approximately 30%. After a median follow-up of 49 months, the investigators reported 88 total DFS events, including 66 that were breast cancer related (8 local, 6 regional, 42 distant, and 10 contralateral breast). The 4-year DFS rate was 91%. The first comparison of outcomes between the two groups will be reported after a median follow-up of 5 years. The overall low event rate in the IBCSG 23-01 trial supports the findings from the Z0011 trial suggesting that ALND can be safely omitted in selected patients with clinically node-negative early stage breast cancer who have a positive SLN.

### Sentinel Lymph Node Micrometastases

One purported benefit of SLND is that it allows more rigorous pathologic evaluation of fewer lymph nodes that are at greatest risk for harboring disease. Whereas lymph nodes obtained during ALND are bivalved and subjected to H&E staining, SLNs routinely undergo serial sectioning with or without IHC. Using these techniques, pathologists can identify small-volume metastases down to the level of isolated tumor cells (ITCs). The clinical relevance of this small-volume disease has been the subject of considerable debate.[53–55]

### NSABP B-32

The NSABP B-32 trial, discussed in detail previously, provided an opportunity to investigate the clinical significance of occult metastatic disease. Tissue blocks from patients with negative SLNs at the local site were sent for central evaluation. Additional sections deeper in each block were evaluated by H&E staining and IHC to identify occult metastases.[56] For the analysis, patients who underwent SLNB plus ALND and those who underwent SLND alone were grouped together and classified according to whether occult metastasis was detected. The primary outcomes were OS, DFS, and DDFS.[57] Because central analysis results were masked, no clinical decisions regarding adjuvant therapy were made based on the knowledge of whether occult metastases were present.

Pathologic material was available for 3887 (97%) patients who were determined at local sites to have a negative SLN. Occult metastases were detected in approximately 16%; 11% had ITCs, 4.4% had micrometastases, and 0.4% had macrometastases. The median duration of study enrollment was 95 months. There were significant differences in OS ($P = .03$), DFS ($P = .02$), and DDFS ($P = .04$) between patients with and without occult metastases. The 5-year OS estimates for patients with and without occult metastases were 94.6% and 95.8%, respectively. Although occult metastases were associated with a statistically significant detriment in OS, the small degree of absolute difference led investigators to conclude that the additional evaluation of initially negative SLNs using IHC yielded no clinical benefit.[57]

### ACOSOG Z0010

The Z0010 trial was designed specifically to evaluate the incidence and significance of SLN and bone marrow micrometastases in patients with early stage breast cancer who underwent breast-conserving surgery and WBI.[32] Briefly, patients with clinical T1 or T2, N0, M0 breast cancer were enrolled and underwent breast-conserving surgery that included lumpectomy and SLND and bilateral anterior iliac crest bone marrow aspiration biopsies (**Fig. 5**). Bone marrow aspiration was initially an optional procedure; however, it was subsequently integrated as a mandatory trial component. Bone marrow aspirates and SLNs that were negative by H&E evaluation at local sites were submitted to a central laboratory for immunocytochemistry (to detect bone marrow micrometasasis) or IHC (to detect SLN micrometastasis). Treating physicians

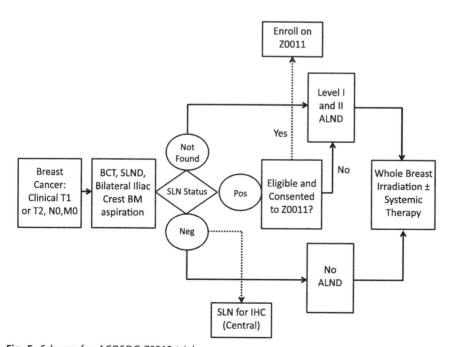

**Fig. 5.** Schema for ACOSOG Z0010 trial.

were masked to the immunochemical status of bone marrow and SLN specimens. The primary end point was OS, and the secondary end point was DFS.

The Z0010 trial began enrolling patients in 1999 with an accrual goal of 5300. The study completed accrual in 2003 with 5538 patients, 5210 of whom were eligible. Of these, 5119 (98%) had an SLN identified, 3904 (76%) of which were negative by H&E staining. Of those that were negative by H&E staining, 3326 (85%) were available to be assessed centrally by IHC, and 349 (11%) of those contained occult metastases.[32] The ages and tumor characteristics of patients with SLNs examined by IHC are shown in **Table 2**. At a median follow-up of 6.3 years, the investigators found no significant association between IHC-detected occult metastases and OS or DFS.[32] The 5-year OS rates for patients with IHC-positive and -negative SLNs were 95% and 96%, respectively ($P$ = .64). The 5-year DFS rates in these patients were 90% and 92%, respectively ($P$ = .82). IHC-positive SLN metastases were not associated with decreased OS on either univariate or multivariate analysis. Occult metastases were identified in 104 (3%) of 3413 patients who underwent bone marrow biopsy. No concordance between the presence of SLNs and bone marrow occult metastases was found. Bone marrow metastases were associated with decreased OS (unadjusted hazard ratio for mortality = 1.94; 95% CI, 1.02–3.67; $P$ = .04); however, this association was not significant on multivariate analysis. The only factors found on multivariate analysis to be associated with decreased OS were age greater than 50 years and

**Table 2**
Age and tumor characteristics of patients in the American College of Surgeons Oncology Group Z0010 trial who had a negative SLN by hematoxylin and eosin staining that was subsequently evaluated by IHC

| Variable | Negative by IHC (N = 2977) | Positive by IHC (N = 349) | P Value |
|---|---|---|---|
| Age in years, median (range) | 57 (23–95) | 54 (27–87) | |
| Tumor size, cm | | | |
| ≤1 | 1260 (45%) | 101 (31%) | <.001 |
| 1.1–2 | 1202 (43%) | 161 (49%) | |
| >2 | 330 (12%) | 67 (20%) | |
| Missing, number | 185 | 20 | |
| Histology | | | |
| Ductal | 2387 (80%) | 262 (75%) | .002 |
| Lobular | 226 (8%) | 45 (13%) | |
| Both | 77 (2%) | 14 (4%) | |
| Other | 284 (10%) | 28 (8%) | |
| Missing | 3 | 0 | |
| ER status | | | |
| Positive | 2225 (81%) | 268 (84%) | .3 |
| Negative | 518 (19%) | 53 (16%) | |
| Missing | 234 | 28 | |
| LVI | | | |
| Absent | 1921 (90%) | 217 (83%) | <.001 |
| Present | 205 (10%) | 44 (17%) | |
| Missing | 851 | 88 | |

*Abbreviations:* ER, estrogen receptor; IHC, immunohistochemistry; LVI, lymphovascular invasion.
*Data from* Giuliano AE, Hawes D, Ballman KV, et al. Association of occult metastases in sentinel lymph nodes and bone marrow with survival among women with early-stage invasive breast cancer. JAMA 2011;306:385–93.

tumor size larger than 1 cm. Bone marrow metastases were not associated with increased recurrence.[32]

The findings from the Z0010 trial therefore support the conclusion that routine use of IHC to detect occult micrometastases in SLNs negative by H&E staining has no clinical benefit. This conclusion is consistent with guidelines from the College of American Pathologists and American Society of Clinical Oncology, which do not recommend the routine use of IHC for SLN evaluation.[42,58] Interestingly, the investigators found no correlation between bone marrow metastases and SLN occult metastases, thereby suggesting that the status of the bone marrow may be a distinct prognostic factor. However, the proportion of patients in the ACOSOG Z0010 trial with bone marrow metastases was low; thus, further investigation is needed before consideration can be given to recommending the incorporation of bone marrow aspiration biopsy into practice for patients with early stage breast cancer.

### Summary and Future Directions: Management of the Axilla

Randomized clinical trials have been instrumental in guiding the surgical management of breast cancer to include using SLND to determine the axillary status of patients with clinically node-negative disease. The status of the SLN accurately reflects the status of the entire nodal basin; therefore, SLND permits accurate staging of the axilla. For patients with a negative SLN, no further axillary surgery is indicated; therefore, patients without axillary metastases are spared the morbidity of ALND. For patients with a positive SLN, standard practice had been completion ALND; however, data from the recently reported Z0011 trial suggest that ALND may be safely omitted in selected patients undergoing BCT that includes WBI.[44,45] Data yet to be reported from the IBCSG 23-01 trial will determine whether selected patients who have undergone mastectomy can also avoid ALND after the finding of a micrometastasis in the SLN. Considering early data from that trial and data from the NSABP B-32 and Z0010 trials showing that occult metastases detected by IHC do not have clinical relevance, one would anticipate that the IBCSG 23-01 trial will confirm that ALND can safely be omitted in patients with micrometastasis in their SLN. However, final results of this trial are not yet known and based on currently available data, standard practice for patients with a positive SLN who have undergone mastectomy is completion ALND.

Because ALND is associated with significant morbidity in a substantial proportion of patients, ongoing work is focused on investigating alternative strategies for axillary management in patients with a positive SLN. As has been discussed in detail, the Z0011 data support omitting ALND in a select group of patients undergoing BCT that includes WBI. Although WBI is designed to treat the breast, a portion of the lower axilla is naturally included in the treatment field. Therefore, among patients enrolled in the Z0011 trial, WBI likely had a therapeutic effect on a portion of the axilla, although data documenting the amount of the axilla that may have been treated are not currently available. This raises the question, however, of whether axillary radiation is a less invasive alternative to ALND for patients with a positive SLN. In the NSABP B-04 trial, described in detail previously, patients with clinically node-negative disease were randomized to radical mastectomy, total mastectomy, or total mastectomy with axillary radiation; the rate of axillary recurrence in the total mastectomy with axillary radiation arm was 4% after 25 years.[11] To further investigate whether axillary radiation is an appropriate alternative to ALND, investigators from the European Organization for Research and Treatment of Cancer are conducting the AMAROS (After Mapping of the Axilla: Radiotherapy or Surgery?) trial. AMAROS is a phase III study comparing ALND with axillary radiation in clinically node-negative patients with tumors smaller than 3 cm who have a positive SLN. The primary objective is to prove that axillary radiation yields equivalent locoregional control and reduced morbidity when compared with ALND. Between 2001 and 2010, the trial accrued 4827 patients.[59] An initial publication from this trial reported the technical outcomes for the first 2000 patients. The SLN identification rate was 97%, and the SLN was positive in 647 (34%), including macrometastases in 409 (63%), micrometastases in 161 (25%), and ITCs in 77 (12%). For patients randomized to undergo ALND, additional nodal involvement was identified in 41% of patients with SLN macrometastases, 18% of patients with micrometastases, and 18% of patients with ITCs.[60] Because the extent of nodal involvement may have implications on adjuvant therapy, the investigators also evaluated the administration of adjuvant therapy in these first 2000 patients. In the ALND and axillary radiation arms, 58% and 61% of patients, respectively, received chemotherapy. Multivariate analysis showed that age, tumor grade, multifocality, and SLN metastasis size significantly affected decisions regarding the use of chemotherapy. Treatment arm was not a significant factor in the decision to administer systemic therapy.[61] Primary outcome data from the trial are not yet available.

Future trials will likely investigate whether there are populations of patients in whom any surgical intervention in the axilla, including SLND, can be safely omitted. A trial randomizing patients to SLND or no surgery seems reasonable in a population of patients with very favorable clinicopathologic characteristics, including postmenopausal women with clinical T1 N0, low-to-intermediate grade, ER-positive tumors. Because of the overall favorable DFS and OS for this population, such a trial may be difficult to conduct in light of the number of patients and length of follow-up time required. Because decisions regarding the use of adjuvant systemic therapy are now made largely based on characteristics other than the nodal status, including patient age and pathologic features of the primary tumor, another potential trial could enroll patients in whom chemotherapy would be administered regardless of nodal status (eg, patients with triple-negative breast cancer or HER2-positive breast cancer) and randomize them to SLND or no surgery. Such a trial is currently being discussed within the newly established Alliance for Clinical Trials in Oncology cooperative group (A.E. Giuliano and K.K. Hunt, 2012, personal communication).

## SUMMARY

Randomized clinical trials have been critical in guiding the surgical management of breast cancer. Breast cancer is no longer a fatal disease or one that necessitates radical surgery with significant associated morbidity. Today, largely because of the efforts of surgeons conducting these trials, most patients receive personalized surgical management of their disease, including BCT with lumpectomy, SLND, and radiation.

## ACKNOWLEDGMENTS

The authors acknowledge that this article only highlights notable trials that have guided the surgical management of breast cancer. Other trials have contributed to the advancement of breast surgical care; however, because of space limitations they are not included in this review.

## REFERENCES

1. Halsted WS. A clinical and histological study of certain adenocarcinomata of the breast: and a brief consideration of the supraclavicular operation and of the results of operations for cancer of the breast from 1889 to 1898 at the Johns Hopkins Hospital. Ann Surg 1898;28:557–76.

2. Fisher B, Redmond C, Fisher ER. The contribution of recent NSABP clinical trials of primary breast cancer therapy to an understanding of tumor biology: an overview of findings. Cancer 1980;46:1009–25.

3. Fisher B, Fisher ER. Transmigration of lymph nodes by tumor cells. Science 1966; 152:1397–8.

4. Fisher B, Fisher ER. Experimental evidence in support of the dormant tumor cell. Science 1959;130:918–9.

5. Fisher B, Fisher ER. The interrelationship of hematogenous and lymphatic tumor cell dissemination. Surg Gynecol Obstet 1966;122:791–8.

6. McWhirter R. The value of simple mastectomy and radiotherapy in the treatment of cancer of the breast. Br J Radiol 1948;21:599–610.

7. Handley RS. The technic and results of conservative radical mastectomy (Patey's operation). Prog Clin Cancer 1965;10:462–70.

8. Fisher B. Laboratory and clinical research in breast cancer–a personal adventure: the David A. Karnofsky memorial lecture. Cancer Res 1980;40:3863–74.

9. Fisher B, Montague E, Redmond C, et al. Comparison of radical mastectomy with alternative treatments for primary breast cancer. A first report of results from a prospective randomized clinical trial. Cancer 1977;39:2827–39.

10. Fisher B, Redmond C, Fisher ER, et al. Ten-year results of a randomized clinical trial comparing radical mastectomy and total mastectomy with or without radiation. N Engl J Med 1985;312:674–81.

11. Fisher B, Jeong JH, Anderson S, et al. Twenty-five-year follow-up of a randomized trial comparing radical mastectomy, total mastectomy, and total mastectomy followed by irradiation. N Engl J Med 2002;347:567–75.

12. Crile G Jr. Treatment of breast cancer by local excision. Am J Surg 1965;109: 400–3.

13. Montague ED, Gutierrez AE, Barker JL, et al. Conservation surgery and irradiation for the treatment of favorable breast cancer. Cancer 1979;43:1058–61.

14. Peters MV. Carcinoma of the breast. Stage II–radiation range. Wedge resection and irradiation. An effective treatment in early breast cancer. JAMA 1967;200: 134–5.

15. Fisher B, Bauer M, Margolese R, et al. Five-year results of a randomized clinical trial comparing total mastectomy and segmental mastectomy with or without radiation in the treatment of breast cancer. N Engl J Med 1985;312: 665–73.

16. Fisher B, Redmond C, Poisson R, et al. Eight-year results of a randomized clinical trial comparing total mastectomy and lumpectomy with or without irradiation in the treatment of breast cancer. N Engl J Med 1989;320:822–8.

17. Fisher B, Anderson S, Redmond CK, et al. Reanalysis and results after 12 years of follow-up in a randomized clinical trial comparing total mastectomy with lumpectomy with or without irradiation in the treatment of breast cancer. N Engl J Med 1995;333:1456–61.

18. Fisher B, Anderson S, Bryant J, et al. Twenty-year follow-up of a randomized trial comparing total mastectomy, lumpectomy, and lumpectomy plus irradiation for the treatment of invasive breast cancer. N Engl J Med 2002;347:1233–41.

19. Veronesi U, Cascinelli N, Mariani L, et al. Twenty-year follow-up of a randomized study comparing breast-conserving surgery with radical mastectomy for early breast cancer. N Engl J Med 2002;347:1227–32.

20. Effects of radiotherapy and surgery in early breast cancer. An overview of the randomized trials. Early Breast Cancer Trialists' Collaborative Group. N Engl J Med 1995;333:1444–55.

21. Mittendorf EA, Buchholz TA, Tucker SL, et al. Impact of chemotherapy sequencing on local-regional failure risk in breast cancer patients undergoing breast conserving therapy. Ann Surg 2013;257:173–9.

22. Houssami N, Macaskill P, Marinovich ML, et al. Meta-analysis of the impact of surgical margins on local recurrence in women with early-stage invasive breast cancer treated with breast-conserving therapy. Eur J Cancer 2010;46:3219–32.

23. Hughes KS, Schnaper LA, Berry D, et al. Lumpectomy plus tamoxifen with or without irradiation in women 70 years of age or older with early breast cancer. N Engl J Med 2004;351:971–7.

24. Hughes KS, Schnaper LA, Cirrincione C, et al. Lumpectomy plus tamoxifen with or without irradiation in women age 70 or older with early breast cancer. J Clin Oncol 2010;28:15s.

25. National Comprehensive Cancer Network. Clinical practice guidelines in oncology: breast. National Comprehensive Cancer Network; 2005.

26. Mamounas E, Wickerham DL. Kuerer's textbook of breast surgical oncology. In: Kuerer HM, editor. The NSABP experience. 1st edition. New York: McGraw-Hill; 2010. p. 627.

27. National Institutes of Health. Cryoablation therapy in treating patients with invasive ductal breast cancer. 2012. Available at: http://www.clinicaltrials.gov/ct2/show/NCT00723294. Accessed August 1, 2012.

28. National Institutes of Health. Radiation therapy in treating women who have undergone surgery for ductal carcinoma in situ or stage I or stage II breast cancer. 2012. Available at: http://www.clinicaltrials.gov/ct2/show/NCT00103181?term=NCT00103181&rank=1. Accessed August 1, 2012.

29. Fleissig A, Fallowfield LJ, Langridge CI, et al. Post-operative arm morbidity and quality of life. Results of the ALMANAC randomised trial comparing sentinel node biopsy with standard axillary treatment in the management of patients with early breast cancer. Breast Cancer Res Treat 2006;95:279–93.

30. Lucci A, McCall LM, Beitsch PD, et al. Surgical complications associated with sentinel lymph node dissection (SLND) plus axillary lymph node dissection compared with SLND alone in the American College of Surgeons Oncology Group Trial Z0011. J Clin Oncol 2007;25:3657–63.

31. Krag DN, Anderson SJ, Julian TB, et al. Technical outcomes of sentinel-lymph-node resection and conventional axillary-lymph-node dissection in patients with clinically node-negative breast cancer: results from the NSABP B-32 randomised phase III trial. Lancet Oncol 2007;8:881–8.

32. Giuliano AE, Hawes D, Ballman KV, et al. Association of occult metastases in sentinel lymph nodes and bone marrow with survival among women with early-stage invasive breast cancer. JAMA 2011;306:385–93.

33. Veronesi U, Paganelli G, Viale G, et al. A randomized comparison of sentinel-node biopsy with routine axillary dissection in breast cancer. N Engl J Med 2003;349:546–53.

34. Cabanas RM. An approach for the treatment of penile carcinoma. Cancer 1977;39:456–66.

35. Morton DL, Wen DR, Wong JH, et al. Technical details of intraoperative lymphatic mapping for early stage melanoma. Arch Surg 1992;127:392–9.

36. Giuliano AE, Kirgan DM, Guenther JM, et al. Lymphatic mapping and sentinel lymphadenectomy for breast cancer. Ann Surg 1994;220:391–8 [discussion: 398–401].

37. Krag DN, Anderson SJ, Julian TB, et al. Sentinel-lymph-node resection compared with conventional axillary-lymph-node dissection in clinically node-negative

patients with breast cancer: overall survival findings from the NSABP B-32 randomised phase 3 trial. Lancet Oncol 2010;11:927–33.

38. Ashikaga T, Krag DN, Land SR, et al. Morbidity results from the NSABP B-32 trial comparing sentinel lymph node dissection versus axillary dissection. J Surg Oncol 2010;102:111–8.

39. Land SR, Kopec JA, Julian TB, et al. Patient-reported outcomes in sentinel node-negative adjuvant breast cancer patients receiving sentinel-node biopsy or axillary dissection: National Surgical Adjuvant Breast and Bowel Project phase III protocol B-32. J Clin Oncol 2010;28:3929–36.

40. Veronesi U, Paganelli G, Viale G, et al. Sentinel-lymph-node biopsy as a staging procedure in breast cancer: update of a randomised controlled study. Lancet Oncol 2006;7:983–90.

41. Veronesi U, Viale G, Paganelli G, et al. Sentinel lymph node biopsy in breast cancer: ten-year results of a randomized controlled study. Ann Surg 2010;251: 595–600.

42. Lyman GH, Giuliano AE, Somerfield MR, et al. American Society of Clinical Oncology guideline recommendations for sentinel lymph node biopsy in early-stage breast cancer. J Clin Oncol 2005;23:7703–20.

43. National Comprehensive Cancer Network. Clinical practice guidelines in oncology: breast. National Comprehensive Cancer Network; 2008. Version 2.

44. Giuliano AE, McCall L, Beitsch P, et al. Locoregional recurrence after sentinel lymph node dissection with or without axillary dissection in patients with sentinel lymph node metastases: the American College of Surgeons Oncology Group Z0011 randomized trial. Ann Surg 2010;252:426–32.

45. Giuliano AE, Hunt KK, Ballman KV, et al. Axillary dissection vs no axillary dissection in women with invasive breast cancer and sentinel node metastasis: a randomized clinical trial. JAMA 2011;305:569–75.

46. Morrow M, Giuliano AE. To cut is to cure: can we really apply Z11 in practice? Ann Surg Oncol 2011;18:2413–5.

47. American Society of Breast Surgeons. Position statement on management of the axilla in patients with invasive breast cancer. 2012. Available at: www. breastsurgeons.org. Accessed August 1, 2012.

48. National Comprehensive Cancer Network. Clinical practice guidelines in oncology: breast. National Comprehensive Cancer Network; 2012. v12.

49. Caudle AS, Hunt KK, Kuerer HM, et al. Multidisciplinary considerations in the implementation of the findings from the American College of Surgeons Oncology Group (ACOSOG) Z0011 study: a practice-changing trial. Ann Surg Oncol 2011;18:2407–12.

50. Gainer SM, Hunt KK, Beitsch P. Changing behavior in clinical practice in response to the ACOSOG Z0011 trial: a survey of the American Society of Breast Surgeons. Ann Surg Oncol 2012;19:3152–8.

51. Caudle AS, Hunt KK, Tucker SL, et al. American College of Surgeons (ACOSOG) Z0011: impact on surgeon practice patterns. Ann Surg Oncol 2012; 19:3144–51.

52. Galimberti VC, Zurrida S, Viale G, et al, International Breast Cancer Study Group Trial 23-01 Investigators. Update of International Breast Cancer Study Group Trial 23-01 to compare axillary dissection versus no axillary dissection in patients with clinically node negative breast cancer and micrometastases in the sentinel node. Cancer Res 2011;71:102s.

53. Dowlatshahi K, Fan M, Snider HC, et al. Lymph node micrometastases from breast carcinoma: reviewing the dilemma. Cancer 1997;80:1188–97.

54. de Boer M, van Dijck JA, Bult P, et al. Breast cancer prognosis and occult lymph node metastases, isolated tumor cells, and micrometastases. J Natl Cancer Inst 2010;102:410–25.

55. Weaver DL. Sentinel lymph nodes and breast carcinoma: which micrometastases are clinically significant? Am J Surg Pathol 2003;27:842–5.

56. Weaver DL, Le UP, Dupuis SL, et al. Metastasis detection in sentinel lymph nodes: comparison of a limited widely spaced (NSABP protocol B-32) and a comprehensive narrowly spaced paraffin block sectioning strategy. Am J Surg Pathol 2009;33:1583–9.

57. Weaver DL, Ashikaga T, Krag DN, et al. Effect of occult metastases on survival in node-negative breast cancer. N Engl J Med 2011;364:412–21.

58. Fitzgibbons PL, Page DL, Weaver D, et al. Prognostic factors in breast cancer. College of American Pathologists Consensus Statement 1999. Arch Pathol Lab Med 2000;124:966–78.

59. EORTC 10981–22023 AMAROS trial website. Cancer E O f R a T o. 2010. Available at: http://research.nki.nl/amaros/. Accessed August 1, 2012.

60. Straver ME, Meijnen P, van Tienhoven G, et al. Sentinel node identification rate and nodal involvement in the EORTC 10981-22023 AMAROS trial. Ann Surg Oncol 2010;17:1854–61.

61. Straver ME, Meijnen P, van Tienhoven G, et al. Role of axillary clearance after a tumor-positive sentinel node in the administration of adjuvant therapy in early breast cancer. J Clin Oncol 2010;28:731–7.

# Miscellaneous Syndromes and Their Management

## Occult Breast Cancer, Breast Cancer in Pregnancy, Male Breast Cancer, Surgery in Stage IV Disease

Alfred John Colfry III, MD

### KEYWORDS

- Breast cancer • Occult breast cancer • Breast cancer in pregnancy
- Male breast cancer • Stage IV disease

### KEY POINTS

- Surgical therapy for occult breast cancer has traditionally centered on mastectomy; however, breast conservation with whole breast radiotherapy followed by axillary lymph node dissection has shown equivalent results.
- Patients with breast cancer in pregnancy can be safely and effectively treated; given a patient's pregnancy trimester and stage of breast cancer, a clinician must be able to guide therapy accordingly.
- Male breast cancer risk factors show strong association with BRCA 2 mutations, as well as Klinefelter syndrome.
- Traditionally, surgical therapy in stage IV breast cancer has been relegated to palliative control of an ulcerated breast wound; however, several retrospective trials have associated a survival advantage with primary site tumor extirpation in the setting of stage IV breast cancer.

## OCCULT BREAST CANCER

### Introduction

Occult breast cancer (OBC) is defined as clinically recognizable axillary metastatic carcinoma from an undectable primary breast tumor. In 1907, Halsted was the first to report 3 cases of "cancerous axillary glands with non-demonstrable cancer of the mamma."[1] The disease is rare, with 0.3% to 1.0% of all patients who present with breast cancer.[2,3] The American Joint Committee on Cancer Staging classifies OBC as T0N1/2M0 stage II. Other adenocarcinomas metastasize to the axilla as well; these most commonly include lung, thyroid, gastrointestinal, ovary, and uterus.[4,5] However,

Department of General Surgery, Atlanta Medical Center, 303 Parkway Northeast, Atlanta, GA 30312, USA
E-mail address: acolfr@gmail.com

Surg Clin N Am 93 (2013) 519–531
http://dx.doi.org/10.1016/j.suc.2012.12.003
0039-6109/13/$ – see front matter © 2013 Elsevier Inc. All rights reserved.

when metastatic adenocarcinoma presents with isolated axillary nodes, the occult primary is most likely to be an ipsilateral breast cancer.[6,7]

## Diagnosis

Patients with OBC typically present with a persistent axillary mass. A thorough history and physical examination should be taken, followed by bilateral mammography, ultrasound, and chest radiograph.[8] Once these preliminary studies are negative for tumor pathology, fine-needle aspiration versus core needle biopsy of the axillary mass should be undertaken; core needle biopsy is preferred because it will provide the pathologist with an adequate tissue sampling for immunohistochemical staining receptor positivity.[8] Ultrasound-guided biopsy of the axillary mass is another valid option.

With negative preliminary imaging modalities and a biopsy-confirmed tissue diagnosis of metastatic adenocarcinoma in the axilla, the patient is now classified as having an occult cancer with unknown primary. As noted earlier, metastatic adenocarcinoma in the axilla with unknown primary is most likely an ipsilateral breast cancer.[6,7] Magnetic resonance imaging (MRI) of the breast has proven a useful imaging modality in OBC. Buchanan and colleagues[9] identified 55 patients with OBC with stage II disease. MRI revealed suspicious lesions in 76% of patients (42 of 55). In this subgroup, 62% of the time MRI revealed the occult primary tumor with a false-positive rate of 29%, and 58% of these patients received breast conservation therapy. Although recently criticized for high false-positivity rates in routine breast cancer diagnoses, MRI clearly has a place in the diagnostic dilemma of OBC.

## Surgery

Beginning in 1909, the standard treatment for OBC was a blind radical or modified radical mastectomy[10]; however, one-third of patients who undergo blind mastectomy will not have any pathologic evidence of carcinoma on serial sectioned analysis.[2] When this is taken into consideration, along with increased sensitivity of imaging modalities, such as ultrasound and MRI, a discussion of breast conservation is warranted. In 1982, Vilcoq and colleagues[11] treated 11 patients with OBC conservatively with whole-breast radiotherapy. At 5 years, only 3 of the 11 patients had local breast recurrences that were managed with salvage mastectomy. In an even larger study by Vlastos and colleagues,[12] 45 patients with OBC were treated with either mastectomy or breast conservation with whole breast radiotherapy. When comparing mastectomy to breast conservation, there was no significant difference in locoregional recurrence (15% vs 13%), distant metastases (31% vs 22%), or 5-year survival (75% vs 79%). Breast conservation is a valid surgical option for OBC, and an informed discussion with the patient regarding surgical options is mandatory.

Management of the axilla does not differ from patients with breast cancer with clinically palpable nodes. All of these patients should undergo an axillary lymph node dissection for locoregional control and staging. The most important determinant of survival in OBC is the number of positive axillary nodes. In the study by Vlastos and colleagues,[12] 5-year overall survival was 87% with 1 to 3 positive nodes compared with 42% with more than 4 positive nodes (P<.0001).

## Adjuvant Therapy

With regard to systemic therapy, patients with OBC should be treated systemically as any other patient with stage II/II breast cancer. There are no specific prospective data on survival benefit with systemic therapy for OBC; however, most investigators agree in recommending adjuvant chemotherapy and hormonal therapy for estrogen receptor/progesterone receptor (ER/PR)-positive.[8,12,13]

## Summary

OBC accounts for fewer than 1% of all breast cancers. Although other cancers metastasize to the axilla, the most common primary source of metastatic adenocarcinoma in the axilla is an ipsilateral breast caner. Core needle biopsy is preferred for tissue sampling in the axilla for hormone receptor evaluation. MRI is warranted for diagnosis of the primary occult cancer. Surgical therapy has traditionally centered on mastectomy; however, breast conservation with whole-breast radiotherapy followed by axillary lymph node dissection has shown equivalent results. The axilla should be managed as in any patient who presents with clinically palpable disease, and an axillary lymph node dissection should be undertaken for all patients with OBC. Systemic therapy follows guidelines similar to stage II/III breast cancers.

## BREAST CANCER IN PREGNANCY
### Introduction

Pregnancy-associated breast cancer (PABC) is defined as breast cancer diagnosed either during pregnancy or within 1 year postpartum. With women increasingly deferring to have children later into their third and fourth decades, there has been a recent increase in the incidence of PABC. After cervical cancer, breast cancer has become the second most common malignancy in pregnancy.[14] The incidence of PABC has been reported as 0.2% to 3.8% of all breast cancers or 2.4 per 100,000 deliveries.[15,16] Because termination of pregnancy does not improve maternal outcome, clinicians need to be familiar with effectively and safely treating PABC.[17]

### Diagnosis

A conundrum associated with PABC remains a delayed diagnosis. Because of estrogen and progesterone surges, the physiologic changes in the breast during pregnancy include glandular hypertrophy, and increased size and density.[18] These changes act to either obscure a new lesion or to provide a false explanation for a newly appearing lesion that needs to be investigated. Older studies from the 1960s to 1970s quote a 6-month diagnostic delay.[19,20] More recent studies by Tretli and colleagues,[21] however, found a delay in diagnosis of 2.5 months in pregnancy and 6 months during lactation.

Clinical presentation in PABC is similar to that in nonpregnancy breast cancer-a painless, palpable mass. The imaging modality of choice in PABC is ultrasonography followed by mammography. Patients with PABC have dense breast tissue, not only because of the physiologic changes in pregnancy alluded to earlier, but also because of the patients' younger age. Ultrasonography is the imaging modality of choice in the workup of dense breast tissue in PABC.[22,23]

If ultrasonography is inconclusive, or if magnification of both breasts is desired, mammography in pregnancy may be indicated. With proper fetal shielding, fetal radiation exposure has been estimated to be 0.4 mrad; the literature quotes a 5.0-rad level to be linked to fetal malformations.[24,25] If a suspicious mass is noted on either ultrasonography or a 1-view oblique mammogram, craniocaudal and mediolateral views of both breasts help rule out bilateral or multifocal disease. MRI of the breasts with gadolinium should be reserved until after pregnancy; gadolinium has been shown to cross the placenta and has the potential for fetal abnormalities.[26]

### Biopsy/Pathology

Core needle biopsy is the gold standard with a sensitivity rate of 90%.[27] Invasive ductal carcinoma is the most common histologic type in PABC.[22,28] Pathology and hormone receptor status is similar to age-matched controls. Patient age and not pregnancy determines the biologic activity of tumors in PABC.[17,29] Estrogen and progesterone receptors are typically absent; whereas HER2/Neu receptors are positive 28% to 58% of the time.[30,31]

### Staging

Appropriate staging of patients with PABC focuses on major sites of metastasis: liver, lung, and bone. Guidelines for staging indicate an MRI of the spine without contrast, chest radiograph with fetal shielding, and liver ultrasound.[32] Sentinel lymph node biopsy has recently been accepted as a safe and accurate means of staging the axilla.[33–35] Because of the risk of anaphylactic shock in the mother, the use of blue dye to aid in identification of the sentinel lymph should be avoided in pregnant patients; however, the use of technetium 99m-labeled sulfur colloid has been proven a safe means for sentinel node identification.[34,35] With technetium 99m sulfur colloid–guided sentinel lymph node (SLN) biopsy, Keleher and colleagues[35] reported a radiation exposure dose of 4.3 mGy, which is below the estimated safe fetal threshold of 0.1 to 0.2 Gy.

### Surgery

After appropriate diagnosis and staging, surgery should not be delayed. If delivery is planned within 2 to 4 weeks, surgical treatment can be delayed.[36] The principles that guide breast cancer surgery in nonpregnant patients should also be followed in PABC. Both modified radical mastectomy and breast conservation surgery, followed by sentinel node biopsy/axillary lymph node dissection, are viable options. At the M.D. Anderson Cancer Center, Dominici and colleagues treated 67 patients with PABC with either mastectomy or breast conservation surgery; they concluded that both surgeries are viable options with low postoperative complications in PABC.[37]

### Radiation Therapy

For patients who pursue breast conservation, radiation therapy remains a mainstay of their treatment. The optimal timing for radiotherapy after breast conservation is 12 weeks or less.[38] Thus, when the diagnosis of PABC is made in the third trimester, delay of radiation treatment until after delivery is an accepted course. The dilemma of radiotherapy in PABC centers on women who pursue breast conservation in the first and early second trimesters. Some of these women will go on to receive either neoadjuvant/adjuvant chemotherapy, and thus their radiotherapy may be delayed until after completion of surgery and systemic therapy. In these patients, the timing is favorable to delay radiotherapy. The dilemma really focuses on a small subset of patients in the first and early second trimesters who pursue breast conservation but will not need systemic chemotherapy. In this circumstance, a thorough discussion with the patient should ensue. The patient should weigh the risk of fetal exposure to radiation with a risk of local recurrence if outside the 12-week window eluded to earlier.[25,39]

### Chemotherapy

Systemic chemotherapy should be avoided in the first trimester of pregnancy because of its detrimental effects on organogenesis and possible fetal death.[40,41] Chemotherapy has been proven safe in the second and third trimesters of pregnancy.

Cardonick and colleagues[17] reported a fetal malformation rate of 3.8% in PABC treated with chemotherapy after the first trimester; this malformation rate is not higher than that observed in the general population. To avoid complications from the hemopoietic nadir associated with systemic chemotherapy, a 3-week interval from the last cycle of chemotherapy until delivery should be undertaken.[32]

### Trastuzumab

Trastuzumab is not recommended for PABC. It has been associated with oligohydramnios, anhydramnios, and fetal death.[42]

### Tamoxifen

Endocrine therapy is not recommended during pregnancy. Tamoxifen has been associated with craniofacial defects and abnormalities of the urogenital tract.[43,44] Aromatase inhibitors are not appropriate because of the patients' premenopausal age.

### Summary

Patients with breast cancer in pregnancy can be safely and effectively treated. The termination of pregnancy does not improve outcomes. Given a patient's pregnancy trimester and stage of breast cancer, a clinician must be able to guide therapy accordingly.

Treatment guidelines for PABC should closely follow established breast cancer treatment protocols. Patients typically present with a painless palpable mass that can be further imaged with ultrasound. With fetal shielding, mammographic views are possible; MRI without gadolinium can be used in select cases in which ultrasound or mammography are inconclusive. Core needle biopsy is the gold standard for tissue diagnosis.

Breast surgery should proceed with either mastectomy or breast conservation with radiation therapy. Sentinel node biopsy with technetium sulfur colloid is an effective means to stage the axilla. If breast conservation is chosen, a discussion with the patient regarding the risks of radiation to the fetus should be undertaken. Patients with PABC who are in their third trimester can delay radiotherapy until after delivery; patients with PABC who are in their first or second trimester will often need systemic chemotherapy and the timing of delaying radiation until after delivery maybe favorable.

Systemic therapy guidelines differ from patients with breast cancer who are not pregnant. During the first trimester, chemotherapy should not be administered; however, it has been proven a safe means of systemic treatment in the second and third trimesters. Neoadjuvant chemotherapy is a viable option for systemic treatment in the second and third trimesters. Both hormonal therapy and trastuzumab are contraindicated in pregnancy.

## MALE BREAST CANCER
### Introduction

In 2012, the National Cancer Institute estimated 226,870 newly diagnosed female breast cancers and 2190 newly diagnosed male breast cancers.[45] Male breast cancer is rare; it accounts for 0.7% of all breast cancer diagnoses.[46] Because of the rarity of the disease, few prospective clinical trials are available; most of the surgical literature is dependent on retrospective reviews. Treatment algorithms for male breast cancer have been derived from the treatment of female breast cancer.

The mean age for male breast cancer diagnosis is 67 years; this is approximately 5 years older than the mean age diagnosis for women.[47] More than 50% of male breast cancers are stage II or greater at the time of initial diagnosis; this compares less favorably to 35% of female breast cancers that are diagnosed as stage II or greater.[47,48] When 5-year survival rates for stages I to IV male breast cancers (96%, 84%, 52%, and 24% respectively) are compared with stages I to IV female breast cancers, there is no significant difference.[47]

### Risk Factors

BRCA 1 and BRCA 2 are tumor suppressor genes that aid in regulating cell cycle control. Unregulated cell proliferation leads to tumorigenesis. BRCA 2 mutations occur more frequently in men with breast cancer than women. It is estimated that 4% to 16% of male breast cancers are associated with a BRCA 2 mutation.[49] These patients with BRCA 2 mutations often present at a younger age, and have bilateral disease and a poorer survival.[49,50] BRCA 1 mutations are associated with male breast cancer to a much lesser extent.

Hormonal imbalances may also play a role in male breast cancer. Klinefelter syndrome (XXY) is strongly associated with male breast cancer.[51,52] This results from the relative imbalance of high estrogen/androgen ratio. Hultborn and colleagues[53] determined that a man with Klinefelter syndrome has a 49% risk of developing breast cancer. With increased estrogen levels, obese men (body mass index >30) have been shown to have double the risk of developing breast cancer compared with nonobese men.[48] Gynecomastia is the enlargement of breast glandular tissue in men. In men older than 50, it is caused by hormonal imbalances centering on a decline in serum testosterone while maintaining estradiol levels. However, the rates of male breast cancer in men with versus without gynecomastia do not appear to differ.[54] Testicular abnormalities are other risk factors for the development of male breast cancer, specifically those disorders that cause a paucity of androgen production.[55,56] These disorders include congenital inguinal hernia, undescended testes, testicular injury, orchiectomy, or orchitis.

### Pathology

Male breast tissue is predominately composed of undeveloped ductal components encircled by connective, adipose, and subcutaneous tissues. As a result of this, lobular carcinoma is extremely rare in male breast cancer. Ninety percent of male breast cancers are invasive ductal carcinomas; 10% are ductal carcinoma in situ of the papillary or cribriform type.[57] Male breast cancers have high rates of estrogen and progesterone receptor positivity. About 90% of men express positivity for the estrogen receptor, and 80% of men express positivity for the progesterone receptor[47]; however, male breast cancers express HER2/Neu positivity less often than female breast cancers (5% vs 15%).[58,59]

### Diagnosis

Male breast cancer typically presents as a painless subareolar mass. Acceptable imaging modalities include mammography and ultrasound. Mammography has a sensitivity and specificity for diagnosing male breast cancer of 92% and 90%, respectively.[60] If a lesion is discovered, stereotactic or ultrasound-guided biopsy should be used.

### Surgery

Although for many years radical mastectomy was the standard treatment for male breast cancer, modified radical mastectomy followed by SLN biopsy/axillary lymph node dissection has become the standard surgical therapy.[48,61] Because of the paucity of male breast tissue and the central location of male breast tumors, breast conservation therapy is rarely an option.

Axillary staging consists of SLN biopsy followed by axillary lymph node dissection if indicated. The first case of SLN biopsy in male breast cancer was in 1999.[62] A retrospective review of the Memorial Sloan-Kettering Cancer Center SLN biopsy database from 1996 to 2005 revealed 78 (1%) of 7315 SLN biopsies performed in men.[63] Of the 78 performed, the SLN was found in 76 (97%) patients. In 37 (49%) of 76 patients displaying node positivity, axillary lymph node dissection was completed either at the initial operation or at a subsequent surgery with no axillary recurrences at a median follow-up of 28 months.

At the M.D. Anderson Cancer Center from 1999 to 2005, Boughey and colleagues[64] compared their SLN experience of 30 men versus 2784 women. In men, the SLN was found in 100% of the cases. Interestingly, the male tumors were larger than women's ($P = .04$), and the incidence of positive SLN in men was higher (although not statistically significant) than in women, at a rate of 37.0% versus 22.3%. In male breast cancers with a positive SLN, the investigators found a non-SLN positivity rate in 62.5% of the cases, with 20.7% of the female cohort ($P = .01$). SLN biopsy can safely and effectively be used as a means to accurately stage the axilla in men with breast cancer.

## Adjuvant Therapy

Because of the rarity of male breast cancer, randomized prospective trials on adjuvant therapy for male cancer is scarce. Typically male patients with breast cancer follow adjuvant therapy guidelines similar to female patients with breast cancer. In one of the largest retrospective trials, Giordano and colleagues[65] evaluated 51 of 156 male patients with breast cancer who received adjuvant systemic therapies (both cytotoxic and hormonal) and found a 43% lower risk of death than in those who did not receive any systemic therapy. Statistically significant improvement was seen in time to disease recurrence and overall survival with respect to adjuvant hormonal therapy. Adjuvant chemotherapy was associated with lower risk of disease recurrence and death, although this was not statistically significant.

Extrapolating the effectiveness of systemic chemotherapy in female breast cancers and adding to that the retrospective evidence referred to previously, chemotherapy is indicated in male breast cancer. Giordano,[66] at the M.D. Anderson Cancer Center, suggests chemotherapy for breast cancers larger than 1 cm or with positive lymph node involvement. Given the high incidence of ER/PR positivity, tamoxifen should be used as adjuvant hormonal therapy in all ER/PR-positive male breast cancers.[67] In male patients with breast cancer with stage II or III disease, administration of tamoxifen resulted in a 56% 5-year disease-free survival versus 28% in historical controls.[68]

Postmastectomy radiotherapy (PMRT) guidelines for male breast cancer also follow female breast cancer guidelines. Yu and colleagues[69] retrospectively analyzed 75 male patients with breast cancer; 29 did not receive PMRT and 46 completed PMRT. PMRT did not demonstrate a benefit to overall survival; however, it did confer better local recurrence-free survival ($P<.0001$). The investigators site node positivity, advanced stage, or surgical margin smaller than 2 mm as risk factors for male patients with breast cancer who may show an improvement in locoregional recurrence with PMRT.

## Summary

Male breast cancer remains a rare diagnosis. Although many characteristics of male breast cancer are similar to female breast cancer, there are a few important differences. Men are typically diagnosed at a later age and stage than women with breast cancer. Male breast cancer risk factors show strong association with BRCA 2 mutations, as well as Klinefelter syndrome. Histologic characteristics show a strong predilection for invasive ductal carcinoma as well as ER/PR receptor positivity.

Surgical treatment centers on modified radical mastectomy followed by SLN biopsy. If the SLN is positive, an axillary lymph node dissection is indicated. Systemic therapy focuses on hormonal and chemotherapy. With male breast tumors correspondingly high estrogen/progesterone positivity rate, tamoxifen is the gold standard for adjuvant hormonal therapy. Radiation therapy should be considered in those patients with risk factors for local regional failure.

## PRIMARY BREAST SURGERY IN STAGE IV BREAST CANCER
### Introduction

In the United States, approximately 6% of newly diagnosed women with breast cancer present with stage IV disease.[70] Median survival for patients with stage IV disease has improved to 29 months.[71] Classic breast oncologic dictum has preferred systemic therapy as the mainstay of treatment for stage IV disease. Surgical therapy of the primary tumor has been reserved for palliation. However, several retrospective reviews evaluating the efficacy of surgical treatment of the primary breast cancer in the metastatic setting have shown an increased survival advantage.[72–74] Critics point to selection bias and stage migration in these retrospective reviews. Prospective randomized controlled trials are lacking. Is there a specific subgroup of patients with stage IV disease who may benefit from surgical treatment of the primary breast tumor?

### Retrospective Reviews

Several single-institution and population-based retrospective reviews have proclaimed an increased survival advantage for primary breast surgery in patients with stage IV breast cancer. The largest retrospective study by Khan and colleagues[72] evaluated 16,023 patients from the National Cancer Database from 1990 to 1993 who were diagnosed with stage IV disease. A total of 9162 women (57%) underwent either partial or total mastectomy. Using a Cox proportional model on multivariate analysis, the investigators identified the following covariates as independent prognostic indicators of patient outcomes: surgical resection of primary tumor, type of metastatic disease, and the number of metastatic sites. Three-year survival rates were 17% with no surgery, 28% for partial mastectomy, and 32% for mastectomy.

Evaluating the Surveillance, Epidemiology, and End Results (SEER) database, Gnerlich and colleagues[73] analyzed 9734 patients with stage IV breast cancer; 47% underwent extirpation of the primary tumor. Median survival was longer in the surgical cohort versus the nonsurgical cohort in patients alive during the study period (36 vs 21 months, $P<.001$), as well as for women who died during the study period (18 vs 7 months $P<.001$).

A single-institution retrospective study from the University of Texas M.D. Anderson Cancer Center evaluated 224 patients with stage IV breast cancer from 1997 to 2002.[74] Eighty-two patients underwent either a partial mastectomy (48%) or total mastectomy (52%) for local control of their primary breast tumor. The surgical cohort was associated with a trend toward improved overall survival ($P = .12$) and an improved metastatic progression-free survival ($P = .0007$).

### Selection Bias

Even though only 3 articles are referenced touting increased survival for patients with stage IV breast cancer with extirpated primary tumors, there is a plethora of literature with the same claims; however, there is inherent selection bias in many of these retrospective single-institution studies. Patients were not randomly assigned to cohorts; rather, surgical candidates were selected by the treating physician.

Cady and colleagues[75] performed a matched pair analysis in an attempt to analyze potential bias in selecting patients for primary site surgery in metastatic breast cancer. Of 622 patients analyzed, 388 (62%) had no surgery and 234 (38%) underwent surgery. Once again, the surgery cohort was associated with an improved survival (P<.0001); however, on case-matched control analysis, the timing of systemic chemotherapy played a significant role in survival. Patients who received preoperative chemotherapy followed by surgery had a 90% survival at 2 years; this differed markedly from those patients who received chemotherapy and surgery simultaneously, as well as those patients who received chemotherapy postoperatively. And thus, Cady and colleagues[75] suggest selection bias can explain much of the survival advantage evident in the previously mentioned nonrandomized retrospective reviews. This calls for randomized prospective trials to evaluate the efficacy of primary site surgery in patients with stage IV breast cancer.

*Stage Migration*

Bafford and colleagues[76] performed a retrospective review from the Dana Farber Cancer Institute at the Brigham and Women's Hospital and the Massachusetts General Hospital evaluating the effect of surgery in patients with stage IV disease. From 1998 to 2005, 148 women presented with stage IV cancer; 61 (47%) underwent mastectomy or lumpectomy. On univariate and multivariate analyses, the surgery cohort versus the nonsurgical cohort had superior overall survival of 3.52 years versus 2.36 years (P = .093) and 4.13 years versus 2.36 years (P = .003), respectively. However, in those patients undergoing surgery, 36 patients (59%) were diagnosed with metastatic disease postoperatively and 25 patients (41%) were diagnosed with metastatic disease preoperatively. Median survival in the patients with postoperatively discovered metastatic breast cancer was 4.0 years; however, median survival in the preoperatively detected metastatic disease group undergoing surgery versus the nonsurgical cohort differed very little: 2.40 years versus 2.36 (P = .18). This clearly demonstrates stage migration bias.

*Targeted Molecular Therapy*

Although acknowledging the aforementioned retrospective reviews, Neuman and colleagues[77] sought to identify subsets of patients who would benefit from surgical resection of the primary tumor in stage IV disease. They examined the relationship between tumor molecular subtype in combination with targeted molecular therapy and surgery. During 2000 to 2004, 186 patients with stage IV disease and an intact primary tumor were treated at the Memorial Sloan-Kettering Cancer Center. Sixty-nine (37%) patients' primary tumors were treated surgically: 34 patients with unknown metastatic disease at the time of surgery, 15 patients for local control, 14 patients for palliation, and 6 patients to obtain tissue. On univariate analysis, there was a trend toward improved survival in patients treated surgically of 40 months compared with nonsurgically treated patients of 33 months. This trend was also evident in the previously discussed retrospective reviews. On further analysis, however, Neuman and colleagues[77] identified tumor molecular subtype as the most significant prognostic factor for surgery as an adjunctive to multimodality therapy in patients with stage IV disease with an intact primary tumor. Surgery of the primary tumor was associated with improved survival in patients who were ER/PR-positive and HER2/Neu-positive (P = .004); however, no survival benefit was seen in patients who were triple negative who underwent resection of the primary tumor. This proposes that the influence of local control is most effective in the presence of appropriate targeted molecular therapy.

## Summary

Stage IV breast cancer has classically been treated with systemic therapy. Traditionally, surgical therapy in stage IV breast cancer has been relegated to palliative control of an ulcerated breast wound. However, several retrospective trials have associated a survival advantage with primary site tumor extirpation in the setting of stage IV breast cancer. Selection bias and stage migration may be contributors to improved survival seen in retrospective reviews of single-institution or population-based trials arguing for primary site surgery in metastatic breast cancer. A subset of patients with stage IV breast cancer who underwent targeted molecular therapy may benefit the most from local control of the primary tumor. Prospective randomized controlled trials are needed to obviate selection bias.

## REFERENCES

1. Halsted WS. The results of radical operation for the cure of carcinoma of the breast. Ann Surg 1907;46(1):1–19.
2. Baron PL, Moore MP, Kinne DW, et al. Occult breast cancer presenting with axillary metastases. Updated management. Arch Surg 1990;125(2):210–4.
3. Patel J, Nemoto T, Rosner D, et al. Axillary lymph node metastasis from an occult breast cancer. Cancer 1981;47(12):2923–7.
4. Copeland EM, McBride CM. Axillary metastases from unknown primary sites. Ann Surg 1973;178(1):25–7.
5. Varadarajan R, Edge SB, Yu J, et al. Prognosis of occult breast carcinoma presenting as isolated axillary nodal metastasis. Oncology 2006;71(5–6):456–9.
6. Abbruzzese JL, Abbruzzese MC, Hess KR, et al. Unknown primary carcinoma: natural history and prognostic factors in 657 consecutive patients. J Clin Oncol 1994;12(6):1272–80.
7. Hainsworth JD, Greco FA. Management of patients with cancer of unknown primary site. Oncology (Williston Park) 2000;14(4):563–74 [discussion: 574–6, 578–9].
8. Brill KL, Brenin DR. Occult breast cancer and axillary mass. Curr Treat Options Oncol 2001;2(2):149–55.
9. Buchanan CL, Morris EA, Dorn PL, et al. Utility of breast magnetic resonance imaging in patients with occult primary breast cancer. Ann Surg Oncol 2005; 12(12):1045–53.
10. Cameron HC. An address entitled some clinical facts regarding mammary cancer. Br Med J 1909;1(2514):577–82.
11. Vilcoq JR, Calle R, Ferme F, et al. Conservative treatment of axillary adenopathy due to probable subclinical breast cancer. Arch Surg 1982;117(9):1136–8.
12. Vlastos G, Jean ME, Mirza AN, et al. Feasibility of breast preservation in the treatment of occult primary carcinoma presenting with axillary metastases. Ann Surg Oncol 2001;8(5):425–31.
13. Abe H, Naitoh H, Umeda T, et al. Occult breast cancer presenting axillary nodal metastasis: a case report. Jpn J Clin Oncol 2000;30(4):185–7.
14. Antonelli NM, Dotters DJ, Katz VL, et al. Cancer in pregnancy: a review of the literature Part II. Obstet Gynecol Surv 1996;51(2):135–42.
15. Guidroz J, Scott-Conner C, Weigel R. Management of pregnant women with breast cancer. J Surg Oncol 2011;103:337–40.

16. Andersson TM, Johansson AL, Hsieh CC, et al. Increasing incidence of pregnancy-associated breast cancer in Sweden. Obstet Gynecol 2009;114(3): 568–72.

17. Cardonick E, Dougherty R, Grana, et al. Breast cancer during pregnancy: maternal and fetal outcomes. Cancer J 2010;16(1):76–82.

18. Ishida T, Yokoe T, Kasumi F, et al. Clinicopathologic characteristics and prognosis of breast cancer patients associated with pregnancy and lactation: analysis of case-control study in Japan. Jpn J Cancer Res 1992;83(11):1143–9.

19. Bunker ML, Peters MV. Breast cancer associated with pregnancy or lactation. Am J Obstet Gynecol 1963;85:312–21.

20. Applewhite RR, Smith LR, DiVincenti F. Carcinoma of the breast associated with pregnancy and lactation. Am Surg 1973;39(2):101–4.

21. Tretli S, Kvalheim G, Thoresen S, et al. Survival of breast cancer patients diagnosed during pregnancy or lactation. Br J Cancer 1988;58(3):382–4.

22. Navrozoglou I, Vrekoussis T, Kontostolis E, et al. Breast cancer during pregnancy: a mini-review. Eur J Surg Oncol 2008;34(8):837–43.

23. Keleher AJ, Theriault RL, Gwyn KM, et al. Multidisciplinary management of breast cancer concurrent with pregnancy. J Am Coll Surg 2002;194(1):54–64.

24. Nicklas AH, Baker ME. Imaging strategies in the pregnant cancer patient. Semin Oncol 2000;27(6):623–32.

25. Mazonakis M, Varveris H, Damilakis J, et al. Radiation dose to conceptus resulting from tangential breast irradiation. Int J Radiat Oncol Biol Phys 2003;55(2): 386–91.

26. Novak Z, Thurmond AS, Ross PL, et al. Gadolinium-DTPA transplacental transfer and distribution in fetal tissue in rabbits. Invest Radiol 1993;28(9):828–30.

27. Oyama T, Koibuchi Y, McKee G. Core needle biopsy (CNB) as a diagnostic method for breast lesions: comparison with fine needle aspiration cytology (FNA). Breast Cancer 2004;11(4):339–42.

28. Parente JT, Amsel M, Lerner R, et al. Breast cancer associated with pregnancy. Obstet Gynecol 1988;71(6 Pt 1):861–4.

29. Amant F, Deckers S, Van Calsteren K, et al. Breast cancer in pregnancy: recommendations of an international consensus meeting. Eur J Cancer 2010;46(18): 3158–68.

30. Aziz S, Pervez S, Khan S, et al. Case control study of novel prognostic markers and disease outcome in pregnancy/lactation-associated breast carcinoma. Pathol Res Pract 2003;199(1):15–21.

31. Scott-Conner CE, Schorr SJ. The diagnosis and management of breast problems during pregnancy and lactation. Am J Surg 1995;170(4):401–5.

32. Loibl S, von Minckwitz G, Gwyn K, et al. Breast carcinoma during pregnancy. International recommendations from an expert meeting. Cancer 2006;106(2):237–46.

33. Gentilini O, Cremonesi M, Toesca A, et al. Sentinel lymph node biopsy in pregnant patients with breast cancer. Eur J Nucl Med Mol Imaging 2010;37(1):78–83.

34. Gentilini O, Cremonesi M, Trifiro G, et al. Safety of sentinel node biopsy in pregnant patients with breast cancer. Ann Oncol 2004;15(9):1348–51.

35. Keleher A, Wendt R 3rd, Delpassand E, et al. The safety of lymphatic mapping in pregnant breast cancer patients using Tc-99m sulfur colloid. Breast J 2004;10(6): 492–5.

36. Jones AL. Management of pregnancy-associated breast cancer. Breast 2006;15 Suppl 2:S47–52.

37. Dominici LS, Kuerer HM, Babiera G, et al. Wound complications from surgery in pregnancy-associated breast cancer (PABC). Breast Dis 2010;31(1):1–5.

38. Whelan TJ, Lada BM, Laukkanen E, et al. Breast irradiation in women with early stage invasive breast cancer following breast conservation surgery. Provincial Breast Disease Site Group. Cancer Prev Control 1997;1(3):228–40.

39. Molckovsky A, Madarnas Y. Breast cancer in pregnancy: a literature review. Breast Cancer Res Treat 2008;108(3):333–8.

40. Doll DC, Ringenberg QS, Yarbro JW. Antineoplastic agents and pregnancy. Semin Oncol 1989;16(5):337–46.

41. Zemlickis D, Lishner M, Degendorfer P, et al. Fetal outcome after in utero exposure to cancer chemotherapy. Arch Intern Med 1992;152(3):573–6.

42. Azim HA Jr, Azim H, Peccatori FA. Treatment of cancer during pregnancy with monoclonal antibodies: a real challenge. Expert Rev Clin Immunol 2010;6(6):821–6.

43. Barthelmes L, Gateley CA. Tamoxifen and pregnancy. Breast 2004;13(6):446–51.

44. Isaacs RJ, Hunter W, Clark K. Tamoxifen as systemic treatment of advanced breast cancer during pregnancy—case report and literature review. Gynecol Oncol 2001;80(3):405–8.

45. National Cancer Institute. Breast cancer. Available at: http://www.cancer.gov/cancertopics/types/breast. Accessed October 2012.

46. Jemel A, Tiwari RC, Murray T, et al. Cancer statistics, 2004. CA Cancer J Clin 2004;54:8–29.

47. Giordano SH, Cohen DS, Buzdar AU, et al. Breast carcinoma in men: a population based study. Cancer 2004;101:51–7.

48. Fentiman IS, Fourquet A, Hortobagyi GN. Male breast cancer. Lancet 2006;367: 595–604.

49. Basham VM, Lipscombe JM, Ward JM, et al. BRCA 1 and BRCA 2 mutations in a population-based study of male breast cancer. Breast Cancer Res 2002;4:R2.

50. Kwiatkowska E, Teresiak M, Filas V, et al. BRCA 2 mutations and androgen receptor expression as independent predictors of outcome of male breast cancer patients. Clin Cancer Res 2003;9:4452–9.

51. Evans DB, Crichlow RW. Carcinoma of the male breast and Klinefelter's syndrome: is there an association? CA Cancer J Clin 1987;37:246–51.

52. Thomas DB. Breast cancer in men. Epidemiol Rev 1993;15:220–31.

53. Hultborn R, Hanson C, Kopf I, et al. Prevalence of Klinefelter's syndrome in male breast cancer patients. Anticancer Res 1997;17:4293–7.

54. Giordano SH, Buzdar AU, Hortobagyi GN. Breast cancer in men. Ann Intern Med 2002;137:678–87.

55. Thomas DB, Jimenez LM, McTiernan A, et al. Breast cancer in men: risk factors with hormonal implications. Am J Epidemiol 1992;135:734–48.

56. Mabuchi K, Bross DS, Kessler II. Risk factors for male breast cancer. J Natl Cancer Inst 1985;74:371–5.

57. Stalsberg H, Thomas DB, Rosenblatt KA, et al. Histologic types and hormone receptors in male breast cancer in men: a population based study in 282 United States men. Cancer Causes Control 1993;4:143–51.

58. Ottini L, Palli D, Rizzo S, et al. Male breast cancer. Crit Rev Oncol Hematol 2010; 73:141–55.

59. Muir D, Kanthan R, Kanthan SC. Male versus female breast cancers. A population based comparative immunohistochemical analysis. Arch Pathol Lab Med 2003; 127:36–41.

60. Evans GF, Anthony T, Turnage, et al. The diagnostic accuracy of mammography in the evaluation of male breast disease. Am J Surg 2001;181:96–100.

61. Contractor KB, Kaur K, Rodrigues GS, et al. Male breast cancer: is the scenario changing. World J Surg Oncol 2008;6:58.

62. Hill AD, Borgen PI, Cody HS III. Sentinel node biopsy in male breast cancer. Eur J Surg Oncol 1999;25:442–3.
63. Flynn L, Park J, Patil S. Sentinel lymph node biopsy is successful and accurate in male breast carcinoma. J Am Coll Surg 2008;206(4):616–21.
64. Boughey JC, Bedrosian I, Meric-Bernstam F, et al. Comparative analysis of sentinel lymph node operation in male and female breast cancer patients. J Am Coll Surg 2006;203(4):475–80.
65. Giordano SH, Perkins GH, Broglio K, et al. Adjuvant systemic therapy for male breast carcinoma. Cancer 2005;104(11):2359–64.
66. Giordano SH. A review of the diagnosis and management of male breast cancer. Oncologist 2005;10(7):471–9.
67. Lanitis S, Rice AJ, Vaughan A, et al. Diagnosis and management of male breast cancer. World J Surg 2008;32(11):2471–6.
68. Ribeiro G, Swindell R. Adjuvant tamoxifen for male breast cancer (MBC). Br J Cancer 1992;65(2):252–4.
69. Yu E, Suzuki H, Younus J, et al. The impact of post-mastectomy radiation therapy on male breast cancer patients—a case series. Int J Radiat Oncol Biol Phys 2012; 82(2):696–700.
70. Ries L, Melbert D, Krapcho M, et al. SEER cancer statistics review, 1975-2004. National Cancer Institute; 2007. Available at: http://seer.cancer.gov/csr/1975_ 2004. Accessed October 2012.
71. Andre F, Slimane K, Bachelot T, et al. Breast cancer with synchronous metastases: trends in survival during a 14-year period. J Clin Oncol 2004;22(16): 3302–8.
72. Khan SA, Stewart AK, Morrow M. Does aggressive local therapy improve survival in metastatic breast cancer? Surgery 2002;132(4):620–6.
73. Gnerlich J, Jeffe DB, Deshpande AD, et al. Surgical removal of the primary tumor increases overall survival in patients with metastatic breast cancer: analysis of the 1988-2003 SEER data. Ann Surg Oncol 2007;14(8):2187–94.
74. Babiera GV, Rao R, Feng L, et al. Effect of primary tumor extirpation in breast cancer patients who present with stage IV disease and an intact primary tumor. Ann Surg Oncol 2006;13(6):776–82.
75. Cady B, Nathan NR, Michaelson JS, et al. Matched pair analyses of stage IV breast cancer with or without resection of primary breast site. Ann Surg Oncol 2008;15(12):3384–95.
76. Bafford AC, Burstein HJ, Barkley CR, et al. Breast surgery in stage IV breast cancer: impact of staging and patient selection on overall survival. Breast Cancer Res Treat 2009;115(1):7–12.
77. Neuman HB, Morrogh M, Gonen M, et al. Stage IV breast cancer in the era of targeted therapy: does surgery of the primary tumor matter? Cancer 2010;116(5): 1226–33.

# Index

*Note:* Page numbers of article titles are in **boldface** type.

Surg Clin N Am 93 (2013) 533–548
http://dx.doi.org/10.1016/S0039-6109(13)00017-0
0039-6109/13/$ – see front matter © 2013 Elsevier Inc. All rights reserved.

surgical.theclinics.com

# Moving?

## *Make sure your subscription moves with you!*

To notify us of your new address, find your **Clinics Account Number** (located on your mailing label above your name), and contact customer service at:

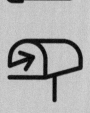

**Email: journalscustomerservice-usa@elsevier.com**

**800-654-2452** (subscribers in the U.S. & Canada)
**314-447-8871** (subscribers outside of the U.S. & Canada)

**Fax number: 314-447-8029**

**Elsevier Health Sciences Division**
**Subscription Customer Service**
**3251 Riverport Lane**
**Maryland Heights, MO 63043**

*To ensure uninterrupted delivery of your subscription, please notify us at least 4 weeks in advance of move.